KEEPING REFLECTION FRESH

Keeping Reflection Fresh

A Practical Guide for
Clinical Educators

Edited by

ALLAN PETERKIN

and

PAMELA BRETT-MACLEAN

THE KENT STATE UNIVERSITY PRESS

Kent, Ohio

© 2016 by The Kent State University Press, Kent, Ohio 44242
ALL RIGHTS RESERVED
Library of Congress Catalog Number 2015036112
ISBN 978-1-60635-283-0
Manufactured in the United States of America

LIBRARY OF CONGRESS CATALOGING-IN-PUBLICATION DATA
Keeping reflection fresh : a practical guide for clinical educators /
edited by Allan Peterkin and Pamela Brett-MacLean
p. ; cm. — (Literature and medicine ; 24)
Includes bibliographical references and index.
ISBN 978-1-60635-283-0 (pbk. : alk. paper) ∞
I. Peterkin, Allan, editor. II. Brett-MacLean, Pamela, editor.
III. Series: Literature and medicine (Kent, Ohio) ; 24.
[DNLM: 1. Education, Medical—Personal Narratives. 2. Teaching—Personal
Narratives. 3. Thinking—Personal Narratives. W 18]
R834
610.71—dc23
2015036112

20 19 18 17 16   5 4 3 2 1

For educators and learners everywhere
interested in the connections between reflection and healing.
And
for Robert (AP),
and
Mel and Caleb (PBM),
with love.

In memory of
L. C. Chan, a kind and generous
pioneer in our field and
contributor to this book.

Contents

Part 5: Ethics and Professionalism

Part 6: Spirituality and Mindfulness

Foreword

Keeping Reflection Beautiful

ALAN BLEAKLEY

REFLECTION

In Book I of Homer's *Iliad,* Agamemnon bruises Achilles's honor and they argue furiously. In the heat of the quarrel, Achilles—famous for his intemperance—contemplates simply running Agamemnon through with his sword and being done with it. His hand is on the hilt, but "while he . . . was pulling the great sword from the scabbard, Athene came up behind him and caught the son of Peleus by his yellow hair," stopping Achilles in his tracks to take a moment to reflect on the possible consequences of his action. Achilles "stayed his massive hand on the silver hilt, and pushed the great sword back into the scabbard."[1]

This famous scene captures what the father of reflective practice, Donald Schön, described as a shift from knowing-in-action to reflection-in-action—cultivating a turn of mind and emotion in the heat of activity that is a contemplative pause unhitching from raw impulse to open up fresh possibilities.[2] It is knowing-in-action that allows us to ride a bicycle without falling off. However, if a unique situation—such as a moment of ambiguity or a conflict of values—arises, then habitual knowing-in-action fails and we must reflect and improvise. This reflective pause turns knowing-in-action into reflection-in-action. We can take the goddess Athena as a metaphor for the reflective pause—the meta-cognitive and meta-affective process that is reflection-in-action.

As you'll see in this book, more than two and a half millennia after Homer, medical and health-care schools across the world have come to see the value—indeed, the necessity—of fostering reflective capacity in their learners. At Peninsula Medical School, UK, where I used to teach, educators placed great emphasis on students developing the attribute of reflection because reflective students take better care not only of their patients but also of themselves. We have found that the capacity for reflection is best learned not as a functional skill but, as Schön described it, as a practice artistry.[3] Schön, however, never progressed the notion of practice artistry to its logical end—that we should teach and learn such artistry through introducing medical and health-care students to reflective capacity through the arts.

The health-care educators who have contributed to *Keeping Reflection Fresh* demonstrate amply how the primary method for establishing reflective practice is arts- and humanities-based learning. These educators further argue for working toward an ideal of core and integrated curriculum provision of the arts and humanities and for promoting a permeating value complex of humane care, creativity, and critical evaluation—focused on the practice artistry of whichever clinical discipline they represent. These future-looking educators draw widely on written and spoken literature, the visual arts, drama, music, and ethics to educate for both sensibility (tuning the senses for "close noticing" and discrimination) and sensitivity (ethical and humane practice). They remind us that we need to listen to our students, who may have become jaded around the hegemony of evidence-based learning but who also increasingly resent being compelled to reflect "on demand" and to be assessed with imperfect tools when they do so.

We need to look for actual changes in attitudes and practices. After a recent humanities workshop in which visual artists taught with clinicians to improve close noticing, one senior medical student said, "Over the last few months I have noticed a change in my approach to patients; I now use my inspection skills more and work around the bedside for visual clues in their diagnoses." Close noticing, greater awareness, and improvement in diagnostic acumen—surely these are important products of a medical humanities curriculum, which brings artists together with clinicians to deepen "looking" into "seeing." And what about the other senses? Numerous entries in this text provide diverse examples of ways in which educators incorporate the senses as a whole to promote learning in students.

My own work while at Peninsula included not only education of the visual but also enabling medical students to work with a perfumier and wine connoisseur to develop smell and taste, and with musicians to attune the ears and hands—so important for auscultation, palpation, and percussion. Importantly, we challenged reductive "hard" science to reveal the intrinsic beauty of the scientific method. Keeping reflection fresh and beautiful also means accommodating aesthetically what is often mistaken as instrumental "reductive" method—for example, situating the classic clinical case presentation within the genre of minimalism, where there is beauty too in stripping back to bare essences. Introducing arts and humanities perspectives and methods into scientific thinking is not about replacing that thinking but about enhancing and enriching it and, again, drawing out the beauty of established methods.

ARTISTRY

Donald Schön suggested that thinking on your feet (as reflective practice) is most potent in the "swampy lowlands" of practice—areas of indeterminacy, uniqueness, and values conflict—rather than in the safe "high ground" of logic and protocols, where technical-rational thinking is the norm.[4] In the swampy lowlands, emotions run high, tinting and saturating rational judgment. But these passions are not always a hindrance; they can fuel innovative lines of flight and other positive outcomes.

Read on for essays by students who have described the personal impact of arts-based reflection. Here's what one of my medical students says of her engagement with the humanities, working with my wife, Sue, a visual artist and educator: "This experience helped me to explore the emotional aspects of medicine . . . to let my feelings guide me and think outside the box, rather than bottling them up. . . . This revelation will help me in my future career." From experiences gained on a cardiology placement, another medical student made a quilt embroidered with images evoking the suffering and complexities of living with heart conditions: "Exploring patients' emotions though their illnesses, as well as my own emotions towards them, has been an enlightening process. . . . I have been able to relate to my patients in a new and unique way, which will undoubtedly benefit me in my future practice as a doctor."

REFLECTION, REFLEXIVITY, AND REFRACTIVE PRACTICE— THE "THREE RS"

While reflection demands an introspective pause that says "think again!" about impulsive actions, reflexivity is a checking of moral and ethical positions, or values, that shape such actions. For example, first-level reflection tells Achilles to pause amid impulse and curb his anger. Second-level reflexivity shows that Achilles's anger is not just personal but driven by a values complex—that of heroic warriors. Don't think that this is a historical oddity of a bygone era—heroic types are alive and well, particularly in surgery and emergency medicine. But what if such types learned to be reflexive about the heroic, individualistic values that drive them—for example, through appreciating the values that shape nursing or social work cultures, which are traditionally about collaboration and collective effort? Such a relativizing of values is best served by feedback from patients, students, and colleagues.

Finally, reflection in, and on, practice does not occur in a vacuum but is situated in social contexts, such as entering a specialty or working on a new team. A third level of reflection is implied by these social contexts—refractive practice.[4] Just as a stick is refracted when plunged into water, so individuals are refracted as they enter the differing media of communities of practice. While adapting to the local rules, new members have the right to resist or challenge those rules. Refractive practice affords students a voice as a fresh and critically aware resource, able to spot what might have become habitual, crystallized, and overlooked by old-timers. At the heart of refractive practice is acquiring democratic habits, challenging stale and morally unjustified authorities. The arts and humanities afford the primary media through which such critical, democratic habits are learned, where the traditional role of the arts is to challenge the crystallized and unproductive habits of cultures and to suggest alternatives. Reflective, reflexive, and refractive practices collectively make up the artistry of caring for patients as aesthetic labor—forming a style of practice that, at its best, is both elegant and beautiful and transcends mere function. This is what shifts merely competent clinical care into excellence. You will find compelling examples of these new "three Rs" within these pages.

METHODS

How then are students to become soaked in the arts and humanities in the health-care "solution," set out above as a complicated conversation between the "three Rs" and arts and humanities educational interventions? First, an arts/ humanities perspective should permeate as much of the teaching as possible, constituting a climate of more feminine values that nourish care (patient-centeredness) and collaboration (effective, democratic teamwork). However, getting students on board with this idea has not been the main challenge for most of the authors of the essays in this book. Rather, it is recruiting and retaining science and clinical faculty with the "right stuff"—a broad, tolerant, humanitarian, and imaginative outlook on clinical education. This outlook needs to be twinned with regular, ongoing faculty development. Many of the essays that follow will provide you with more than enough tools to inspire your teachers.

Second, processes of learning must be valued as much as content. Students learn to learn, and learn to reflect through a core values climate of other-directedness, patient-centeredness, and tolerance of ambiguity. The authors in this book invite readers to move from a "problem-based" to a "patient- and population-based" curriculum. Patients are not "problems" to be solved but persons to be appreciated.

Ideally, compulsory arts and humanities content—tailored, assessed, and evaluated— should be designed throughout the curriculum, with a broad base of arts- and humanities-based offerings. Many of the authors here take an important second step by publicly exhibiting projects as creative works that fully honor the creative output and risk taking of students through public engagement. In this move, laypersons engage democratically with the wide spectrum of professional clinical education. I suggest that, whenever possible, workshops be facilitated by clinicians in collaboration with artists or humanities scholars—and there are many good examples of this in the book. Students then see differing ways of knowing modeled and debated. One student, who made a short film about a patient's journey through a hospital, said, "This . . . has given me the chance to talk to patients about their lives rather than their diseases. . . . I hope this journey and this lesson never stop, because if they do I think I will have lost something more important to being a doctor than knowing which muscle of the hand may or may not flex that metacarpophalangeal joint!"

SNAGS

As readers of and contributors to *Keeping Reflection Fresh*, we clearly value the approaches described above, but not all of our colleagues do. We are always at the whim of changes in the Deanery. As many of the authors in this book remind us, we need to carefully research, evaluate, and situate our work in the developing cultures of interprofessional humanities in health care nationally and internationally—through academic papers, conferences, networks, meetings, and public exhibitions. Books like this help to do just that. While we need to build an evidence base to demonstrate the value of educating the "three Rs"—reflection, reflexivity, and refractive practice—and to keep them fresh, we must not become slaves to evidence-based practice when narrative-based practice also has so much to offer.

Designing, implementing, and evaluating complex educational interventions involving the arts and humanities are fraught with difficulties. This book provides inspiration, encouragement, and troubleshooting in this field. Our informing philosophy for the humanities in health care should and must be challenging—we need to promote both "critical" health humanities and inspiring avant-garde forms of art as primary media for teaching and learning, while resisting evangelicalism—despite our fervor. In this way, our work in fostering reflective, critical, and creative capacities in our learners positions the humanities in health care as a core, pervasive democratizing critique, not only of potentially reductive biomedical science and dehumanizing life sciences, anatomy, and clinical skills, but also of poorly conceived and badly taught communication skills. We can convincingly argue that the critique offered by both the humanities in health care and more radical, challenging art forms better tests the limits of tolerance of ambiguity in the world of health care (and the world at large), however risky. For example, evaluations of graduates at Peninsula exposed to arts- and humanities-based education have subsequently shown relatively higher levels of tolerance of ambiguity and practice artistry, supporting the approaches detailed by the innovative educators showcased in this book.

CONCLUSION

The humanities in health care educate for practice artistry in all clinical disciplines through personal reflection, values reflexivity, and refraction within a community of practice. Education in these "three Rs" links to increased tolerance of ambiguity, empathy, and emotional intelligence or fluency. We need to provide the hottest kinds of learning environments embodying the uncertainties, idiosyncrasies, and values conflicts that students will face when working in clinical teams with complex technologies and patients who deserve empathic, mindful care.

NOTES

1. Homer, *Iliad,* lines 193–94, 196–97, 219–20.
2. Donald A. Schön, *Educating the Reflective Practitioner: Toward a New Design for Teaching and Learning in the Professions* (Oxford: Jossey Bass, 1991).
3. Ibid.
4. Alan Bleakley, "From Reflective Practice to Holistic Reflexivity," *Studies in Higher Education* 24 (1999): 315–30.

SUGGESTED RESOURCE

1. Bleakley, Alan, Robert Marshall, and Rainer Brömer. "Toward an Aesthetic Medicine: Developing a Core Medical Humanities Undergraduate Curriculum." *Journal of Medical Humanities* 27 (2006): 197–213.

Foreword

Keeping Reflection Poetic

JACK COULEHAN

Nothing will sustain you more potently than the power to recognize in your humdrum routine . . . the true poetry of life—the poetry of the commonplace, of the ordinary man, of the plain, toil-worn woman, with their loves and their joys, their sorrows and their griefs.

—WILLIAM OSLER, FROM *THE STUDENT LIFE*, IN *AEQUANIMITAS*

In "Transplant," cardiologist-poet John Stone evokes the scene of a medical miracle. As a recipient lies waiting in an operating room, a donor heart arrives by helicopter from Wisconsin. Surgeons remove the recipient's diseased heart ("Within the green purpose of the room / there were ten beating hearts, but now are nine") and insert the silent, motionless replacement. The poem concludes with the miraculous moment when the patient's new heart comes alive: "And then the shock, the charmed expectant start, the last astonished harvest of the heart."[1]

When I teach this poem, students readily appreciate the amazing technological feat of heart transplantation. They can also understand how moving it must be for a physician to see his patient reborn in such a fashion. However, those who have had experience with patients respond to "Transplant" with additional insight. They often relate stories of seemingly mundane episodes when a patient said this or did that, small encounters that had nothing to do with technology, but which caused them to experience moments of fulfillment or astonishment. These moments, I suggest, are the astonished harvest of medical practice.

As a junior faculty member in Pittsburgh, I worked at a community health center in Terrace Village, the city's largest public housing project. With its institutional buildings and drab, cracked streets, the place looked nothing like a village, and the only place resembling a terrace was a huge slab of broken concrete in front of the housing office. The clinic was one of the few safe places to socialize. I remember one woman who had lived in the "projects" since the day President Roosevelt cut the ribbon at their opening in 1943. This lonely widow had multiple medical problems and lived in constant fear of the hoodlums in her building. I hated to see her name appear on my office schedule because her symptoms never improved, her medications always caused side effects, and, according to her, I was too young to know anything. Yet she never missed an appointment, if only to tell me that she had been carried to the emergency room, where they did special tests and gave her new prescriptions.

One day just before Easter, Celia Houston[2] appeared in my office wearing a childlike white lace dress and carrying a small potted plant that she brought for my office. "An act of Christian love," she said, "not a sign of being personal." I was stunned by the unexpected gesture of gratitude from this chronically dissatisfied woman and afterward wrote a poem called "The Act of Love" that ended like this: "As for me, I'm stunned / out of the ordinary anger / at failing to help her / by the waxy-leaves of her gesture / and I receive this wafer of the season, / heartbroken for no reason." It was a moment of astonishment.

I began to use poetry in teaching medical students and residents because poems can capture in a direct way the joys, uncertainties, and emotional distress of medical practice. The American poet Rafael Campo hit the nail on the head when he wrote, "Many of us find ourselves looking instinctively to the humanities as a source of renewal, reconnection, and meaning."[3] In my mind, these three words—renewal, reconnection, and meaning—summarize the yearnings of many clinicians who daily face the existential demands of medicine while often moving too fast or becoming too detached to experience its existential rewards. I love poetry and literature and history and the visual arts for many reasons, but in teaching future practitioners the art of healing, I value these disciplines as catalysts for reflection and self-discovery. Although making poems is a major part my own process of renewal and reconnection, I'm quick to reassure students that many pathways are available for them to move toward reflective practice.

Encounters with patients have always engaged my emotions. From the beginning I resisted the idea that doctors should foster detachment in order to achieve objectivity. For me "detached concern" is an oxymoron. What can empathy be, if not a form of human connection? How can a person be caring or compassionate in the context of emotional distance? At the same time, I often found myself frustrated, dejected, and angry, sometimes even wanting to run away from it all. While "Transplant" may open the door to astonishment, reflective practice must lead us to these darker doors as well.

This was the case when I took care of Ronald Colman some years after I had left the neighborhood health center and was practicing in a university setting. Mr. Colman was a proud and aggressive man from a distinguished local family. He made me feel defensive. At times he would exude hearty camaraderie, but I sensed his arrogance beneath. At each office visit he would brag about his success in the market and drop the names of famous acquaintances. On one occasion I ordered an MRI to investigate Mr. Colman's "it's probably nothing" abdominal pain. It turned out to be carcinoma of the head of the pancreas. The day he returned for follow-up, Mr. Colman was full of himself as usual, remarking that he planned to visit a well-known diagnostic clinic, but he needed a script for Vicodin until he could get there. Later, I tried to capture my conflicted feelings in a poem called "The Words," which ends "I want to escape from the room, / to leave him with his power / and run from mine, the words that cut / to his core: *Behold the pancreas!* / He looks at me with faint unease / rising in the creases of his eyes— / My words will make him mortal, he will die." I don't think my strong aversion to sharing the bad news with him resulted only from a desire to avoid causing distress. Rather, it was also fed by a subversive fear that I might actually *enjoy* giving him pain, I might somehow compensate for my feelings of inferiority by knocking this "Olympian father of the gods" down to size. Poetry provided me with a way of coming to understand and cope with these very human feelings.

We often attribute detachment and burnout in today's physicians to the rapid pace and dehumanizing features of our health-care system. Yet, long before medicine became a roiling pressure cooker, teachers like John Gregory, Thomas Percival, William Osler, and Francis Peabody warned their students that a life in medicine could foster emotional distress and insensitivity. Although these physicians wrote in a language of moral sentiment that seems archaic to us, in many ways their expressions capture our existential concerns more vividly than does today's aseptic language of medicine. For example, students often complain that they are being dehumanized by their training, or they find themselves morally conflicted about the way one of their patients was treated, or they feel abused, but powerless to do anything about it. In these situations, they can more easily relate to metaphors like "hardness of heart" and concepts like balancing steadiness and tenderness than to ethical principles like autonomy and beneficence.

I began using poetry in clinical teaching some years before it entered my preclinical repertoire. I occasionally brought a poem to read toward the end of rounds. I distributed copies to students, and we sat and discussed the poem for a few minutes. My objectives were originally focused on behavior, such as helping them become better observers or more careful listeners. Topics like grief or the psychology of chronic illness, which would fall flat when discussed as "issues," were enlivened when they appeared in Denise Levertov's "Talking to Grief" and James Dickey's "Diabetes." Poems appeared to provide these trainees with a more humane way of understanding and responding to their work. Later, when I became responsible for an extensive medical ethics and humanities curriculum, I smuggled poetry into preclinical teaching. Not surprisingly, many students responded with comments like "I don't understand poetry" and "I don't see how poetry is relevant." For most, this attitude changed when they realized our focus was on personal experience and self-discovery, rather than literary analysis.

In a journal entry, one of my fourth-year medical students described the practice of medicine "as simply poetry in motion. The art of medicine is the validation of everything that makes the human experience. I learned more about myself than I ever imagined." It took me a while to realize that the real value of poetry in medical education is just that: self-discovery. Attentiveness, careful observation, empathic responding, and the other clinical skills are desirable but secondary phenomena. The primary process involves mindfulness, self-awareness, and the moral imagination, a process in which reflective reading and writing, especially of poetry, may play a significant role.

In her essay "Metaphor and Memory," Cynthia Ozick claims that doctors cultivate a detached concern for patients because they are afraid of finding themselves "too frail . . . to enter into psychological twinship with the even frailer souls of the sick."[4] All of us, not just physicians and other health-care professionals, fear this vulnerability. Acknowledging frailness is a step toward resilience, just as discovering tenderness is a step toward steadiness. In 1990 I visited the Oglala Sioux Reservation at Pine Ridge, South Dakota, as part of a study of coronary artery disease among Native Americans. While there, I was invited to observe a Sun Dance near the site of the 1890 Massacre at Wounded Knee, when the Seventh Cavalry shot and killed about two hundred defenseless Sioux men, women, and children. In the Sun Dance, young men and women seek to restore harmony in their lives by communing with their totemic spirits. At one point during the several-day ceremony, participants invite spectators to pick up a stone and bring it to a great circle. I did so. The dancers and medicine men moved around the circle, stopping to bless each supplicant with sage branches and a medicine pipe. I was moved to tears by this ceremony. Back at home, I put my little stone in a buckskin pouch that I still carry in my briefcase. Later, I tried to evoke the healing power of that experience in a poem that concluded: "This stone is an aspect of soul that lasts. / I call it my friend, my black stone friend."

Poetry speaks for the art in healing, for the "aspect of soul that lasts," for meaning and value in medical practice. As Gregory, Percival, Osler, and Peabody knew, the risk of losing heart, or of hardening one's heart, is always present in medicine. In pursuing objectivity, we are tempted to neglect the more difficult project of nourishing tenderness in our relationships with patients and with ourselves. However, taking this path prevents us from reaping John Stone's "astonished harvest of the heart." Poetry bids us to consider taking a different path in our professional lives.

NOTES

1. John Stone, *Music from Apartment 8: New and Selected* (Baton Rouge: Louisiana State Univ. Press, 2004), 157.
2. In this essay, all names of patients have been replaced by pseudonyms.
3. Rafael Campo, "'The Medical Humanities,' for Lack of a Better Term," *Journal of the American Medical Association* 294, no. 9 (2005): 1009–11.
4. Cynthia Ozick, *Metaphor and Memory: Essays* (New York: Knopf, 1989), 278.

Preface

Extend a Broad, Global Invitation.
Court Innovative Thinking. Be Open to Surprise

ALLAN PETERKIN AND PAMELA BRETT-MACLEAN

Extend a broad, global invitation. Court innovative thinking. Be open to surprise. We had these guidelines in mind when we drafted the call for submissions for *Keeping Reflection Fresh*. We wanted to be open to all health professions, so we invited submissions from a wide range of contributors—from students, practitioners, and educators, as well as artists and humanities scholars—anyone engaged in the education of health professionals.

Our goal was to inspire readers interested in reinvigorating their own approaches to reflection and teaching in health professions education. Therefore, we looked for creativity, innovation, passion, and provocation. We welcomed anecdotes as well as hard evidence that the innovative methods described resonated with students and colleagues. We specifically asked for "eureka moments" in teaching, personal stories of projects undertaken or lessons learned. As a bold step for an academic book, we limited the word count of submissions and the number of references allowed. This decision allowed us to accept a wider range of truly refreshing, even unexpected submissions than would otherwise have been possible. We were interested in the story of how an idea for reflective learning came about, a "how-to" of practical steps for implementing it, along with iterative reflections on the experience of doing so. Recognizing the growing role of the visual arts and new media in promoting reflective capacity, we welcomed those submissions as well. As curators of this collection, we wanted to recognize the wide-open opportunity that exists for joining together as a community and learning from each other. We thus anticipated a broad readership consisting of educators, practitioners, and lifelong learners across the healing professions, social sciences, humanities, and artistic media.

To our surprise and gratification, we received many more submissions than we could accept (enough for a full second volume), suggesting that our invitation had resonated across an extensive range of learning communities. At the same time, we had to make difficult decisions to ensure the presence of a wide range of approaches and voices from different disciplines and across different geographies. We included newcomers to the field, as well as numerous educators and scholars recognized for their long-standing and significant contributions. By simply flipping through the pages of this book or scanning the table of contents, you'll find contributors hailing from regions across the world—from the United States, Canada, the United Kingdom, Switzerland, Israel, Australia, New Zealand, and Hong Kong.

What is most evident throughout *Keeping Reflection Fresh* is proof of a growing community of educators, scholars, researchers, and artists collaborating across disciplines who recognize reflection as integral to personal and professional development. All of the submissions offer impressive insights and suggest a flourishing range of approaches to teaching and modeling reflection in both education and clinical practice. We made a deliberate decision not to emphasize formal evaluation strategies in this collection, recognizing the many challenges associated with assessing reflective capacity in a manner that positively promotes the ongoing development of authentic self-awareness and relational responsiveness. However, we do encourage all readers to contemplate new, respectful, and creative ways of demonstrating the value of the teaching approaches represented here, especially their contributions to the personal and professional formation of caring, compassionate, resilient, and effective health practitioners.

We are delighted to have Alan Bleakley open the book with a discussion of the importance of creativity in our shared work and to have Jack Coulehan draw our attention to the poetics involved in healing. We conclude with a contribution by Louise Aronson, who urges us to remember that any innovation in teaching must always be directed at improving patient care and well-being. Together their reflections on the urgent need for beauty, poetics, and accountability in our shared work will stimulate many important conversations over time. Most importantly, they remind us that we are accountable not only to the scholarly enterprise and to those we teach but, above all, to those we serve and care for. These themes are addressed passionately and imaginatively in the collection's lead essay, "Writing toward Self, Other, and Health" by Rita Charon. That her work is the most frequently cited throughout the collection provides evidence of her contribution to narrative medicine and reflection.

We are profoundly grateful to all those who accepted our invitation to have their work included in *Keeping Reflection Fresh*. In the dozens of essays included in this volume, over 170 authors outline a dazzling array of approaches, techniques, and exercises they have used to nurture reflection and personal growth in clinical curricula. In addition to narrative, visual, and performative approaches to reflection, other important pedagogical themes are included, such as learning from patients and clients, unpacking contemporary challenges to ethics and professionalism, appreciating the role of new media and other technological innovations in curriculum design, and honoring the personal and spiritual dimensions of reflection on teaching and clinical practice.

In each essay, the authors concisely outline a compelling idea or approach they have found useful. As editors, we most often offered a light touch as we did not want to introduce a tone of academic detachment or impose uniformity in style. Rather we wanted to preserve the voice of each author (idiosyncrasies included). Interested readers may want to follow up with authors whose work they find particularly interesting or useful. In their short biographies, we encouraged each author to include information about the organization with which they are affiliated in order to assist in making these connections (see Contributors). We believe *Keeping Reflection Fresh* will inspire new imaginings, connections, and conversations, which may in turn serve to enrich practices and stimulate scholarly inquiry in this area. We imagine that all the resulting adaptations, applications, and improvisations offered here will not only deepen and enhance our understanding of our current efforts but may also help us face the challenges of coordinating multimodal, developmental approaches to teaching reflection to professionals throughout their careers.

The commitment of the contributing authors to *Keeping Reflection Fresh* through the long and at times complicated process of preparing this manuscript was more than appreciated; in fact, it deeply inspired us as editors. We were reminded again and again about the importance of wholeness (and integrity), connection, and the valuing of personal and professional growth both of our students *and* of ourselves as educators. All of the wonderful forms of reflection described in this collection offer opportunities for revitalizing our teaching practices by encouraging us to take better care of ourselves and to recharge our sense of connectedness and meaning in the challenging work we do.

Reflective practice invites us to inquire into our own thoughts, biases, assumptions, feelings, and behaviors and to reconnect with our own sense of purpose and commitment to our work. Just as we endeavor to make sense of our own complex experiences, we are also obligated to reflect on our experience of teaching. Our students deserve to be taught and mentored by truly reflective educators. It is helpful to be reminded (with a strong dose of humility) that we are involved in learning journeys focused on enhancing clinical education that have the potential for influencing the culture of biomedicine and influencing health care. Indeed, we would like to recognize all *we* have learned from our students and collaborators over the past many years. Ultimately, *Keeping Reflection Fresh* has enriched our own thinking and teaching and shown us the importance of contributing to a wider conversation that will in turn inspire new innovations in this area.

In closing, we are grateful to all those who guided and supported us in completing this collection, including our students, trainees, and colleagues within our academic departments and programs at the University of Toronto and University of Alberta. In particular, we would like to thank Michael Black-ie, editor of the Literature & Medicine series, and Joyce Harrison, acquiring editor at the Kent State University Press, who saw the potential in this project from the beginning. We thank Lynn Kavanagh, Elizabeth Ludwig, and Nicole Schafenacker for their assistance in helping us prepare the manuscript for submission, and we also thank those who were involved in reviewing and copyediting the text prior to publication. And, finally, we thank those we love for their patience and support during this deeply rewarding process.

PART 1

Narrative Approaches—
Reading, Writing, and Reflecting

Writing toward Self, Other, and Health

RITA CHARON

Early in the day before the workplace starts to hum, I welcome eight men and women into a quiet, high-windowed room to read and write. Today, we start with two paragraphs from William Maxwell's novel, *So Long, See You Tomorrow.* Twelve-year-old Cletus enters the kitchen of the Illinois 1930s farmhouse he lives in, taking it in, with its "wooden surfaces that have been scrubbed to the texture of velvet.... The wood box, the sink, the comb hanging by a string, the roller towel . . . The smell of Octagon soap."[1]

We notice how the young boy is shaped by those spaces and silences and smells. No other kitchen, the narrator writes, "would have been waiting in absolute stillness for Cletus to come home from school, or have seemed like all his heart desired when he walks in out of the cold."[2]

We talk about the style and the rhythms of Maxwell's lean prose, about the congruities between the novelist's own life and the lives of his protagonists, about the governing images that emerge from these short excerpts. We notice how his sensory-rich sentences enable us to imagine Cletus's situation, how they admit us into the inner world of this young boy. We see, suddenly, how the miracle of reading leads us to care about this boy.

We move next to a later paragraph in the novel, after terrible things in Cletus's life have forced him and his mother to move out of the farmhouse into town:

Take away the kitchen—the smell of something good in the oven for dinner. Take away the patient old horse waiting by the pasture fence. Take away the cow barn where the cats, sitting all in a row, wait with their mouths wide open for somebody to squirt milk down their throats. Take all this away and what have you done to him? In the face of a deprivation so great, what is the use of

3

asking him to go on being the boy he was. He might as well start life over again as some other boy instead.[3]

Now we talk about deprivation. We readers feel sorrow in the face of the inexorable diminishment of this young boy. We notice that care—the attention of the patient horse, the nourishing of those open-mouthed cats by the cow milkers—is part of what's been stripped away. Twenty minutes of close reading have gathered us around a life exposed, a life from which the veil has been lifted. Cletus becomes visible and maybe even comprehensible to us by virtue of 350 words of great prose.

Together, now, in the shadow of these paragraphs, the students and I begin to write. We have four minutes to respond to my writing prompt: "Write about the things you cannot do without." After writing, we take turns reading our pieces to one another. The woman from Dublin, who knows sorrow up close, describes life without her passport, which expired, how she felt captured, restricted—her freedom of movement, which she didn't even know she treasured, taken away. The solemn, bearded man writes about standing at his kitchen sink scrubbing a potato, imagining the future for his children, sensing their impending adulthood, treasuring their time together, refusing to squander it. The intense young man, long hair, bottomless eyes, writes not of time but of space—the empty horizons of early morning runs, his lone figure moving against the river and the sky, the magnitude of the space, his own insignificance and necessity in the face of the cosmic sublime.

No onlooker would know that we readers are doctors or that this class has anything to do with health care. We are gathered in the pediatric conference room for what we have come to call Narrative Peds. Once a month, we carve out an hour before the start of clinic to write about our lives, which are filled with sick and struggling children.

These doctors know that what they do matters for their young patients. They watch over their patients' physical health. They help them get into good high schools, stay out of jail, or dream of a bright future. They have also come to know things about the world that they'd rather not know—how some parents abuse their children, how random unfair cancers end young lives, how some children give up. They hold within themselves these secrets about the world, finding somewhere alongside the despair the surprise that leads to hope. Writing helps them do this.

As we bend over this novel, our heads touch. We leave at the hour's end, having made authentic contact with one another, contact that is not otherwise encouraged in big academic medical centers. Having written about our own possibilities of deprivation simply makes more likely that we will see—or rather wonder about and then see—the things our patients cannot do without.

This hour of Narrative Pediatrics expands the capacity of these doctors to imagine, learn about, and care about the situations of their patients. The hour also gives these doctors, struggling against a high tide of suffering and shipwrecks, some communion with one another, some time to tell the truth, to talk of self, to hear one another out. Members of this group have described how their reading and writing have shifted the balance of their own curiosity in clinic, how they feel grateful for the chance to hear patients' stories in practice, how they find themselves hungry to learn about their patients' lives.

The woman from Dublin is a neonatologist in charge when parents in the NICU learn that their tiny premature baby might die. The bearded man at the sink envisioning the future for his own children is the pediatrician who directs pediatric training for Columbia medical students, envisioning a future medicine on their behalf. The intense young runner has committed his life in pediatrics to international health care driving toward health-care justice, able to envision a form of care that reaches those horizons he imagines.

We have learned in the twelve years since originating narrative medicine that close reading and creative writing encourage clinicians and trainees to behold the realities they encounter in their practice, to take them in, to wonder about them. This monthly seminar for pediatricians is one of many narrative medicine seminars offered at Columbia in a variety of clinical departments and training settings. Unlike conventional medicine's reductions, narrative medicine expands. Instead of cataloguing the typically seen, this medicine discovers the never before seen, widening the possible meanings of what is suffered. Perhaps those who care for the sick can perceive and then recognize the scenes, spaces, silences, and designs of mortal life. Perhaps this is what health care is for.

Our narrative work exposes and influences the culture of our institution. We have gradually accrued credibility by funding our work, studying its outcomes, working with faculty and student allies, and publishing studies of the consequences of our narrative medicine teaching in good medical and medical education journals.

Our work has come to matter to the institution. Narrative methods and practices now underlie major faculty development efforts, externally funded teaching and research in interprofessional education, curricular innovations, and novel clinical routines on the wards and in the clinic. Within our highly research-oriented academic institution, our work has steadily illuminated the importance of patients' and staff members' lived experience. The scholarly attention we have paid to reflection and creativity has enabled these concepts to be seen, more and more, as an established part of our institution's culture.

In the end, our work is done on behalf of the patients who come to us for care. If there is a bonus of clarity and pleasure and beauty for the clinicians, if an outcome of our narrative work is greater collegiality and greater skill in the acts of reading and writing, the undeniable goal of this work is to improve the health care for the sick. By welcoming beauty and the imagination into its midst, our medical center is coming to understand that creativity is required of effective care, that the art can improve the care, that the care of the sick is a work of art.

NOTES

1. William Maxwell, *So Long, See You Tomorrow* (New York: Random House/Vintage, 1996), 58.
2. Ibid., 59.
3. Ibid., 113.

SUGGESTED RESOURCES

1. Charon, Rita. *Narrative Medicine: Honoring the Stories of Illness.* New York: Oxford Univ. Press, 2006.
2. Miller, Eliza et al. "Sounding Narrative Medicine: Studying Students' Professional Identity Development at Columbia University College of Physicians and Surgeons." *Academic Medicine* 89, no. 2 (2014): 335–42.

Decentering the Doctor-Protagonist

Personal Illness Narratives in the Narrative Medicine Classroom

SAYANTANI DASGUPTA

Who is the hero of the medical story? To whom does an illness story belong? Disciplines alternately called humanities and medicine, or narrative medicine, seek to bring patient stories to the fore—to listen to them, teach with them, honor them. Yet the tradition of "doctor stories" being told by and about doctors/ clinicians remains. Patients—and more often, their diseases, families, and bodily idiosyncrasies—may be objects in most medical stories, but clinicians are their active subjects. Most often, doctors are the protagonists of medical tales, their stalwart heroes; they drive the story and enact change. Patients, on the other hand, do not act but are acted upon. These narrative understandings are more than merely scholarly; they have deep impact on the way that clinicians and patients think about themselves and each other, while ultimately undermining the potential for real mutuality and partnership in the medical relationship.

Reflective writing by physicians, nurses, and other clinicians deepens insight into the clinical relationship with the patient, the medical team, and the self. However, these practices rarely challenge the seemingly fixed categories of "clinician" and "patient," "health" and "sickness," categories that inevitably suggest a hierarchy of power favoring the medical professional. Yet reflective writing holds the potential to destabilize these binaries and, in doing so, contribute to a more just practice of medicine. In a "Narrative, Health and Social Justice" seminar I teach in Columbia University's master's program in narrative medicine, I often ask my students to analyze written, visual, and oral narratives about health and embodiment, to ask themselves if these stories are socially just or unjust. Parts of these discussions inevitably focus on the issues of the protagonist—who acts and who is acted upon, who speaks and who is spoken for. Indeed, the question that drives much of our work is "Whose story is it?"

One type of narrative I often examine with my students is film about global health issues, documentaries such as *Born into Brothels* (2004) or the more recent *Blood Brother* (Hoover, 2013). Despite being moving, award-winning stories, our critique of these films inevitably lands upon the issue of the Western protagonist, the "white savior" who arrives in an impoverished developing country and not only changes local lives but is emotionally and spiritually changed in the process. The roots of this sort of neocolonialist "rescue" narrative are multiple. One issue is that of reader/viewer entry point. For example, two-time Pulitzer Prize–winning *New York Times* columnist Nicholas Kristof, who often writes about human rights and health issues in developing countries, is frequently criticized for portraying the "rescuer" as a white Westerner. Kristof has responded to critiques that he often portrays "black Africans as victims" and "white foreigners as their saviors" by saying that he believes readers need a foreigner as a "bridge character," someone they can "identify with" in order for them to care about the problems of "distant countries."[1] The implicit assumption here is that all of Kristof's readers are white, privileged, and situated in the Global North. Anyone else, whether reading the *New York Times* or not, is not an actor, but someone to be acted *upon*.

A second, more subtle, reason for this phenomenon of the white "rescuer" is the tradition in Western narratives of having one fixed, central protagonist rather than multiple, or shifting, centers of narration. The expectation is usually that there will be one central character whose inward journey parallels the journey of the story's plot. Yet this is not the only way a story can unfold. Consider the film *Revolutionary Optimists* (2013), another documentary about health and illness in an impoverished Indian community. The directors of *Revolutionary Optimists* do not make central a Western or foreign protagonist. Nor do they privilege one person's voice or narrative, but they create multiple entry points with multiple points of view and multiple protagonists, therefore perhaps telling a more socially just tale.

What is the impact of such understandings on clinician reflective writing? In another class I teach (Illness and Disability Narratives) at both Columbia's narrative medicine program and the graduate program in health advocacy at Sarah Lawrence College, I ask that, in lieu of weekly "reaction papers," my students write a "dynamic personal illness narrative." This exercise seeks to destabilize the clinical protagonist in the medical story.[2] I ask my clinicians- and advocates-in-training to write on a weekly basis not about the professional work of healing or advocacy but about a personal or familial experience of illness, disability, or caregiving. My students choose one experience—a spouse's cancer, a personal operation, a child's mental illness—and write about that same experience all semester long. Based on our topics of study, I give the students weekly prompts—ways to change the point of view, the genre, or the frame of the narrative—but these prompts ("write from the point of view of your clinician," "write from the point of view of the body," "create a visual narrative or collage," "write a poem or play") are suggestions only. What is important to me is not that students follow my prompts, or even produce work of publishable quality (although they often do). Rather, the goal is to give the students a sense of their own personal frames of listening—the experiences, prejudices, and expectations they bring to any listening encounter with future patients. The exercise also allows students to write about their own bodies and families rather than the bodies and families of others, thereby breaking down the "us" and "them" binary of "well clinician" and "ill patient" on which so much of medical power is predicated. This binary is so strong it often pro-hibits students, particularly already practicing doctors or nurses, from even *remembering* personal moments of vulnerability. "I have never been ill," claim many such students, only to discover, through the process of writing, a host of personal experiences that have remained buried in the face of the invulnerable facade so necessary to their medical professional cultures.

Yet the "personal illness narratives" exercise is not therapy, and I am ex-tremely conscious of issues of safety in the semester-long classroom. When students share their work, I reiterate rules of respect and confidentiality. I only require that students share one narrative aloud per semester, one of their own choice and timing. The exercise works because of the clear boundaries and the sense of safety that is created. Within the parameters of this safe community, the personal illness narrative exercise allows health-care professionals in training to see themselves as "patients" as well as "professionals," and in doing so, it effectively decenters the position of the singular clinician protagonist in the medical narrative. As philosopher Judith Butler has asserted, this kind of decentering of the protagonist-self is an act of profound social justice, which leads beyond an egocentric, binary understanding of the world ("us" vs. "them").[3] Although Butler is meditating on American fantasies of national invulnerability and global "mastery" that crumbled after 9/11, her words can be applied to the fantasies of professional invulnerability that are so common in medical culture: "We cannot, however, will away this vulnerability. We must attend to it, even abide by it, as we begin to think about what politics might be implied by staying with the thought of corporeal vulnerability itself."[4]

Like narratives in which a foreign protagonist "rescues" helpless others, medi-cal narratives have the potential of being deeply neocolonialist stories—earnest tales of intrepid heroes solving mysteries and saving lives in the impoverished landscapes of their patients' embodied experiences, even as they are spiritually transformed in the process. Engaging health-care professionals in personal illness narrative exercises, like the one described here, challenges the seemingly fixed categories of clinician and patient, making clear that there breathe vulnerable bodies on both sides of the stethoscope, while allowing for a mindful attention to the category of corporeal vulnerability itself. The dynamic nature of the seminar, the fact that students approach and reapproach the same topic through different points of view and genres all semester, simultaneously allows students to break free of the expectation of the singular narrative protagonist and to recognize that there are shifting, multiple understandings of any one story.

Clinicians must decenter themselves from the medical narrative to achieve any real sense of collaborative partnership, mutuality, or power sharing in the health-care relationship. They must accept that they are not present for every part of the medical story's plot; nor are their recommendations and actions always the driving force of every health-care outcome. Attention to clinicians' own physical and emotional vulnerabilities may allow room for a different sort of medical politics. Reflective writing such as the personal illness narrative exercise can allow this shift to take place, making room for more than one hero in the medical story.

NOTES

1. Nicholas Kristof, "Youtube Question on Africa Coverage," *The New York Times,* July 9, 2010, http://kristof.blogs.nytimes.com/2010/07/09/youtube-question-on-africa-coverage.
2. Sayantani DasGupta and Rita Charon, "Personal Illness Narratives: Using Reflective Writing to Teach Empathy," *Academic Medicine* 79 (2004): 351–56.
3. Judith Butler, *Precarious Life: The Powers of Mourning and Violence* (London, New York: Verso, 2006).
4. Ibid., 29.

Holding a Mirror to Reflective Writing and Discourse

LINDA S. RAPHAEL

Reflective writing and *reflective thinking* are buzz terms in medical humanities these days. Yet we may be mistaken if we assume that we are all talking about the same thing when we use the terms. What do we mean when we talk about *reflection?* The first thing that comes to mind is the reflection in a mirror, and while an object and its mirror image may seem to enjoy a simple relationship, literary critic Stephen Greenblatt challenges such an undemanding interpretation of mirror images with a conclusion that has relevance to our use of reflection in medical education.[1] Referring to Hamlet's lines about the play within the play—that the mirror shows "virtue its feature, scorn his own image, and the very age and body of time his own form and pressure," Greenblatt explains that this notion of the mirror as an image "of instantaneous and accurate reproduction [that] takes nothing from what it reflects and adds nothing but self-knowledge," while "convenient and self-protective," obscures the reality that "something was actively passing back and forth in the production of mirror images." He concludes that "only if we reinvest the mirror image with a sense of pressure as well as form can convey something of its original strangeness and magic."[2] Pressure and form—the demands of medical education, clinical experience, our students' own diverse backgrounds, and personal experiences—inevitably influence their reflective writing and thinking in ways that surpass any simple notions of a "mirror image."

In relation to pressures bearing on medical educators, Ruth Cigman argues that teaching students how not to think and how not to act so that they may avoid lawsuits passes as a rationale for teaching ethics in medical schools.[3] Citing the work of Atul Gawande, she recommends that students learn about "ethical thinking as the appropriate management of doubt."[4] In reflecting on a patient's experience, an attending's "modeling" behavior, a peer's actions, or one's own behavior, doubt and ambiguity must play a significant role. Attempts to discourage doubt, or to deny ambiguity, ignore the multifaceted nature that medical situations share with most human experience. Reflective writing can be an effective way for students to explore doubt and "locate themselves" at various stages in their medical education.

Reflective writing and discussions in the medical humanities courses I teach at the George Washington University School of Medicine and Health Sciences fall into two broad categories: reflections on, or responses to texts (films, graphic medicine texts, fiction, essays, and poetry), and reflections on experience. The former provides the basis of elective courses offered in the first, second, and fourth years of our undergraduate curriculum. The latter are introduced as components of required humanities sessions in our third-year clerkships and involve our students' response to texts and reflection on their own personal experience. While there are a number of objectives that reflective writing might accomplish, I concentrate on three: to encourage students' awareness of their values, attitudes, beliefs, and emotions; to articulate their expectations about what it will mean to be a physician (including what they believe a doctor's care and advice, medicines, and procedures can do to prevent or cure illness); and to appreciate the dialogic nature of their interactions with patients. One of the important benefits of narrative reflections aimed at these goals, which cannot be underestimated, is that they stimulate a more dynamic class discussion, and allow me to develop a fruitful relationship with students.

The above are ideals; the reality sometimes falls short. For example, how does one explain the contradiction in the following responses to a short reflection exercise in the third-year medicine clerkship? In the first instance, a student commented that the discussion of reflections in the previous session did not result in answers to problems: "It was like an AA meeting," she concluded. Two weeks later, in a session with a different group, a student read his reflection about a patient who, he wrote, "could be me." He imagined details in the life of the young man whose gastric cancer had returned. During the discussion, he repeated, with dismay, the gastroenterologist's brief words to the patient as she left the room, "Did anyone tell you the cancer has come back?" A few days later, the student sent me a poem he had composed about the patient, using the ideas and some of the phrases from his reflective writing.

It is tempting to dismiss the comment that reflective writing and discussions are like AA meetings, that reflection which is primarily descriptive may be a way of looking in the mirror only to see that which is "convenient and protective," as Greenblatt warns. However, we need to keep in mind the "pressures and forms" that motivate the student. One pressure comes from the rigorous testing for right answers in the science courses and board examinations during the first two years of most medical schools in the United States and Canada. Another comes from the form, or practice, which students look forward to and which involves curing, or at least alleviating, health problems. In clerkship, students' aspirations may crash on the rocks of reality, at least temporarily. Most students do not enter medical school to learn to cope with doubt and ambiguity. It takes skill, practice, and sometimes more time than allotted in the curriculum to deal effectively with their frustrations and disappointments. Yet it is important that students who are inspired to write poems about patients and students who resist the complexity of reflection feel that their concerns are being understood. Occasionally, we may be able to do no more than acknowledge someone's disappointment with the clerkship medical humanities sessions; "to acknowledge" is what we advise them to do in their interactions with patients when there is no answer to the patient's mental or physical pain.

Although elective courses in the humanities attract students who are typically willing and even eager to write about and discuss readings and films, a few challenges worth noting occur in these classes. Approximately one in ten students writes a summary rather than a critical or contemplative reaction to the assigned reading or film. Somewhat surprisingly, there does not seem to be much correspondence between their superficial writing and their contributions to class discussion, which are often enthusiastic and introspective. It seems that we ought to be careful not to privilege writing to the extent that we overlook the value of oral communication. On the other hand, students occasionally write deeply personal responses that give one pause. I can recall one student's response to readings on obesity that raised important questions about a physician's personal reactions to patients, which divulged her feelings about her own body. She considered herself to be obese and believed she was the only obese female in her year. I do not assign readings that would be difficult for an obese student, but she had not impressed me as obese. While I was forewarned about her feelings in a way that was helpful in guiding the class discussion, I was uncertain about my role as interlocutor for this reading. I decided to express my regret at having assigned a reading that was painful for her. Her appreciation of my concern and her desire to further discuss her feelings indicated that I was right in offering the chance for more discussion. However, this sort of situation could develop in a different direction.

Another student wrote in response to readings in a session titled "Illness and Identity" that her "family had recently experienced a death from cancer." She did not say who had died, and she did not speak of the matter in class.

She seldom participated in discussions, but her reflections on readings were thoughtful and engaged. In the course that immediately followed this one, a student asked if I would substitute other films for two about a cancer because both her father and the father of the student referred to above had died of cancer in the last few months. What did it mean for this student to write a reflection, leaving out any expression of the loss she had just experienced? I assume that she found the class meaningful, or she would not have enrolled in the next one, but I cannot say more than that.

These cases call attention to how sensitive we need to be when we ask students to read and discuss reflectively. The student who writes a summary may be eliding personal matters he or she is not ready to express or to confront. One of the criticisms of reflection among students comes from their sense that they are being forced to "emote." Although educators whose goal is to lead students to more self-understanding and compassion for others are likely to be skilled at handling delicate situations, we need to remind ourselves that students are responding to pressures and forms that affect their mirror image and our ability to understand their reflections.

NOTES

1. Stephen Greenblatt, *Shakespearean Negotiations: The Circulation of Social Energy in Renaissance England* (Berkeley: Univ. of California Press, 1988).
2. Ibid., 8.
3. Ruth Cigman, "How Not to Think: Medical Ethics as Negative Education," *Medicine, Health Care and Philosophy* 16 (2013): 13–18.
4. Ibid., 13.

Enhancing Learning Cultures across Campus

An Interdisciplinary Reading Group

DOROTHY WOODMAN AND TAMAR RUBIN

Our individual associations with the Arts & Humanities in Health & Medicine (AHHM) program at the University of Alberta brought us—an instructor in English and Film Studies (EFS), and a medical resident—together. Dorothy's participation in medical humanities events and Tamar's experience in a narrative reflective practice group were essential experiences for developing an interdisciplinary reading group pilot project. We both grappled with diverse influences on representation and interpretation in our work, including complex patterns, symbols, and structures of meaning, along with their often uncomfortable ambiguities. One of the many challenges in our respective specialties is developing an appreciation and acceptance of such irresolvable complexities.

We each hoped to create a group that could enhance interdisciplinary learning cultures, promote reflection, and inspire lifelong practices in diverse professional lives. Participants could recognize and collaborate on challenges common to both disciplines. Our primary goal was not to have those trained in literary and cultural studies teach medical professionals how to analyze a range of medical texts or write reflective narratives. Nor was it to have medical professionals instruct humanities experts in the specialized technologies or experiences of medicine. Rather, both disciplines would have the opportunity to engage their respective training in a shared study of interpretation and representation. By developing insights into human experiences represented in literary imaginaries we could gain understanding of each other's approaches to interpretation and responses to human experiences. This would foster a learning culture recognizing the strengths of our separate disciplines and encouraging diverse viewpoints.

A reading group could offer a range of discussion not always possible in other academic contexts. We anticipated that there would be differences in reading styles, practices, and disciplinary investments, and that individuals would bring unique amalgams of cultural and social backgrounds to the discussion. Moreover, a group such as this could represent a range of affiliations and investments. By reading, critiquing, and expressing our feelings, we could become further sensitized to the ways in which culture shapes medical experiences and our bodies' changes engage with our sense of identity. Furthermore, interdisciplinary discussions would expand knowledge, understanding, and even the nature of the questions we could ask. In a reading group context, our intellectual, ethical, and affective reflections would be unconstrained by pressures to achieve consensus, closure, or measurable outcomes.

Our pilot project was simple. We invited medical students, medical residents and fellows, and EFS graduate students and instructors. A maximum of twenty participants would represent the disciplines equally. With just four meetings during one academic term for the pilot, we let textual selections emerge in a brainstorming session. Our only criterion for selection was that the works have a medical theme. Once texts were chosen by consensus, participants volunteered to facilitate the discussion. The facilitator would simply open up the conversation, offering prompts if the conversation lagged and encouraging all individuals to participate. The discussion could then develop responsively to the interests of the group.

We chose the university hospital's public art gallery as our meeting place. Its exhibits represent multiple perspectives and experiences within medical encounters and also the larger cultural contexts in which medicine, as both a discipline and a practice, is situated. Symbolizing the interconnections between medicine and humanities, academic study and public service, such a space would emphasize the interdisciplinary nature of our meeting. Its wall of windows opens to a central passageway leading into the hospital; a photo exhibit on the walls and upholstered armchairs arranged in an informal circle offered a neutral, comfortable, and inspiring venue conducive to open and egalitarian conversation. This space foregrounded our ongoing relationships with public life. It reminded us that the work on which we had embarked was also a practice: crossing the threshold into the gallery brought us into a discursive and aesthetic space that became so much more.

Meeting together as a group, we were reminded that representation and interpretation involved more than intellectual work carried out in isolation. Our past and present contexts, our professional investments, and the environment in which we shared our reading experiences also shaped them. Within the circle of participants, the text became both the focus and background for multiple interpretive and experiential intersections. These might occur within the text, between reader and text, and among the participants gathered together. Crossing back into the trafficked hallway of the hospital's entry we were reminded that representation and interpretation are already material practices—they were worked out through our embodied experiences in the world. Leaving the gallery invigorated, we then reentered our lives on the larger campus—our professional and academic practices—and then those spilling over beyond its perimeters.

The first half hour was given to sharing a meal and informal discussion. This preliminary activity promoted discussion of both formal knowledge and personal experience among the participants, who also shared their emotional responses to the texts. It would, we hoped, minimize academic anxieties about reporting, competing, and performing. An hour was dedicated to close readings of characters, plots, settings, and form, modeled on Rita Charon's work on close reading. First we focused on literary elements in the text. Then discussion expanded to reader response and personal reflections. We first excavated meaning in the text and then explored what emerged from our engagements with it and those in the group, thereby expanding the meaning of text to include participants' stories as well as words on the page. In our first year, our chosen texts included Margaret Edson's fictional play *Wit* and Clem Martini and Olivier Martini's coauthored memoir *Bitter Medicine: A Graphic Memoir of Mental Illness*. These texts varied greatly in genre and style. Sharing critical perspectives of medical culture, they explored the effects of power, privilege, and medical science on patients who were treated, respectively, for terminal ovarian cancer and schizophrenia and who inhabited differing social and cultural contexts.

This pilot project became the foundation for a second iteration in the following academic year. We decided to dedicate the series to exploring one elusive theme: the meaning of healing. We again invited students, faculty, and staff at the University of Alberta, but this time included those working in Alberta Health Services professions in another set of four evening sessions. This more diverse group of participants—from yoga instructors to English professors, to medical doctors—shared a common interest in exploring medical themes. Again drawing from texts chosen by participants, written from different perspectives and in a variety of genres (for example, short stories, readers' theater, and memoir), participants explored the thorny issue of healing, with its diverse meanings and manifestations.

The texts sparked discussions guided by prewritten prompts provided by the coordinators. This new format enabled a less guided approach than the prepared facilitation tended to produce in the pilot, and it allowed discussion to develop more organically, whether in small groups or a single, large gathering. The reading quickly became both the focus and background for multiple interpretive and experiential intersections between reader and text, and among the participants gathered together. The final part of each meeting was devoted to journal writing and reflection, followed by large group sharing. At the last meeting in the series, participants discussed future possibilities for this reading and writing group.

In conclusion, the pilot project and subsequent year-long program offered opportunities to develop connections among disciplines that, especially on large campuses, might otherwise have little or no formal interaction. In an environment of mutual respect and interest in disciplinary perspectives, individuals can learn more about shared concerns and become better acquainted with disciplinary differences and commonalities. An enhanced comfort with ambiguity and "irresolvable problems" is beneficial to individuals in all fields that deal broadly with humanistic issues and could be further developed in a setting such as these reading groups.

SUGGESTED RESOURCES

1. Charon, Rita. *Narrative Medicine: Honoring the Stories of Illness.* New York: Oxford Univ. Press, 2006.
2. New York University School of Medicine. Literature, Arts and Medicine Database. Accessed June 5, 2015. http://medhum.med.nyu.edu/.

Medicine as a Second Language

ELIZABETH GAUFBERG, RACHAEL BEDARD,
AND MAREN BATALDEN

The first time, they crowded around you. Doting grown-ups and older siblings, smiling and pointing. Chair . . . book . . . nose. They clapped and cooed and corrected. Later, there was fine-tuning of grammar, vocabulary lists to memorize. When you started medical school, new words came. You paired *-itis* and *-osis* and *-ectomy* with a pantheon of Latin roots. You understood that these new expressions would be grafted onto your first language: the language of campfires and s'mores, your first love, your grandmother's death. You couldn't wait to use the official vocabulary. When you finally got to the wards, you found that the new words were embedded within entirely new forms of speech, replete with acronyms and slang: the H&P, orders, D/C summaries, rounds. These forms allowed you to see patterns and make connections. They marked the rhythm of your day and helped you get the work done. Some things didn't make sense at first. Why do we say ambulate rather than walk? Why do we wedge in brief notations about alcohol and tobacco use and label it "social history"? But you didn't wonder for long. Pretty soon, every one of your patients complained. Never once did you fail them, but many failed treatment. When the stories your patients told about their own lives didn't fit, they became poor historians. You learned a host of shorthand notations. Just one symbol—ψ—covered every form of emotional distress. You learned to speak about the unspeakable—death, deformity, unbearable loss—in an efficient monotone. Maybe you even began to notice things about yourself. Perhaps, when your best childhood friend was in tears over a breakup, you automatically ran through a list of neuro-vegetative symptoms rather than ranting about the jerk who dumped her. Your Aunt Millie's colorful tales became harder to take—what is her point and when will she get to it? But then maybe you stopped noticing. The new speech simply became part of you, or perhaps you figured out how to switch it on when you entered the world of fluorescent lights and beeping monitors. Perhaps you learned to leave the words on the wards when you went home.

We suspect this happened to you, dear resident, because it happened to us. Developing true fluency in the language of caring is a lifelong learning endeavor. In learning the language of doctoring, you have spent years making the strange familiar. We now invite you to make the familiar strange. In our monthly reflective practice session, "Food for the Soul," we will remove the words from the pockets of our white coats, turn them around in our hands, and run our fingers over the rough edges. We'll roll them back and forth across the table and maybe learn to juggle, tossing in words from our first language.

We might compose found poems. Starting with a standard admission note, we will cross out text until only the essence is left—like liberating a sculpture from granite. When we are done, we will have something we can set on the table and look at together. The Admission H&P did not move us, but surprisingly the poem does. We may return to our notes and the act of writing them with a new consciousness.[1] We may even find that the exercise opens our ears to listen differently as well. We consider anew a complex history recorded in the chart of a seventy-seven-year-old woman with CAD, DM2, HTN, and COPD who awoke at home with trouble breathing and acute abdominal pain and who calls 911 for transport: Old woman awoke in trouble / Alone and in pain / She calls / Receives IV and IV and IV and no solution.

We'll spend another session crafting haiku in response to common prompts from the world of medicine. Each resident will pull from a basket a phrase written on a piece of paper: "Discharge," "Diurese," "Short call," "Duty hours," "Length of stay." We'll read our haiku poems out loud and try to guess each other's prompts. Can you guess what prompts inspired your peers to write the poetry lines below?

> You should go outside / It will make you feel better / But I can't prove it
> Excruciating! / She says as she smiles at me / And asks for morphine
> Someone is afraid / A color in the rainbow / Swallowed by themselves
> I have five minutes / So, small seed, what would it take / For you to flower[2]

We may ask you to bring beginner ears to work rounds and assign you as a "designated listener." We'll ask you to jot down words or phrases that strike you as meaningful or evocative. Then you'll arrange those phrases on a page, attending to order and line breaks, in the form of a poem. Your recitation at the end of the meeting becomes a sort of community echo, an auditory mirror that reflects the conversation back to the participants and helps them to listen to themselves differently.

At first it may feel awkward to move like this back and forth between your native tongue and your adopted language. These stretching exercises can be uncomfortable. But we believe this attention to language has the power to make you a better doctor. Good communication requires this bilingual fluency. This fluency permits you to listen simultaneously as a doctor and as a human being; it permits you to be simultaneously effective and kind with your speech. You need to be able to translate patient stories into differential diagnoses and treatment plans, but you also need to be able to translate differential diagnoses and treatment plans back into patient stories. Do not abandon your native tongue—the language of campfires and s'mores, your first love, and your grandmother's death. You need it as much as your patients do.

This is the first of three related essays we have authored as co-facilitators of "Food for the Soul," a Cambridge Health Alliance (CHA) Medicine Residency reflective practice seminar. Collectively, these essays describe the main organizing principles and several of the exercises used in this seminar.

NOTES

1. Loreen Herwaldt, ed., *Patient Listening: A Doctor's Guide* (Iowa City: Univ. of Iowa Press, 2008).
2. Line 1 was inspired by evidence-based medicine; line 2, a pain scale of 1 to 10; line 3, Code Purple (psychiatric emergency); line 4, motivational interviewing.

A Surgeon's Reflections on Reflection in Surgery

KAREN DEVON

September 19—Reflective writing? But I'm a surgeon. What am I doing here? I joined this educational program for faculty to learn to become better educators (and because it is part of my contract). Of course I think about my experiences and how I felt. I so-called "reflect" while driving home or when I can't sleep after completing a difficult case in the operating room. I reflect over drinks with my colleagues. In fact, I pride myself on being a compassionate and empathetic physician. I respond thoughtfully to breaches of professionalism and even obtained additional training in ethics. When I write, it needs to be serious and scholarly work. This is definitely a waste of my time, but I suppose since I'm in this program thirty minutes a week I should try to make something of it. So I have this difficult learner . . .

October 2—Was what happened last night an error or a complication? It's not always so easy to tell the difference and that uncertainty continues to plague me. It was torture for the process to go so slowly. Frankly, I'm not sure who suffered most: me, my resident, the patient, or their family. It is never supposed to be about me; however, I was there too! For years as a resident, the hidden curriculum taught me to respect, or even fear, death and dying, but not use it as a way to understand the human condition or myself. People often ask if I disconnect from people in order to deal with their serious illnesses. I always replied that I do not. I want to believe that it is the opposite. I think you need to connect with people even more deeply to be able to make any sense of the pain and suffering. But I wonder if I have been fooling even myself. Is the fact that I find it extremely difficult to write about critical incidents in my life evidence of my personal disconnection from those situations? When I have to respond to the scenario beyond the moment in which it occurred, it really forces me to reconstruct the experience and think critically. It's not that I don't have enough support or people to talk to. Rather, my friends and colleagues do not necessarily have more insight than I do. They can't tell me what my response was or why I acted that way. Although I am writing to no one in particular, I feel it decreases my isolation and stress. Thirty minutes goes quickly.

October 25—OK. My apologies to the family practitioners who have been espousing reflective practice for years. I performed a Medline search on "reflection in surgery." "Peritoneal reflection" and "reflection spectroscopy" were not exactly what I was looking for. Surgeons are not different from other doctors. Why have we not embraced reflective practice? We are usually natural innovators ahead of the curve. And the surgeons I work with are some of the most thoughtful people I know. We have the operating room team perform a "debrief checklist" after every case for the benefit of current and future patients. Written reflective practice is simply an extension of that established exercise and allows me to discover more possibilities and explanations. Had I begun reflective writing when I was younger, would it be easier now that I'm a surgeon? I imagine that even if I'd engaged my teachers after every operation, all of the educational dead space I encountered would have been transformed into learning opportunities. I think I am going to try this with my residents—a not-so-hidden curriculum.

November 1—Today I spoke with Bryan, the elective resident who just joined me for the month. I explained that the purpose of this exercise is not to create more work but to transform his experience into learning, growing, and developing more skills. In fact, looking back to how I felt while training, let alone only a few months ago, I decided it was important enough to trade work. I promise to dictate the necessary operative notes after our cases, while the resident reflects. I've asked to see, but not read, the journal. I'm convinced that such mindfulness is a key step in the process of becoming a professional, and not merely a technician. Of course, it was not part of my own routine, but I think I've matured into an enhanced practitioner in a short time. Like in yoga, the aim is to practice just a little better every time. I provided some guiding questions taped to the inside cover of the journal: *Describe your expectations and experience. What were the best parts, what were the worst? How did those make you feel? Why do you think it happened? Have you challenged any previous assumptions? What gaps have you identified and how will you fill them? What will you do differently next time?*

November 20—Today was disappointing yet significant for me. Bryan asked me to read a page of his journal to ensure he understood me correctly. I should have done this earlier than the end of his month-long rotation. He is eager to learn, as well as to please me, but I failed in my instructions. Furthermore, I'm learning that the residents have to feel as responsible for this aspect of learning as they do for reading the medical science. I hope that I don't misguide learners in other ways. I will have to think back to other scenarios where I may have been hasty. Perhaps I assumed everyone has the same style as I do. I even wonder if this goal is realistic, given the group of learners I am faced with. I know now that worthwhile reflection goes beyond simply thinking out loud. Bryan is describing operations in a "he said, she said" format. I would have liked to see him to grow past being a technician. I had hoped I could help him realize learning through his own experiences. Ironically, I thought it would make him a better technician as well.

December 5—I'm adjusting my approach with Arthur, my next student. The learners need more direction. I am not sure I have the skill set to steer reflection in my learners but I shall try. Firstly, I gave him the example we discussed in class that demonstrates different levels of reflection. I encouraged him to write about things that he does not like about my teaching style. I have also asked him to show me one page weekly that is not about me, just to make sure he's on the right track. We'll see how it goes. In the meantime, I am exposing myself. I am showing residents a completely different side. I wonder why this feels so important to me. Surprised even. Maybe I am doing this for personal gains. I imagine using an innovative educational strategy successfully will be rewarded.

December 13—What's the best thing that happened to me this week? Asking Arthur how the reflection is going. "Actually, I really like it and think it helps. Instead of doing it only after the OR on Wednesdays, I am doing it every day," he says. He showed me an excerpt where he describes how it feels to verbalize the things "we never get to talk about." I feel like I won a little prize. And that prize is not a promotion. My own doubts about the motivations and inherent conflict of obligations I face as an academic surgeon are lessened as my joyful response to this little victory proves that I am seeking meaningful rewards. That is good.

January 16—What's the worst thing that's happened to me this week? How disappointed I am in some of my colleagues and their unfounded assumptions. A committee's feedback on the idea of reflective practice as part of my new rotation was less than favorable. "If they have time to do this, they are not busy enough." Even though it is not dissimilar to my own initial response, I feel anger. Is that fair or am I now the one being judgmental in return? I am angry that no one actually spoke with me directly or with my trainee. I'm unsure if it is truly anger at a small group of surgeons on a committee, or the realization that I have been missing out on a great tool for all of these years.

The problem feels insurmountable. How do I channel this? Perhaps I can look at how my own bias affected my response. Was it just practice itself that got me over the hump? What they need is an intervention by way of reflective experience, but it is going to be much more challenging for me to prescribe this treatment to them. And certainly it cannot work with everyone. Like with all methods, there is a number needed to treat. What has become obvious to me is that our clinical training is largely experiential, and so examining those experiences serves to multiply the learning. I will persist.

March 12—Medicine is an art and a science. Both need practice. This journal has become my studio: a creative space for expression of new ideas and a safe one for learning the art of medicine. We are experts at examining the beliefs and values of our patients but also need to reflect on our own. It's akin to expecting physicians to make the healthy lifestyle choices they recommend to others. But of course my bias has changed. I need to be aware of it as I proceed on this new journey. See you next week.

Imagining Problem-Based Learning Cases as Real People

Creative Reflective Writing in Medical Education

JEANNE BEREITER

Medical educators struggle to integrate psychosocial, public health, and reflective components into the medical school curriculum in a way that is meaningful to medical students who are preoccupied with learning the science of medicine and passing high stakes examinations. Problem-based learning (PBL) is a key component of medical education during the first and second years of medical school. It allows medical students to learn biomedical content knowledge and clinical thinking through solving problems as a group, with the help of a faculty facilitator.[1]

At the University of New Mexico School of Medicine we have added psychosocial and public health components to the PBL cases. Students research treatment resources available in the community, role-play clinical interactions, and so on. They comply with these parts of the case but see them as soft, and they dislike role playing.

I teach a reflective writing course in a premedical enrichment program (PrEP), offered annually to seven educationally disadvantaged New Mexican students who exhibit exceptional nonacademic characteristics. Two years ago, our faculty team decided to integrate the concepts the students were learning in biochemistry with those studied in their PBL cases and their reflective writing and society and medicine classes. I first considered having students write reflective pieces about the biomedical content they were learning but struggled to link biomedical content to my goals for reflective writing, such as giving medical students greater insight into themselves and their future patients as people who interact together in different roles.

Each PBL case is constructed around a patient story that illustrates medical concepts. Cases open with a brief history, such as "Steve was a 27-year-old married Caucasian male accountant, who developed chest pain." As the case unfolds, Steve sees a physician, undergoes medical tests, and receives a diagnosis and treatment for his condition.

I asked my students to write approximately a page about Steve from Steve's point of view. They were allowed to begin and end wherever they chose. The students weren't allowed to alter the facts presented in the case, but I invited them to invent any details that weren't provided.

As students read their reflective pieces aloud the next week, I was astounded at the richness and diversity of their writing. Students easily imagined themselves into Steve's mind, providing him with a history, work life, community, interpersonal relationships, and reactions to his illness and the medical care he received. They listened deeply to their peers' renditions of the patient's story, each with its similarities to and differences from their own versions. Pieces were humorous, sad, and very moving. And they were all different.

For the next case—a homeless man, Mr. Jones, who dies due to a medical error—I asked the students to write from the point of view of Mr. Jones, or of someone else involved in the case. Several students wrote from the patient's point of view but picked different time periods in the case. One wrote through the eyes of the emergency medical technician who brought the patient in to the hospital, one, the nurse, and one, the intern whose medical error killed the patient. As the students read their pieces aloud, each piece reflecting and adding to the last, we realized they had created a coherent dramatic presentation. After the last student read, we sat in awed silence.

The fact that each student was able to pick a part of the story that felt important meant that students reflected on something meaningful to them individually. The listening experience was powerful because we heard pieces that resonated emotionally with their authors and stimulated their moral imaginations. The students were pleased with whom they had created and even prouder of their group creation. The whole was definitely greater than the sum of its parts, giving a more complete picture of what happened to poor Mr. Jones than any of them would have been able to create alone. The students went on to perform their Mr. Jones piece in several venues and it was published in our online medical literary journal, the *Medical MUSE*.[2]

Student groups are not all alike. The next year's PrEP group didn't function as harmoniously. It was a class of distinctly different personalities. So I modified the reflective writing exercises to encourage my new students to examine different points of view, looking for sources of tension and what can be done to lessen it.

Students were tasked to write Steve's case from three different points of view: Steve, his wife, and the doctor. What they wrote was rich with detail. As they went through the same events through the eyes of the different characters, they identified places where it would have helped if the doctor explained something in more detail, or if the husband and wife had communicated more. They spiritedly discussed how to improve communication between doctor and patient, the effect of marital tensions on seeking health care, and what it means to be ill.

The PrEP students have engaged in the writing and discussions of their PBL cases in ways I never experienced with medical students, who ironically saw the psychosocial issues in their PBL cases as artificial add-ons. The creative reflective narratives written by the PrEP students allowed them to imagine the cases more fully. The characters became real, because the students inserted something of themselves into their stories.

Creative reflective writing about a PBL case also provides a layer of insulation between the student and the personal topics being discussed. My students were not asked to write or talk about their own experience, but they clearly put their own experience and personal projections into their creative writing. Imagining PBL cases as real people made writers out of students who don't usually write or who believe they cannot. The challenge now is for the University of New Mexico School of Medicine to adopt this creative reflective writing process.

NOTES

1. Diana H. J. M. Dolmans et al., "Problem-Based Learning: Future Challenges for Educational Practice and Research," *Medical Education* 39 (2005): 732–41; Gillian Maudsley, "Do We All Mean the Same Thing by 'Problem-Based Learning'? A Review of the Concepts and a Formulation of the Ground Rules," *Academic Medicine* 74 (1999): 178–85.
2. See "James Jones—Creative Reflections," *Medical Muse* 17, no. 1 (Spring 2012): 13–14, http://hsc .unm.edu/medmuse/docs/MedMuseSpring12.pdf.

Team Writing

A Narrative Approach to Team-Building Skills and Enhancing Competencies in Health-Care Professions

JENNIFER ADAEZE ANYAEGBUNAM, JENNIFER SOTSKY,
AND BRANDON SULTAN

Increasingly, medical schools are emphasizing interdisciplinary teamwork skills with the goal of enhancing patient care and safety. A relatively new approach, team-based learning (TBL), involves small groups of students collaborating on multiple-choice problem sets based on clinical vignettes. These exercises are intended to foster discussion and problem solving with the objective of helping students to work together and achieve greater mastery of the material. In our experience, however, we have found that the rigid nature of a multiple-choice format can limit the creativity and level of collaboration that occurs. Even when the process focuses on subjects such as biomedical ethics, there are a finite number of possible solutions, which restricts discussion and debate. While there may be a variety of correct answers, it is often implied that some answers are "more correct" than others. As a result, there is little originality inspired by the group process, and students are denied the opportunity to develop a sense of ownership in their clinical reasoning.

As premedical students in Columbia University's Program in Narrative Medicine, the three of us wrote a single reflective essay on a passage drawn from Virginia Woolf's *To the Lighthouse.* Comparing our recent experiences with TBLs to this writing exercise, we have concluded that team writing offered us an unparalleled opportunity to triangulate our diverse insights. Through this exercise, we produced a richer, more comprehensive analysis of the Woolf text than each of us could have achieved individually. Furthermore, while TBL has been shown to enhance academic performance,[1] team writing allowed us a unique opportunity to practice empathic listening, giving and receiving feedback, collaboration, compromise, and accountability—all necessary skills for successful teamwork in the health-care setting.

As students bend their heads over a common text, they must look beyond the obvious facts to draw higher order connections and create arguments rather than regurgitating information based on rote memorization. Collaboration requires that students refine and strengthen their arguments—they must take their colleagues' critiques into account in order to ensure the development of a cohesive essay. The American Association of Medical Colleges argues that physicians in training must learn to "provide care in the context of coordinated multi-disciplinary health care delivery teams and must demonstrate that they can work with such teams to make effective use of the group's collective knowledge and experience. Physicians should possess a deep understanding of the fundamental biomedical scientific principles needed to deal with the unexpected; they should not rely solely on algorithm-based practice."[2] Team writing better mirrors the collaborative nature of both the doctor-patient and doctor-colleague relationships than traditional medical school exercises. In this essay, we propose a team writing activity for students of pre-health and health professions, which is designed to facilitate the development of interpersonal skills and team competencies deemed necessary for health care today.

This exercise in team writing, which requires only reading a literary text and writing a short reflective essay, can be easily implemented in health professions or medical humanities curricula for students at or above college-level education. It can be effective in small seminars or large lectures because the functional work takes place in teams of two or three students. In our medical school experiences, despite the presence of team-based initiatives such as TBL, we have observed that many students study alone because they are ultimately evaluated alone, leaving few opportunities to explore group dynamics and practice collective accountability. In team writing, each member of the team is actively engaged in both self-directed learning and peer collaboration. Students enter medical school with the goal of seeing, treating, and healing patients, but the pre-clerkship years are so heavily focused on the molecular foundations of health and disease that it is easy to lose sight of the human side of medicine. Individuals can easily "burn out" from the workload and lack of academic camaraderie with peers. This environment can perpetuate the development of habits that foster feelings of isolation and disconnectedness from the ultimate objective of becoming a physician. Team writing projects reinforce the development of interpersonal skills and allow students to connect with their colleagues in a meaningful way, enhancing the collegiality of the medical school experience.

In our own team writing exercise, the assignment prompted us to "choose a few inches of text" from Woolf's *To the Lighthouse*, "perform a close reading of it," and write a five- to seven-page reflective essay in a small group. Close reading entails analyzing factors including but not limited to plot, syntax, diction, imagery, metaphor, and ambiguity in the text.[3] Our reflective writing drew on this close reading to generate a comprehensive analysis of the text. Any work of literature, especially one rich in figurative language or imagery, that inspires different interpretations of the text and engenders the spirit of discussion would lend itself well to this assignment.

Although we had all done group work before, this assignment was unique because we were asked to craft a single cohesive essay with a unified voice for which we would all be evaluated. Unlike a laboratory report, for example, in which one student might handle the hypothesis and another, the methods section, it is nearly impossible to "split up" the work for this type of essay. Tasks could not be merely divided and recombined since individual ideas and arguments had to be metabolized by the entire team and worked into the essay. Although we did each attempt to write a two-page version of the essay and then integrate the parts, we faced the challenge of conversing about our disparate ideas, establishing connections between them, reconciling conflicting views, and synthesizing a coherent paper. This team writing process required each author to verbally articulate ideas and therefore develop more sound arguments based on the team's feedback—an opportunity not afforded to a student working independently.

Working together in close proximity facilitated familiarity, collegiality, and respect among the members of our group. Our strengths and weaknesses quickly emerged, resulting in augmented situational and self-awareness. This allowed for a fluid leadership that shifted onto different members, depending on the task and our individual strengths. As such, we were able to "make effective use of the group's collective knowledge and experience."[4] Ultimately, this collaborative process allowed us to engage with the assignment on a deeper level and to interact with our classmates in a more meaningful way than we have experienced in medical school thus far. This exercise was particularly rewarding because it enhanced not only academic performance but also knowledge of ourselves and our team members. We became collaborators with a common goal, which allowed us to educate and learn from each other. Team writing may generate new and exciting learning opportunities for students as well as help to develop the competencies required for successful teamwork in the health-care professions.

As future physicians, we have learned that hospitals and other health-care institutions are becoming increasingly focused on training effective teams as a means to improve the quality of patient care. Since people in these fields are jointly responsible and accountable for patients, many medical schools teach students in groups and encourage cooperative learning. Yet as students we are mostly evaluated as individuals rather than as teams. While traditional medical school exercises allow students to work together, the aim is to arrive at the correct answer predetermined by evaluators. A team writing exercise, on the other hand, better mirrors the experience of working with a health-care team to create a cohesive management plan among an infinite pool of solutions. Furthermore, it offers health professions students the opportunity to practice skills such as perception, empathy, and self-reflection, which are critical for competent, compassionate health-care practice.

NOTES

1. Paul G. Koles et al., "The Impact of Team-based Learning on Medical Students' Academic Performance," *Academic Medicine* 85 (2010): 1739–45.
2. AAMC-HHMI Committee, "Scientific Foundations for Future Physicians," Washington, DC: Association of American Medical Colleges (2009), accessed Aug. 31, 2015, www.aamc.org/download/271072/data/scientificfoundationsforfuturephysicians.pdf.
3. Rita Charon, *Narrative Medicine: Honoring the Stories of Illness* (New York: Oxford Univ. Press, 2006).
4. AAMC-HHMI Committee, "Scientific Foundations for Future Physicians," accessed Dec. 18, 2015, www.aamc.org/download/271072/data/scientificfoundationsforfuturephysicians.pdf.

Letters to a Third-Year Student

THERESE JONES AND ANJALI DHURANDHAR

Finding opportunities to integrate reflective and creative writing in a meaningful yet enjoyable way for overworked and overwhelmed medical students can be challenging. The publication project we describe below consists of selected writing by fourth-year students, which is printed and bound in a single volume and distributed to third-year students at the outset of their clerkship rotations. Not only is this assignment easily implemented as a part of a required reflective writing exercise, it also serves as a memorable part of a typical orientation week to the third year. The recipients look forward to submitting their own words and wisdom to the next class, and the contributors are rewarded with a publication credit on their CV—right before interviewing for a residency.

The inspiration for this project is Rainer Maria Rilke's small volume, *Letters to a Young Poet*. Composed from 1903 to 1908, the ten letters are arguably the most famous ever written, serving as the prototype for a brand-new genre. They have inspired many writers, teachers, and professionals to share their own observations and insights with other young readers embarking on a life in the arts, in religious and public service, and in law and medicine. Basic Books, for example, published individual works from 2001 to 2008 as part of a series called "The Art of Mentoring." It included such titles as *Letters to a Young Jazz Musician* by Wynton Marsalis; *Letters to a Young Conservative* by Dinesh D'Souza and its counterpart, *Letters to a Young Contrarian,* by Christopher Hitchens; and *Letters to a Young Lawyer* by Alan Dershowitz.

There are two collections of *Letters to a Young Doctor;* the first, published in 1996 by surgeon and writer Richard Selzer, is, in his words, meant to be "pedagogical and comradely—a reaching out to share."[1] The second, Perri Klass's *Treatment Kind and Fair,* is meant to be "a combination of maternal and

33

medical wisdom."[2] Her letters are addressed to her son in medical school—the very child born during her own education at Harvard in the 1980s, where she was one of only four women in her medical school class. Writing about and across their respective lifetimes, both Selzer and Klass not only reveal the compelling mysteries of the world of medicine but also represent the tedious challenges of the job of medicine.

Because of the emotional truth and profound wisdom contained within, readers of Rilke's letters have often assumed that he—much like Selzer, Klass, and the majority of writers who follow—was an older man looking back on the struggles and the mistakes of his youth. But, in fact, Rilke wrote the letters between the ages of twenty-eight and thirty-three—a time when he himself was beginning a career, embarking on a new marriage, and restlessly traveling the world. Thus, his insights about life, love, and art are immediate and authentic to his young readers because the feelings behind them are still alive and present rather than detached and distant.

Several years ago, Therese Jones, coauthor of this essay, began inviting fourth-year medical students to write letters to rising third-year students, providing them with practical advice, helpful suggestions, and personal reflections about the year ahead, which would be one of the biggest transitions in a medical student's life.[3] Working on the wards and in the clinics during the clerkship year is like traveling to a different country with its own language, customs, and etiquette. However, the rules are not written down, and sometimes the only way to learn about them is by breaking them. Consequently, the clerkship experience is often fraught with anxiety—fear of doing the wrong thing and breaking an unwritten rule—and full of emotions—anger, embarrassment, exhilaration, and sadness.

Since the "Letters to a Third-Year Student" project began, we have had the opportunity to marvel at the writers' courage and creativity, to applaud their stamina and resourcefulness, and to bear witness to their pain and joy. Just as these letters provide a mirror for the experiences and emotions of all third-year students, they also provide a window for the rest of us looking in at them and looking out for them as they make the journey.

Rilke encourages that very first reader to experience and express all that is happening around him, to him, and because of him: "Turn to what your everyday life affords; depict your sorrows and desires, your passing thoughts and beliefs in some kind of beauty. Depict all that with heartfelt, quiet, humble sincerity."[4] The students who have written letters have met the challenge—sometimes brilliantly, sometimes not, but always with heart.

In 2014, fourth-year student Kristin Scott-Tillery considered the all-important question of what (and what not) to wear. Besides reminding readers to launder their lab coats ("It's a white coat not a brown one!"), she lists the essential items to fill their pockets:

> With teamwork: "It's a little bulky, but you will use it all the time, and the more you use it, the less room it seems to take." With patience: "You will wait on everyone, and no one will wait on you. Remember that in the grand scheme of things, your time is not valuable, and that's okay. Just smile and maybe try whistling." With a mirror: "See what your patient sees when you walk into the room. Do you look confident? caring? or bothered, tired, exasperated, and stressed? Worse, do you look judgmental?" With tissues: "You will see things that break your heart. You will lose your first patient, you will tell someone he has cancer, you will see a child battle leukemia, you will swear you are not cut out for medicine. But know that you are." With ears: "Patients will tell you things about yourself, about how they see you in your make-believe role as 'doctor.' If you listen well, you will slowly change the way you carry yourself and the way you wear that coat until it is a part of you and a seamless fit."

In 2011, Mycroft Smith wrote about the white coat and its symbolism in his published letter:

> Wearing my "tighty whitey," I always felt like an imposter. For me, the problem was that I saw the coat not only as the symbol of a physician but of all the clinical knowledge a physician is supposed to command. When I wore the coat, I felt as though I were pretending to possess knowledge far beyond what I had really acquired. But when a sweet little old lady called me, "Baby Doc," she somehow released me of the guilt that I felt for impersonating someone with all the answers. I felt proud to be a baby doc. . . . She reminded me that we all start as baby docs, and it is okay not to know the right answer, even if your white coat suggests to others that you should.

A final example, excerpted from a letter by student Dorothy Dow, recommended that every third-year student actually begin with Rilke:

> My first piece of advice is to pick up a copy of this thin yet powerful tome. There are great parallels between you and this young poet, as your third year is also about finding yourself and your place on your chosen path. You will have your share of feeling alone, feeling confused, feeling challenged by the personalities you encounter and the poverty and pain you never really, really knew existed. If you will write your own letters to yourself in solitude and honesty, you will

form your own definition of a great doctor, recalling with clarity what made you happy, what made you sad, the demeanor of those you admired, the lessons you learned and the mistakes you wish never to repeat. There is a reason you are here. It is no longer about passing the test, or getting through the material twice. It is about finding the healer within and figuring out the burning question . . . with which medium, in what field, will you practice your art of medicine[?]

While the creativity and skill of student writers vary considerably across these letters, there is one commonality among them: sincerity. In essence, students express respect, compassion, and concern for their patients, their colleagues, and their experiences in the clerkship year—the best that we, their teachers, can hope for.

NOTES

1. Richard Selzer, *Letters to a Young Doctor* (San Diego: Harcourt Brace, 1996), i.
2. Perri Klass, *Treatment Kind and Fair: Letters to a Young Doctor* (New York: Basic Books, 2007), xi.
3. The 2011–14 publications are available electronically on request to the coauthors.
4. Rainer Maria Rilke, *Letters to a Young Poet,* trans. J. M. Burnham (Novato, CA: New World Library, 2000), 11.

Haiku It!—Reflection in Seventeen Syllables

BETH PERRY, MARGARET EDWARDS,
AND KATHERINE J. JANZEN

Poetry potentially conveys human emotion, vague ideas, and complex feelings within the limitation of a few words. As is said of poems, they do not require a summary because "the poem is the thing."[1] When student reflections are related to human interaction, poetry provides an avenue to capture and share these experiences and recollections using a specific form.

To challenge students to drill down to the essence of course concepts and their experiences, we developed a teaching strategy called Haiku It! We use Haiku It! as a reflection activity in graduate and undergraduate nursing and health discipline courses in both online and face-to-face learning environments.[2] The idea for Haiku it! came to us after reviewing the website "Dissertation Haiku," which includes a collection of haiku created by doctoral students summarizing their dissertations. Our thinking was that if three-hundred-page dissertations can be captured in seventeen syllables, then so can complex course concepts and experiences.

Many learners remember Japanese haiku poetry from their grade school English courses. With a few instructor-provided triggers, students quickly recall that unrhymed haiku consist of three lines: the first line having five syllables, the second line featuring seven syllables, and the remaining line containing five syllables. It is helpful for the instructor to provide samples, either written by other students or by the instructor. Examples give students confidence in their writing while also providing a refresher in haiku format. Haiku It! may not appeal to all students. Some may have an aversion to writing poetry. Consequently, this activity should be optional.

However, even those who do not write a haiku may benefit from reading poems created by others. In our experience, once some students have taken a risk and shared their haiku the activity takes on momentum and others participate. Since only seventeen syllables are required, the activity is deceptively easy, making it less threatening to attempt. However, considerable reflection is required to limit an experience or concept to a few carefully chosen syllables.

The activity proceeds in this way. Once students are confident in the haiku form, they are invited to reflect on a specific clinical experience or course concept and record their thoughts in a haiku. Learners are reassured that their haiku will not be graded or formally evaluated. Sharing their poem is optional and can be done in a classroom, online post, or webinar session.

The form and framework of the haiku encourages students to be concise and requires a clear understanding of key elements related to a given concept. Additional benefits of writing haiku include developing further academic literacy as well as finding one's inner voice.[3] Further, writing and sharing reflective haiku often provides an avenue for fulfilling affective domain learning outcomes as personal attitudes and feelings are self-assessed and then revealed through the poems.

Two nursing students pursuing master's degrees wrote the following haiku as reflections on their learning in a course on teaching health professionals. These sample haiku demonstrate that the learners grasped essential understandings related to course learning outcomes. Haiku 1: "Vision and purpose. / A pledge to excellence made. / Successful students." Haiku 2: "Successful outcomes? / Assess students' needs and plan. / Triumph will follow."

The following is a sample haiku provided by the professor in an online graduate course about research dissemination strategies. This poem motived learners to create their own haiku to summarize their reflections related to publishing research findings. Haiku 3: "Sharing our discoveries. / Worlds extend further. / Others listen and respond."

Haiku It! is a learning activity that can stimulate reflection and help define what reflection actually is. The succinctness of the poetic form causes learners to focus their reflection on the most salient point, image, feeling, or idea. The novelty and challenge of the activity creates energy in the class and motives learners and instructors. Haiku It! can be used as a stand-alone activity or at the beginning or the end of a reflection session. This versatile learning activity can be used to inspire reflection related to almost any subject matter in online or face-to-face classrooms. Haiku expresses much and suggests more within a very few words.

NOTES

1. Atsushi Iida, "Poetry Writing as Expressive Pedagogy in an EFL Context: Identifying Possible Assessment Tools for Haiku Poetry in EFL Freshman College Writing," *Assessing Writing* 13, no. 3 (2008): 171–79.

2. Beth Perry and Margaret Edwards, "Interactive Teaching Technologies that Facilitate the Development of Online Learning Communities in Nursing and Health Studies Graduate Courses," *Teacher Education Quarterly, Special Online Edition* 37 (2010): 148–72, accessed June 5, 2015, http://teqjournal.org/perry_edwards.html.

3. Max van Manen, *Researching Lived Experience: Human Science for an Action Sensitive Pedagogy* (London, Ontario: Althouse, 1990).

The Reflecting Poem and the Use of Poetry in Health-Care Education

RONNA BLOOM

The Canadian poet Phil Hall wrote in his award-winning book *Killdeer* that he no longer refers to his poems as "tools," though he once did. Does this mean he's realized they aren't? Or has he simply chosen to let them be themselves?

What is a tool? What do I intend, as poet in residence at Mount Sinai Hospital in Toronto, if I say "I use poetry as a tool"? Certainly poems are not corkscrews or can openers, though they do appear to pry things open. They activate something. Perhaps it's the intentionality that Hall objects to. Whatever the case, I write poems for their own sake, as well as to stir empathy, reflection, compassion, writing, and awareness. Here are four directions in which poetry has taken me: the poem that prompts reflection; the poem written as a reflective response; the poem offered at the "Spontaneous Poetry Booth"; and, lastly, the poem that is no tool at all.

POEMS TO PROMPT REFLECTION

One of the main ways I engage people with poetry is to offer one-hour workshops, and the first thing I do is write a description, a "blurb" of the workshop. The description brings people to the workshop. It is an offering. And this description, like a poem, begins working on people so that when they arrive, something is already fizzing. If I give you the title "Awake at Work" and you take it in, something happens. Perhaps a question—"Am I awake at work?"—or an irritation—"What do you mean? Of course, I'm awake!" The theme is activated.

Within this context, my aim in the workshop is to hold out a poem in one hand, and with the other invite the person to come forward with whatever they are bringing and meet it. This meeting is a kind of alchemy between poem and person.

For the writing, I tell participants they don't have to be writers; they only have to want to explore something through writing. I give five rules for writing. These rules are an amalgam of Natalie Goldberg's books[1] and my own writing practice: (1) keep your hand moving, (2) don't think, (3) don't censor, (4) you are free to write the worst crap ever, and (5) you don't have to share.

Then I offer a poem as prompt. One poem I use in "Awake at Work" is "The Red Wheelbarrow" by William Carlos Williams. It lays out in eight short lines a meticulous and clear observation. I offer it in this workshop, which was originally designed for nursing students who are observing patients for the first time. With the workshop, they are relearning to see, touch, hear, and smell. The senses of the nurse practitioner become their tools, and the poem offers a way to activate these. I ask them to attend to something in the room with that kind of focused, acute observation. I say, "Get quiet in your chair. Find two things to look at nearby. Hear two things. Be curious. Pick one of the sounds or sights, and using the rules, write for five minutes."

Several things happen. First, as some participants have never written this way before, the process can be a stunner. They are surprised to see how easily they write and how much they write, or they are surprised at how censored they are or how their minds wander. They begin to attend to their experience through the writing. Second, the prompt directs them to focus on something they see or hear. This heightens their sensual awareness, an awareness that often gets dulled by activity so that assumptions are taken for actual experience. The aim is to foreground the use of their senses in conjunction with what is being learned intellectually. Third, people begin to attune to how much is happening inside them, as humans and as practitioners. And by extension, they realize how much is also happening inside their patients.

When participants write in response to their observation or to the poem, a creative space is opened up in time, in the room, and on the page. This space is neither graded nor supervised, but it's guided. It allows participants to reflect on personal, professional, and academic responses and especially on where they intersect. In this structured space of "not knowing," new learning can happen and unexpected links be made.

Try it now.

Read "The Red Wheelbarrow" and then reread the five rules. Now look at two things where you're sitting. Really look at the details, colors, associations. Now hear two things. No rush. Pick something that has your attention. Write.

POEM AS REFLECTIVE RESPONSE

The intention in this writing is for individuals to find the language that allows the fullest expression of their experience. Interestingly, in many workshops, students often express judgment initially. They're critical of their own writing. One woman called the process "flaky" and the result "cliché." This method is often so new to people that it violates what they've come to think of as "the way to write" academically, scientifically, or professionally. And this stirs them up.

In this same class, students acknowledged being surprised that their compassion had grown for their patients, but not for themselves and their own risk taking. They became aware of how they lacked self-compassion and judged themselves harshly. As with any flash of awareness, this reflective response of seeing can point us toward clarity and presence.

THE REFLECTING POEM

What if, in the middle of a lobby, a person seated at a table asked you what you needed a poem about, wrote it for a dollar and gave it to you? This is what I do. It's called the "spontaneous poetry booth."[2]

My aim in the booth is to hear both the content of what people are saying and who is saying it. I have worked as a psychotherapist so this method has gone into my listening. But when I'm the poet, my aim is not only to listen but to respond to whatever the request is and to come up with a poem.

In writing workshops, the rules for writing are geared toward optimum freedom, including "you don't have to share." In the spontaneous poetry booth, sharing is the goal.

The poem acts as a reflection of what the person has asked. "I need a poem about being more powerful in my job." "I need a poem about my sister's illness." The poem is an articulation of a constellation of events, emotions, and experiences. The poem—when it works—distils and touches the complexity of the moment.

Poetry, whether it's spoken or written, offers a chance to experience, know, reflect on, and express our daily truths from a different angle. "Tell all the truth, but tell it slant," writes Emily Dickinson.

Once, a student said she needed a poem about her father who was ill with dementia. I wrote "Swim" for her: "The threads of you / drift away / like ink secreted and dissolving / I can't hold them / and whatever Octopus sent out this ink / is floating too away / I watch you go and what I say goes too and I don't know / what, if anything, there is to keep / or whether all there is to do is watch / the ink colour the water/ we're in / and just swim."[3]

So try this right now. What do you need a poem about? Write it in one sentence. "I need a poem about . . ."

Take a minute to look at the sentence and see what that's like to have written it down. Now write the poem. If you can do this with a friend or colleague and share your responses, even better.

WHAT ABOUT BEAUTY?

What about the poem that doesn't reflect us back, like a rider on a bicycle in dark clothes who we come upon in the night? We don't see her until suddenly she's there and we're faced with her existence. The poem awakens us, refusing to reflect or be anything but what it is; it absorbs us.

We contemplate it because its presence is strong enough to make us come out of ourselves to meet it. It is a freedom from ourselves that somehow makes us more ourselves.

In that awe is the possibility that we will respond with fresh attention and care.

The poet C. K. Williams wrote, "Beauty won't save the world from the depredations with which it's already been savaged, but it can save us from the enervating despair that is the outcome of panic, that paralysis that might keep us from doing what we can to confront what's before us."[4] A poem sometimes offers an experience of beauty amid despair, an unexpected opening, the way a reflecting pool is a place that arrests turbulence, allowing us to pause before moving again.

NOTES

1. Natalie Goldberg, *Writing Down the Bones: Freeing the Writer Within* (Boston: Shambhala Publications, 1986).
2. Ibid., 121.
3. Ronna Bloom, *Cloudy with a Fire in the Basement* (St. John's, Newfoundland and Labrador: Pedlar Press, 2012).
4. C. K. Williams, "Nature and Panic: Can Beauty Save Us?" *Poetry Magazine,* Oct. 2012, www.poetryfoundation.org/poetrymagazine/article/244608.

"Like a Page Waiting for Music"

Nursing, Poetry, and Autonomy

JOY JACOBSON

Cerasela Shiiba was a senior nursing student in the RN-to-BSN program, a baccalaureate track for licensed RNs at the Hunter–Bellevue School of Nursing in New York City, when she took a writing course for nurses in the fall of 2012. My colleague Jim Stubenrauch and I were her teachers. We're not nurses; we're editors and creative writers. We had created a fifteen-week curriculum centered on reflection, narrative, and poetry, which was aimed at actively and creatively engaging nursing students in fulfilling the school's clinical writing requirements and providing reflective tools for managing stress and preventing burnout.

During the first class of the semester, we asked students to keep a daily journal and to think about topics they might pursue in a narrative essay. Cerasela approached me afterward and asked, clearly caught off guard, "You want us to write a story about ourselves?" Yes, I told her, but she would determine her topic, and her journal writing would be for her eyes only.

The next week Cerasela told me she was uncomfortable journaling about her own life. I suggested she read and write about poetry and lent her a copy of *The Night Path*, a book of poems by Laurie Kutchins. In the beautiful opening poem, "Prelude," a pregnant woman maps out the human and natural worlds for her soon-to-be-born son: "The snow worked hard to cover wheel and animal tracks, / to make the road and the hills look as if no one / had ever passed here. They were getting ready for you, / like a page waiting for music."[1]

Like a page waiting for music, or a writer listening for words.

Having been an editor at a nursing journal for many years, I came to the classroom intimately aware of how much we need to hear from nurses in discussions on health care. I also knew the range of problems that can plague nurses' professional writing—jargon, poor organization, lack of originality, even plagiarism. The need seemed urgent, and I was excited to undertake this experiment with Jim and our colleague, nursing professor Dr. Diana Mason.

Hunter College is a part of the City University of New York, one of the most diverse university systems in the country. But the nursing workforce overall does not reflect the diversity of the population of the United States: of the three million registered nurses, 90 percent are female and 83 percent are non-Hispanic white. Hunter's twenty thousand students hail from 147 countries on six continents. More than half of our undergraduate and graduate students grew up speaking a language other than English. Many work full-time as nurses, often twelve-hour shifts, and at home tend to young kids or aging parents. When asked to synthesize a study's findings, even for a brief assignment, more than a few plagiarize—a survival tactic, I believe—copying from government sites, studies, newspaper articles, blog posts, Wikipedia. Even when told that we use plagiarism-detection software and that penalties may be severe, still some of them will copy and paste.

While preventing the unwanted action of copying, we must also encourage original thought. Poetry makes the mind pause, just as a startling piece of music or a painting does. It's in the pause, the rest stop on the mind's congested highway, that someone alienated from her own writerly voice—even terrified of it—can get excited about language again.

All of us were secretly in love with words when we started out. As poet Marie Ponsot writes in her poem "Language Acquisition," "The delicious tongue we speak with speaks us. / A liquor of sweetness where its root cleaves / ripens fluent, as it runs for the desirous / reason, the touching sense. The infant says 'I' / like earthquake and wavers as place takes voice."[2]

That *liquor of sweetness,* that *desirous reason,* that *earthquake.* Ponsot has depicted how we humans come to discover ourselves through language, an earthquake of self-identity brought on by speech. That's the sort of self-discovery, more than mere self-expression, that I'm trying to spark in nursing students.

I begin each semester by asking students to respond to a poem written by a nurse, in two drafts, between which students meet with me in conference. The drafts encourage them to begin thinking of writing as a process of discovering their own thoughts. In conferences we look at the big picture: What have you managed to say? Is it what you really believe? Is there a personal story you can tell in your second draft to back up your opinion?

Such creative prompts can't do everything for a student whose writing challenges are severe. But they don't have to. In his 2011 guide to writing as a means of encouraging critical thinking in the classroom, John Bean acknowledges the difficulties of helping students to improve their "grammatical competence." Run-on sentences, noun-verb disagreements, and sentence fragments compel many teachers to line-edit students' papers, hoping to aid them in correcting their own flaws. But such efforts largely fail. As Bean writes, "It may well be, in fact, that competence in editing and correctness is a late-developing skill that blossoms only after students begin taking pride in their writing and seeing themselves as having ideas important enough to communicate."[3]

So much of what needs remediation in nursing students is a lack of confidence. And that can be addressed directly by teaching writing as a process, one that involves a step-by-step discovery, through writing and deep revision, on a topic they have chosen. The tools of the poet—metaphor, rhyme, rhythm, compression of story and language—can be useful to the nonpoet as well. By bringing poems to nursing students, I hope to prompt them to speak with a new tongue, and to write with less fear.

ONE STORY

Cerasela Shiiba, a 42-year-old single parent and psychiatric nurse, came to the United States from Romania and began learning English fifteen years ago. Cerasela's progress in developing her narrative essay over the semester shows a mind eager to grapple not just with language but with her life.

Step 1. In the third week of the semester, Cerasela posted on an online course discussion board the following topic for instructor feedback: "I will write a story about training for my first Paris Marathon three years ago. It was a time when I experienced complex feelings about what I can do and who I want to become, despite what others say. . . ."

Step 2. Next, Cerasela presented her topic on the discussion board for student response: "One aspect I will be writing about is how it feels to be a single mother and the challenges that come with it; how mothers feel empowered by their children. . . ."

Step 3. Students then posted a short introductory narrative on their chosen topic for response from peers. Cerasela wrote about a visit to our classroom by Karen Roush, a nurse who shared her writings about domestic violence: "I am also a survivor of domestic violence but never thought that I can speak about it in public. I do understand the pain, embarrassment and guilt that women feel while society points out: 'It is your fault . . .'"

Step 4. In the first full draft of the narrative essay, Cerasela went in a new direction, a lyric evocation of a painful childhood episode involving a game of hopscotch:

I raised my eyes and saw my mother coming slowly up the hill. I saw her step becoming smaller and heavier. She stopped and looked back over the village and sighed. Usually she would go directly into the kitchen through the big green gate. I saw that she turned and passed through the black round gate, which took her longer. Next, I saw her turning and walking toward the twelfth circle of my new pretend game. She tried to jump but her foot would not leave the ground. She took a wooden stick and softly drew a bird outside the circle. She walked slowly around the rim of the circle. Her footprints were covering the edge. I was looking at the bird's wings.

"Cera, it will rain soon. Your aunt will take you to the city so you can start school there. You will come home on vacations." I hit the rock with the side of my foot. It felt hard and cold.

Step 5. For the final draft of the essay, Cerasela continued in the lyric mode, finding the roots of her love of literature and learning in the difficult move to her aunt's: "Her apartment was filled with books that overshadowed the modest furniture she inherited from my grandfather. . . . Soon I found myself spending hours reading. A new book represented a new adventure."

Cerasela's progress as a writer shows a lively, creative mind at work. She has since graduated and recently entered graduate school. I look forward to reading more from her.

NOTES

1. Laurie Kutchins, *The Night Path* (Rochester, NY: BOA Editions, 1997), 11.
2. Marie Ponsot, *Easy* (New York: Random House, 2011), 40.
3. John C. Bean, *Engaging Ideas: The Professor's Guide to Integrating Writing, Critical Thinking, and Active Learning in the Classroom* (San Francisco: Jossey-Bass, 2011), 3.

Making Patient Safety Resonate with, and Relevant to, Trainees Using Narrative

AMY NAKAJIMA

"Life can only be understood backwards; but it must be lived forwards."

—SOREN KIERKEGAARD

In March 2011, I attended The Hospital for Sick Children Medical Education Day in Toronto. Dr. Richard Frankel, a professor of medicine and geriatrics and senior research scientist at the Indiana University School of Medicine, presented grand rounds on "Making Professionalism into a Lifelong Voyage of Discovery." Following rounds, he conducted a workshop during which he shared his students' narratives, describing their experiences and observations relating to professional behaviors.

I was struck by this use of narrative, wherein students explored and questioned how health-care professionals treated patients, students, and each other. Within their narratives, students were developing their own professional identities and trying to make sense of their learning and working environments, and their places within them. In many stories, students identified, and occasionally struggled to articulate, their understandings of "the way we do things around here"—the hidden curriculum of values, attitudes, and behaviors of their faculty and other health-care professionals, and the organizational culture of the environment. The students' stories, my own experience of reflecting on these narratives, and the thoughtful and lively group discussions persuaded me to develop a similar type of exercise, focusing on patient safety.

At the time, I was involved in the development of the Canadian Medical Protective Association (CMPA) Good Practices Guide, an online patient safety and risk-management resource for trainees and faculty. This curriculum is organized along the framework of The Safety Competencies developed by the Canadian Patient Safety Institute. I was convinced that a narrative exercise on patient safety should be included in this curriculum, given that yearly an estimated 7.5 percent of hospitalized patients in Canada experience a serious patient safety incident, with higher rates in teaching hospitals, and yet clinician-teachers and educators struggle to embed patient safety into curricula in practical and meaningful ways.

Narrative and reflective discussion have been used to successfully engage and enable truly relevant learning about patient safety. A small number of published studies looks specifically at the use of trainees' and junior doctors' narratives as a platform to discuss patient safety principles and practices, and to explore how and why "things went wrong." For example, Rick Iedema and his colleagues conclude that the "negotiation of affect through shared or 'dialogic' narrative is central to enabling doctors to deal with adverse events on a personal level, and to enabling them at a collective level to become attentive to threats to patients' safety."[1]

Alexis Ogdie and her colleagues conducted a reflective writing and narrative discussion session among second-year internal medicine residents.[2] The residents were asked to write about a specific incident of diagnostic error with a cognitive or contextual component that they had either witnessed or participated in. They were also asked to describe what they learned from the experience and how this might influence their future practice. Narratives were shared in a group setting with faculty facilitation, which revealed the residents' abilities to thoughtfully reflect on their experiences and identify the personal and team factors, system and environmental factors, and patient factors that contributed to their error stories.

Martinez and Lo reviewed essays written by medical students as a component for a required course in medical ethics.[3] In 9 percent of the essays, students were unsure if an error occurred; these students questioned the appropriateness of actions and management of the patient. Discussion, through one-on-one feedback from an instructor or through a facilitated group setting to clarify the uncertainty of whether an error occurred, could help trainees understand the principles of patient safety, such as the balance between system failure and personal accountability. Through such dialogic exploration, faculty could teach trainees about patient safety, a composite science, which includes contributions from cognitive psychology, human factors engineering, and risk assessment and management, among others. Students could begin to appreciate how this science is embedded (or *not* embedded) in our daily practice of clinical care, including the impact of organizational culture on promoting patient safety;

effective teamwork and communication; approaches to assessing, managing, and anticipating clinical risk; the interfaces between technology and people in health care; and the real meaning of patient-centered care.

Even as trainees learn about the science of patient safety through this instrumental use of narrative, perhaps even more importantly, these narratives and ensuing discourse afford trainees opportunities to help them process their affective experiences. Studies indicate that clinicians suffer doubt and distress when involved in a patient safety incident, and Martinez and Lo suggest that this "distress may extend beyond doctors who commit errors to students who observe them."[4] Iedema et al. discuss how "affect is at once constitutive of clinicians' concern for the patient, of their moral impulse to deal with incidents, and of their own ability to reflect on and learn from adverse outcomes . . . narrativizing the affective dimensions of doctoring and medical failure . . . is central and constitutive [to patient safety]."[5]

Trainees have incomplete knowledge and are dependent on those more senior to themselves. When involved in an event, either as an active contributor or as an observer, they will benefit from the opportunity to make sense of the event, both cognitively and emotionally, through facilitated feedback and guided reflection. Cognitively, reflective discussion provides a venue for trainees to learn about patient safety principles and to enable them to contextualize an event, as the ability to provide care is dependent on multiple factors, many of which they have little influence over, while still realizing their duty of care. Reflective discussion will also help trainees process strong emotions in the wake of an event, including uncertainty, doubt, distress, and guilt.

After reviewing and discussing published literature, the CMPA's Risk Management Services Education Department agreed to include narrative exercises in their *CMPA Good Practices Guide.* My intention was to develop a structure for the narrative exercise that would be applicable to a variety of teaching settings, from in-person interactive group sessions to a non-face-to-face, one-on-one situation (e.g., an ePortfolio venue). I also wondered if the instructions given to the students in the Martinez and Lo study would be sufficient to stimulate the kind of narrative and depth of reflection for which we were hoping: "On one page, prepare a description of an important mistake you have made or observed during medical school."[6]

And so I began looking at narrative exercises and interviews in ethics and professionalism literature and at unpublished sources. Through an iterative process, with the members of CMPA's Risk Management Services Education Department, we developed both instructions to trainees and teaching tips to faculty, the latter including suggestions on how to effectively facilitate trainees' sharing of their stories; encourage discussion of identified patient safety concerns; and enable trainees to consider how to potentially address those concerns.

As a component of these teaching tips, we developed a number of "trigger questions," or probes, that we hoped would provoke the writer (and the other members, in the case of a group exercise) to further consider the experience, would encourage discussion (in the forms of self-reflection and dyadic or group discussion) by trainees, and would prompt both facilitation and guided reflection by faculty. We invited the medical students doing summer student-ships at the CMPA to pilot the narrative exercises. Interestingly, the students shared narratives that included a spectrum of patient safety themes, including disrespectful behavior by faculty toward a standardized patient during a teaching session, and policies regarding equipment maintenance.[7]

We hope these narrative exercises will be utilized by faculty as part of formal patient safety curricula at the undergraduate and postgraduate medical education levels, and potentially integrated into e-portfolio initiatives. They can also be used in lifelong learning of all health-care providers as a form of continuing professional development. We hope that the use of narrative and reflective discourse will enable patient safety to become more relevant to trainees and faculty and will promote a culture of patient safety in both working and learning environments.

NOTES

1. Rick Iedema, Christine Jorm, and Martin Lum, "Affect Is Central to Patient Safety: The Horror Stories of Young Anaesthetists," *Social Science & Medicine* 69 (2009): 1750–56.
2. Alexis R. Ogdie et al., "Seen Through Their Eyes: Residents' Reflections on the Cognitive and Contextual Components of Diagnostic Errors in Medicine," *Academic Medicine* 87 (2012): 1361–67.
3. William Martinez and Bernard Lo, "Medical Students' Experiences with Medical Errors: An Analysis of Medical Student Essays," *Medical Education* 42 (2008): 733–41.
4. Ibid., 738.
5. Iedema, Jorm, and Lum, "Affect Is Central to Patient Safety," 1755.
6. Martinez and Lo, "Medical Students' Experiences with Medical Errors," 734.
7. The set of patient safety narrative exercises is available through the CMPA Good Practices Guide website at www.cmpa-acpm.ca/serve/docs/ela/goodpracticesguide/pages/index/index-faculty-e.html.

Reflection as Side Effect

Use of Creative Writing Exercises in Medical Education

JAY BARUCH

To appreciate my take on reflective writing, I'll ask you to consider the patellar reflex. Years ago, as a beginning medical student tapping my rubber-headed hammer against a patient's knee, I discovered how the word "relax" can work against itself, resulting in paradoxical and unintentional tension. This inhibits the spinal reflex. To overcome this resistance, there was a tendency to drum harder; but the knee never kicked out. Then, one day, I was taught a trick to achieve disinhibition, one that didn't make intuitive sense even if it prevented a lot of bruised knees. Have the patient hook the fingertips of their hands together and pull. Whether it worked through distraction or indirection, focused tension elsewhere created a receptive deep tendon more effectively than all my appeals for the patient to relax.

If I teach reflection in writing, the process is notable for not teaching it.

My perspective on the role of writing in medical education is influenced by my own idiosyncratic struggles as a creative writer. I don't always succeed, but at the most basic level, what I aspire for in my work is what the poet Tess Gallagher described in an interview with Jay Woodruff as entering "emotional spaces on terms that are original."[1] She's alluding to poetry, but she's getting at something that applies to prose. Drill into material that might be emotionally demanding, and then find a responsive voice. This can be a grinding process, questioning unsupported ideas and assumptions, sharpening broad and cliché-riddled language, and dissecting predictable or inconsistent motivations. Rewriting is the key, but each new draft flies under a banner of impatience and false satisfaction, a hidden impulse to believe that I've "finished."

I've learned to distrust this good feeling. Because lurking in those middle drafts sits an unexpected thought, piece of language, image, or tone of voice.

This detail might be tiny, appear unimportant, or feel like a side dish, but it has a pulse and often opens up to the heart of what I was really after, usually truths I was afraid to admit or emotions too volatile to play with. Sometimes intuitive readers point them out, or I stumble upon them through the rewriting process. These vulnerable spaces are often protected by hedges, fences, or even steel walls, with the occasional moat stocked with ninja goldfish. Breaking through requires recognition of those defenses at work, then finding the right language and structure that captures what wants to worm away, or explode in my hands.

Only by writing can I discover what I'm writing about.

The process of genuine reflection must be differentiated from the alleged products of reflection. Years ago I attended a reflective writing workshop for medical educators run by well-respected colleagues, where the group read a few examples of student essays. As it would happen, I later learned the identity of one of the students, someone I knew, and congratulated him on a thoughtful piece of writing. He chuckled, but it wasn't modesty flicking away a compliment—it was a confession. He knew exactly what was expected in his response to the prompt, and he aimed to please. I've heard similar admissions from other excellent, caring medical students, many of whom are writers, who question and sometimes resist the reflection methods imposed upon them.

I'm not saying all students take an assignment approach to reflection in their writing or that medical educators are unknowing conspirators in a well-intentioned practice that's become a ubiquitous check box required of doctors in training. I simply want to emphasize this point. The ability to dig into these deep interior places and then express it on the page requires work, imagination, and the willingness to rewrite again and again. It's a skill, a temperament, a habit, and a muscle. These muscles atrophy or become spastic when I'm away from the page for a spell. Colleagues have shared similar frustrations. If practiced writers experience this difficulty, are we expecting too much from medical students when it comes to their reflections? Are so-called reflections closer in spirit to answers, efficient and mainstream narratives that students know will be received with heart-warming smiles?

I champion writing in medical education, reflective or otherwise, because through the physical act of writing we discover how we think. In his essay "Thank you, Esther Forbes," writer George Saunders said that honing sentences to describe the world changes our perceptions of it, and by working with language—struggling to choose the right words, not only what we say but how we say it—we learn to identify the bullshit within ourselves and others.[2] For me, even the specific writing tool holds a strange influence on what I say and how I say it. Moving a pen across the page opens different access roads into my mind, creates sentences with different rhythms, than tapping a stream of words across my laptop.

Once, while I was running a writing workshop at another medical school, the group reviewed a student's work that was intense and cryptic, the product of great effort and a mind that had important things to say; but the group couldn't figure out what exactly that was. I asked the writer to simply explain a passage, and he could do it beautifully. When asked why he couldn't just say that in the piece, he grinned in bashful retreat and nodded. "I can't go there."

That's what writing is all about. Going to those places that are most uncomfortable, where you feel most vulnerable. Those places easily avoided by masks of language. To quote Saunders once again, "False prose can mark an attempt to evade responsibility."[3] My work with medical students and undergraduates emphasizes creativity, which I think is the best way to go about achieving honest reflection. Writing exercises appropriated from creative writing workshops serve a purpose similar to asking patients to hook their fingers when eliciting a knee reflex—which was more than a trick, but known as the Jendrassik maneuver, named for a nineteenth-century Hungarian physician. By asking students to use their imagination, to turn their focus elsewhere, they lower their guard. Reflection becomes a necessary side effect. By sidling up to tender issues or emotions under the cover of a safe harbor—the creative work—and not steering too stiffly, writing becomes a process for discovering what they're writing about.

Writing and emergency medicine are vastly different enterprises with distinct practical pressures, but these two experiences share a core dependence on language, story, and a focused imagination.[4] In a health-care system undergoing a transformation, physicians need to be creative and flexible, critical thinkers and expert communicators, clinicians who can recognize when they're settling for superficial satisfactions and scripted responses in their work and instead risk confronting ambiguity and uncertainty on terms that are fresh and original.

Writing in the classroom should emphasize openness and perseverance, the importance of probing small details and quiet moments. This can't happen if students write with tense muscles, or kick their knees out because that's what is expected of them. Many students wear creative accomplishments as well as brilliance in the sciences, and what I offer is nothing more than permission to tap into these innate gifts, not by claiming humanistic aims or promoting traits of well-rounded physicians, but by shining a bright light on the craft of writing and the application of student creativity in the clinic.

I'm cautious about working the values and purposes of reflective writing too hard, teaching with themes and virtues on my sleeve. Consider what Tess Gallagher said about expectations of poetry and poets: "People ask quite a lot of a poet these days. They seem to want every poem to be an orchestra, when sometimes you wanted only to hear a sad melody played on the flute."[5]

NOTES

1. Jay Woodruff, ed., *A Piece of Work: Five Writers Discuss Their Revisions* (Iowa City: Univ. of Iowa Press, 1993), 68.
2. George Saunders, *The Braindead Megaphone: Essays* (New York: Riverhead Books, 2007).
3. Saunders, *The Braindead Megaphone*, 64.
4. Jay M. Baruch, "Creative Writing as a Medical Instrument," *Journal of Medical Humanities* 34 (2013): 459–69.
5. Woodruff, *A Piece of Work*, 67.

Critical Incidents in Clinical Teaching

Using Expanded Storytelling to Reflect on Practice

PAM HARVEY AND NATALIE RADOMSKI

The Nigerian writer and poet Ben Okri has observed, "We live by stories, we also live in them."[1] Stories help shape meaning from our experiences, assisting us in sense making. We listen to the stories others tell us, and we have our own to tell, particularly once we have lived and worked in a particular landscape for a while. Stories reveal our experiences but are framed within the scope of our knowledge. Stories are part of practice, arising from a need to share and explore what has happened. The processing of these stories—the reflection and understanding—is not always attended to, especially if time is limited or the listeners have their own tales to tell. Writing a story can enable deeper understanding, as the story is reexperienced and "becomes the avenue toward knowing about it."[2]

At our small regional clinical school, we have a dedicated team of clinical educators who are involved with our medical students. Most are clinicians who teach medical students as part of their clinical workload, and many have had no formal learning about teaching practice. To assist our clinical educators, our educational unit offers various programs and resources, which range from a quarterly published booklet on teaching topics to an accredited graduate certificate in health professional education. Our faculty development sessions are often the only shared opportunities clinical educators have to talk theoretically and practically about their teaching. Many have anecdotes to tell about successful and not-so-successful teaching events but, as is the case for many stories, they are told yet never actually deconstructed for learning purposes. To help clinical educators reflect on their learning and teaching experiences, we have utilized a written template suggested by Janice McDrury and Maxine Alterio.[3]

When clinical educators are asked to reflect on critical incidents (or a significant event that raises issues about professional performance or learning), they usually immediately recall clinical practice experiences. With guidance on thinking about moments of their teaching as critical incidents—defined by us as an event that creates uncertainty associated with a teaching session—the clinical educators often had stories to tell about defining experiences in their own professional formation as teachers.

We start our reflective sessions with clinical educators telling their stories to each other in a conversational way, with the prompt "share your story with another person," and giving the listener permission to ask clarifying questions. This proves to be a key point: asking people to write the story of their clinical incident without discussion is too challenging for most. Oral storytelling assists in developing the story in a chronological fashion, especially when prompted by the listener for details not immediately related. We allow about fifteen minutes for this telling process, with participants swapping roles from storyteller to listener so that each has a chance to construct and share their anecdotes. The purpose of the oral storytelling activity is to process the reflections and outcomes of the event.

After the initial storytelling, the concept of story writing is introduced. We use a template as a guide for this process. For some clinical educators, the task remains challenging, but this type of "telling" is for their own reflection. Completing the areas of the template guides their writing and creates a structure for the reflection activity. Some people write in whole sentences and others use bullet points—for the purpose of the activity, any method of writing the event chronologically is accepted.

The writing process starts with the chronological events of the story. For the major components of the story, the clinical educators are asked to list the key people involved at the time and to reveal how the storyteller felt. Annotating the story in this way allows the writer to see pivotal moments within the critical incident, highlighting points at which the teller had a realization or impediment that affected their teaching. After considering these insights, the storyteller then describes what they learned from the event as a whole, by deconstructing it. These reflections provide the educator with an action plan for future episodes.

Perhaps the ultimate reflection occurs in naming the story. McDrury and Alterio suggest that the title of the story should be written last so that it serves as a reflective label; written first, it may name only the crisis of the story and not its resolution. This is another challenging but very worthwhile component of the exercise.

This reflective storytelling mechanism has also been utilized by our clinical educators in classroom-based sessions with their medical students. The activity requires time for telling and writing and time for constructing, processing, and deconstructing the story. This time is not always available in typical teaching sessions at our clinical school but even so has been taken up by some clinical educators who realize the benefits in linking teaching content with structured opportunities to reflect on clinical practice.

Offering this reflective opportunity to our clinical educators gives them a chance to consider their teaching in a different way, helping them analyze moments of uncertainty in order to strengthen their professional development. We have been surprised at some of the informal feedback we have received about being able to move into the creative space that storytelling allows, giving weight to the lived experiences of teaching.

Stories are the foundation of many professions, including clinical teaching. Using stories to critically reflect on practice is an extension of what often occurs between practitioners—the telling and retelling of experiences. Using storytelling and story writing to further examine the "learnings" of the experience expands the reflective process, enabling overt recognition of how living by and in stories can change practice for the better.

NOTES

1. Ben Okri, *A Way of Being Free* (London: Phoenix, 1997), 46.
2. Rita Charon, "Our Heads Touch: Telling and Listening to Stories of Self," *Academic Medicine* 87 (2012): 1154–56.
3. Maxine Alterio and Janice McDrury, *Learning through Storytelling in Higher Education: Using Reflection and Experience to Improve Learning* (London: Kogan Page, 2003).

PART 2

Visual Reflection—
Learning to See

The Art of Assessment

MARTINA KELLY, SIUN O'FLYNN, AND DEIRDRE BENNETT

Medicine, art, and assessment—unhappy bedfellows or a marriage made in heaven? The *art of assessment* is a term used to capture the complexity of the current assessment of medical students. That one might apply the metaphor in its literal sense is likely to surprise. Yet that is what we did. This is the story of how we did it, why we did it, and how it worked.

In the late 2000s, the Irish government introduced a "graduate entry" pathway to medical school in addition to the traditional route of entrance directly after high school. Students with a prior degree were able to apply to complete an accelerated four-year medical program. As part of this new curriculum, we introduced a community-based placement with a multidisciplinary primary care team. Our students included graduates of health care, science, and liberal arts courses. To widen our assessment modalities and to make the latter group of students feel more included, we developed an assessment that involved art.

"Huh?" That was the initial reaction of our students. Lots of anxiety—how will it be graded? What type of art? Would the assessment be "objective"? We sought advice from a colleague in our education department, who suggested Project Zero. Project Zero is an educational collaborative, established and supported by Harvard Graduate School of Education. It hosts a range of projects, research and educational initiatives aimed to foster crossdisciplinary work. Within this resource we encountered Gardner's idea of "entry points" as a framework to engage with a piece of art.[1] These include the following:

- The "aesthetic entry point"—learners respond to formal or sensory qualities of a subject or work of art (for example, line, color, expression, composition of a painting, or the alliteration or meter of a poem)

- The "narrative entry point"—learners respond to the narrational element of the subject or piece of art (for example, the legend in the painting or the story behind the construction of a skyscraper)
- The "logical/quantitative entry point"—learners respond to the aspects of the subject, or piece of art, that invite deductive reasoning or numerical consideration (for example, what decisions may have led to the creation of the art object, calculation of dimensions?)
- The "foundational entry point"—learners respond to the broader concepts, or philosophical issues, raised by the subject or piece of art (for example, whether metaphors depict or defy reality, why a painting of soup cans can be considered art)
- The "experiential entry point"—learners respond to the subject or piece of art by doing something with their hands or bodies (for example, drawing, or setting a poem to music).

In terms of our own educational innovation, graduate entry, second-year medical students (n = 45) were given the following assignment: "You are asked to submit a piece of work demonstrating the application of your learning to date on interprofessional care to a case you have seen. You can submit this as an essay. We also encourage a creative piece (for example, a poem; piece of music or artwork) which you feel encapsulates your learning. Interprofessional learning refers to learning from and with other health-care professionals." At the end of the module, twenty-two students submitted essays and twenty-three submitted art.

Artwork comprised music, poetry, sculpture, collage, drawing, painting, and photography. We were surprised with by diversity of modalities and student effort. The challenge was how to assess this work. We independently examined student work. Each piece of art was considered in relation to the five entry points that helped us to differentiate the student's level of engagement with, and reflection on, the topic. We met to discuss our findings, and disagreements were resolved by discussion leading to consensus.

We considered and reflected on the impact of students' work. Their work provided us with new perspectives on our students as learners, how they engaged with patients, and their critical appraisal of interprofessional work. Some of the work was deeply moving. One student wrote a poem about a man with Huntington's chorea, a rare genetic condition that affects movement and mind. He drew a picture of a skull, the brain represented by the chromosomal repeat CAG, the repeating gene sequence that causes Huntington's. It was accompanied by a poem expressing the patient's dilemma: fearing death but welcoming it as a release from a future of uncertainty and dependence. He referenced the skull as an icon of death and the patient's inability to recognize himself anymore and his loss of humanity. This submission integrated all entry points (aesthetic, narrative, quantitative, logical, and foundational).

A piece of music inspired by a woman recovering from a stroke was also very poignant. Although none of us was familiar with electronic techno music, the repeating theme was like a fugue; the patient repeatedly fell and stood again before finally walking a few precious steps. (Entry points used: aesthetic, narrative, quantitative, foundational, experiential.) Other pieces showed evidence of creative synthesis, as demonstrated by a sculpture made out of straw and silver wire. The piece was accompanied by directions on how to read the piece according to the time of day. As the lighting changed, the shadows cast by the structure and light reflecting off the silver wire represented the shifting fortunes of the primary care team against the everchanging conditions of providing individualized patient care. (Entry points used: aesthetic, narrative, foundational.)

Metaphors of communication and teamwork were represented by the use of images of hands, puzzles, and interlocking diagrams (for example, the branches of a tree, building blocks). Students reflected on how patient care is impacted when health-care professionals work together; the impression that the sum was more than the parts was prevalent. The effect of the student work spread into the community. Students gave their permission for presentation of their work to the primary care teams they had been placed with. Demonstration of student learning stimulated the group to reflect on their collaborative role as teachers, a new experience for the team. Presentations of the students' work secured assistance from our local health service to coordinate the student placements and extend our work to three additional areas. We have presented and published descriptive accounts of this work, increasing awareness in our institution and beyond.

Can art be used for student assessment? Yes, it can. In our example, students chose diverse means to express their learning and demonstrated Bloom's higher-order objectives (synthesizing, evaluating) as they did so. We did not formally evaluate students' reactions to this task. Anecdotally, they said they participated because it was fun, and it was fun for us too. This project has stimulated our creativity. If we were to repeat this assignment, we would evaluate more systematically. With the students' permission, we would like to present their artwork to the wider community or within an exhibition space within our medical school.

NOTE

1. Howard Gardner, *The Unschooled Mind: How Children Think and How Schools Should Teach* (New York: Basic Books, 2011).

Linking Self-Reflection to Clinical Practice

CAROLINE WELLBERY AND MELISSA CHAN

Caroline: As a trained literary professional—I actually earned a PhD in comparative literature before attending medical school—I have lived most of my life immersed in texts. When I began teaching medical students, I used prose and poetry to explore themes I felt essential to medicine, mostly centered on the simultaneously unique and universal suffering of patients. In recent years, though, I have gravitated toward the visual arts as a teaching tool, a discipline I know very little about and for which I have no personal talent. I explain my attraction to art as a variation on "telling it slant"—the undefined wedge of my ignorance actually carves out a metaphorical space in which creative teaching ideas can germinate. But, as important as this "wedge of ignorance" is to my own evolution, the creative space it opens up is really only a manifestation of the larger potential of the visual arts—the freedom that comes in general with the nonverbal suggestiveness of images.[1]

As John Carey polemicizes in *What Good Are the Arts* (unfairly dismissing the visual arts for this very reason), there is a fundamental difference between literature and art.[2] Literature uses words, and words hold you accountable in particular ways. While art has its own accountability, requiring careful looking, it also frees the imagination—a flight often untethered to specific ideas or explanations, and especially to the facts and figures of doctoring. In medical education, students and residents are starved for this untrammeled exploration. That is how I have come to incorporate a variety of visual arts activities in my work with students and residents, including the activity described here: making self-portraits as a path to self-reflection. I should add that without expert collaboration, I could not have moved from the realm of inspiration to project execution. One important precondition for the success of this work has

64

been the cultivation of relationships with seasoned artists and art educators. Health humanities work is strengthened enormously through collaboration.

Melissa: I am Georgetown's Arts-in-Medicine Fellow 2012–13, working under Dr. Wellbery's supervision. Dr. Wellbery tasked me with developing a self-portrait activity with the family medicine residents.

STRUCTURE OF THE ACTIVITY

We have twenty-one residents who meet Thursday mornings for lectures. Once a month, residents participate in a "well-being" session. Our arts activities have fed into the well-being time slots. For our reflection activity, we allotted two on-site sessions. During the first session, we introduced residents to the concept of self-portraiture. In preparation for the second session, residents were given some preparatory assignments to complete at home. They then convened for the second session to create their own self-portraits.

For the first, introductory session, we recommend consultation with a studio artist to select examples of self-portraits, explain how they are created and used, and impart a basic understanding of contour drawing. We showed twenty examples of self-portraits to illustrate motivations behind self-portraiture, including biographical information on the artists and, to a small extent, their historical context. We explained the method behind blind contour drawing and then ended the session with residents completing blind contour drawings of their hands.

We recommend preparing trainees for the second session by providing them with some background on why self-reflection is important and what the project is meant to achieve prior to the active session. One week prior to the second session, we disseminated a thirteen-minute slide-show video with audio explaining our hypothesis: that a project promoting self-reflection would help providers facilitate self-reflection in their patients. We included examples of self-portraits to help the residents get ideas for their own self-portraits. The video ended with reflection questions often used in classroom art activities[3] that the residents were to complete prior to the session: "Who am I?" "What are the distinctive things that make me 'me'?" "How do I want people to see me?" "How can I express my many different sides?" "How can I reinvent myself for various purposes or times in my life?" "How am I changing from day to day or year to year?" "What do I want to become?" The residents then were requested to bring three items that represented themselves along with a photograph of themselves to work from for the second session.

For the actual self-portrait session, we recommend a two-hour slot, during which residents first execute a blind contour drawing of their own photograph, and then, using the three objects they brought, complete a self-portrait. After the self-portrait session, we recommend breaking into small groups to allow participants to discuss the meaning of their portraits. After our session, all residents hung their self-portraits on the wall of their workroom.

Caroline and Melissa: There has been a great and spontaneous demand for a follow-up self-portrait session, suggesting that residents are willing to give up their formal well-being sessions in favor of this art activity. Many of the residents commented that this activity was the first time they truly evaluated their identity; they felt this activity allowed them time to reflect, providing an outlet for creativity and self-expression. Up to this point, many of the residents had written numerous admission essays and personal statements, but using art allowed them to step beyond the often-limiting realm of words into a space they create. Several residents commented that such an activity provided a sense of camaraderie among participants; they saw themselves and each other with new, more observant and understanding eyes. Additionally, an unexpected consequence was that the self-portraits became a focus of interest for residency applicants during the interview season, and thus fostered a sense of arts and wellness culture associated with our program.

Caroline: Art can free the imagination and allow for a creative and mental health release so necessary to counteract the rigid thought patterns straitjacketing medical trainees. But that is not to say art education is a free-for-all. I strongly feel that reflective practice must be embodied. By *embodied,* I mean preferably, a physical enactment of what is learned—for example, through movement and mindfulness activities or, at the very least, through action and interaction. Sitting in a classroom and interpreting a text is all very well and good, but this is what medical trainees do all the time, and it is too easy for them to divorce themselves from lived meaning. Application and relevance are key. This can be achieved not through any one particular arts or humanities area but always by attention to method and approach. Trainees gain practical skills in healing by experiencing an activity's relevance firsthand and recognizing its relevance to patients under their care. I believe all medical arts and humanities education at the professional level should integrate reflection with action.

Just as art observation activities have gained acceptance as a means of honing clinical observation, this self-portrait exercise is intended to give residents a tool for communicating with patients who may be difficult to approach in traditional ways. Asking a depressed patient, a patient with low literacy, or even a hostile patient to bring with them a self-portrait is one means through which residents could apply their own self-reflection experience to patient care.

Currently, we plan to carry forward the project to teen mom group visits, using self-portraits and journaling as novel avenues through which these patients can reflect productively on their roles and responsibilities. We envision a research project that would not only evaluate the impact of self-portrait reflection on resident well-being but would document through relevant clinical measures how self-portraiture can help patients. In the case of teen moms, such measures might include adherence to medical advice, infant milestones, growth, and breastfeeding rates.

NOTES

1. Khaled Karkabi, Hedy S. Wald, and Orit Cohen Castel, "The Use of Abstract Paintings and Narratives to Foster Reflective Capacity in Medical Educators: A Multinational Faculty Development Workshop," *Medical Humanities* 40 (2014): 44–48.
2. John Carey, *What Good Are the Arts?* (New York: Oxford Univ. Press, 2006).
3. National Endowment for the Humanities Curriculum Development Project, "Rembrandt and Collections of His Art in America," accessed June 5, 2015, http://eev.liu.edu/nehrembrandt/activities/portraitsSchools.htm.

Examining the Body

Fostering Reflection among Student Nurses about "the Body" in Practice

D. STEWART MACLENNAN AND ERIKA GOBLE

In about the fifth week of a health assessment course, I (Stewart) was called to assist a group of nursing students who were struggling with a specific area of the abdominal examination. I waited by the curtain and asked if I could enter. Hearing no objection, I proceeded into the curtained area. There I found three female students sitting topless on the bed. Paying no attention to their state of undress, they casually asked their question. Only a few weeks earlier these same students had been lamenting how embarrassing it was to examine each other's backs for unexpected skin lesions. Concerned, I asked, "Where are your shirts?" to which they responded, "We're comfortable without them." Wanting to draw their attention to what was obvious to me, I queried, "What would it be like for a patient to be topless and exposed in front of other people? Or to be cared for by a topless nurse?" After a moment's reflection, the young women quickly donned their shirts. This incident proved quite harmless, but one can imagine the multiple potential boundary issues inherent in it and it left us wondering: How is it that nurses can examine and overlook the body simultaneously? Further, given how common this type of occurrence is in health assessment courses, how do we, as educators, prepare future health professionals to be attentive to the importance of the body—that of their patients and their own—in the provision of care?

The body is one of the most present and yet least attended aspects of existence. Sartre writes that our bodies are largely "passed over in silence."[1] We tend to take note of them only when something out of the ordinary occurs, such as when they cease to move as they should or when we experience physical pain. And even then, our bodies quickly adjust. Our aching back may be forgotten amid the flurry of a busy day and only recalled when we stop for

68

the evening. Such acclimation is readily evident in the student nurses' obvious lack of discomfort at their own nudity. Within mere weeks, what had once been unthinkable—undressing in front of fellow students—had become the new norm. Perhaps even more surprising, the normalcy of nudity extended beyond their immediate group to include their male instructor.

While we recognize that it is pedagogically important for students to be comfortable in their learning environments, a thoughtlessness regarding comfort with the naked body can have adverse effects in nursing practice. As educators we want our future nurses to be comfortable attending to and caring for patients' naked bodies, but it is equally important that they recognize that their future patients may not share their comfort. Patients may feel awkward, embarrassed, or even ashamed at exposing their bodies. For nursing care to be "good nursing care," a nurse must be respectful of and, more importantly, cognizant of these possible responses.

From the students' actions, it became readily evident that learning how to "attend to the body" was an important, but neglected, part of the health-assessment course. Health assessment in nursing is often taught within a well-defined and prescribed curriculum. Instructors, however, rarely explicitly engaged in a discussion about the body as embodied. And yet, can we consider students "knowledgeable" or even "competent" if they fail to be reflective about the body they are learning to assess?

To address this gap, we devised an hour-and-a-half workshop. Considering how quickly students become accustomed to touching and seeing the body in a clinical manner, the workshop was scheduled to fall immediately after the students' first lab. It is the time when they are most aware of their discomfort with the body and before the body has once again slipped from their attention. Through a series of exercises, we sought to bring to the students awareness their own bodies so that we could collectively discuss and reflect upon the centrality of the body—from the points of view of both the patient and nurse.

We began with a simple mindfulness exercise—asking students to close their eyes and, for two to three minutes, pay attention to how their bodies felt. Did their shoes feel tight on their feet? Were their chairs uncomfortable? Perhaps they felt the pull of their clothing as they sat. This eagerly anticipated activity was designed for students to develop an awareness of their bodies.

With students now focusing on their own bodies, we moved on to explore the experience of the clinical gaze—how practitioners commonly look at patients. Students were paired; one was designated "the nurse" and the other "the patient." The nurse was then told to observe (not touch or talk to) the patient for two minutes in an attempt to mimic an actual clinical encounter. We then asked nurses and patients what their experience was like. Patients, both male and female, reported feeling "examined" and "judged." They worried about "what the nurse saw" and felt they were being "assessed" and "measured to some norm." They described becoming acutely aware of their bodies and being looked at as if they were specimens. Most nurses initially felt comfortable examining their patients but then began feeling like "voyeurs" when they became uncertain "what to look for," reflecting both an already existing comfort with the notion of the clinical gaze but an uncertainty as to its enactment. In debriefing the exercise, we discuss why such a gaze might be important for clinicians, what it allows us to see (for example, injured bodies in trauma settings), and what it enables us to do (invasive procedures, for example). We also discuss why the clinical gaze can become problematic if it becomes the only way practitioners engage with patients. A central message for the students was that their ability to move in and out of the clinical gaze is central to providing good nursing care, but they must also remain aware of the discomfort such a gaze can cause patients.

We next asked the students to view a series of images and consider their personal, gut responses. Each image was shown for approximately twenty seconds and a total of ten images were used. The images presented a range of individuals, from the conventionally beautiful to "ugly," from emaciated to healthy looking, and from "average" in appearance to those with significant body modifications, such as extensive tattooing, body piercings/implants. In our subsequent discussion, students were initially unwilling to speak about their physical reactions to any of the pictures. They kept claiming that "looks do not matter—they are all people." To deny reacting was, in their minds, the appropriate nursing response—until we asked them to consider what they thought of having one of these individuals as their nurse. A collective gasp ensued.

Their gut reactions were now undeniable and proved to be the opening for a discussion about the ethics of responding to another's body. Two possibilities emerged: the nurse reacting to the patient's body and the patient reacting to the nurse's body. We asked students to consider how they might act when faced with caring for a person whose face or body they find different, unacceptable, repulsive, or extremely attractive, and we discussed how fully acknowledging one's discomfort creates the possibility of a thoughtful response and can open the space for ethical practice to occur. Moreover, in having the students consider their reactions in terms of being patients, we were able to draw out an embodied understanding of the importance of "professional dress" and its contextual nature. Rather than seeing the dress code they were expected to follow as some arbitrary set of rules established by elderly and no longer fashionable faculty members, the students understood their uniform and physical presentation as an important component of nursing care.

Lastly, the exercise enabled us to introduce the notion of the nurse's body as facilitating or impeding the healing of the patient's body. To bring this point home, we concluded with a seven-minute video about how the clinicians themselves can act as either a placebo or nocebo, contributing to both positive and negative health outcomes. Students were amazed to learn that the very presentation of their bodies can either heal or harm. By the conclusion of the workshop, the nursing students could readily articulate that how best to be a nurse is to be embodied in a particular caring, healing, and reflective way—to be fully present with one's *embodied patients.*

To date, we have offered the workshop three times, with each session being well received by the students. Because this type of workshop, however, departs from traditional approaches for teaching health assessment in undergraduate nursing programs, it has raised some eyebrows. Nonetheless, we maintain that a reductionist approach to physical assessment fails to foster a reflective understanding of human bodies as *embodied,* an understanding that is necessary to empathic nursing care. And we do not seem to be alone in this: one faculty member observing our workshop stated that it gave her a touchstone that she would refer to in future clinical teaching "when the skill was right but the tact was wrong."

NOTE

1. Jean-Paul Sartre, *Being and Nothingness: A Phenomenological Essay on Ontology,* trans. Hazel E. Barnes (New York: Philosophical Library, 1956), 63.

Cultivating Fresh Eyes

An Arts-Based Workshop Series for Clinical Faculty

ALEXA MILLER, WARREN HERSHMAN, AND GOPAL YADAVALLI

Clinical educators must engage with fundamental problems endemic in medicine. Clinical ambiguity, the decline of physical diagnostic skills, and communication breakdown within care teams are all complex issues that make up the ground underfoot for all practitioners. Yet it is educators who are uniquely responsible for providing pedagogical guidance to students; it is educators who must look up to identify the mountains looming high and close while preparing others for the path ahead. To implement improvements in medical education, we must first step out from the shadow of the mountains; we require renewal, new perspectives, and tools from unexpected sources. How can clinical educators cultivate fresh eyes?

We describe here an innovation piloted at Boston University School of Medicine (BUSM), the Art Practicum, a three-part faculty development workshop series. Designed to allow faculty to revisit long-standing teaching challenges from new vantage points, the program promotes personal and programmatic renewal, offers tools from across professions, and cultivates an atmosphere of interprofessional exchange. The series provides a visual arts–based framework for teaching, practice, and understanding clinical skills. In three areas—observation, navigation of ambiguity, and teamwork—we adapted a tool used broadly in the arts, Visual Thinking Strategies (VTS).[1] Created by Abigail Housen and Philip Yenawine, VTS is a research-based teaching protocol for engaging students in discussion based on a deep examination of art. Its companion professional development model—in which Alexa Miller, coauthor of this essay, is formally trained—is designed to transform teacher practice. Twenty-eight clinician-educators, from all levels of experience and with different specialties, participated. Engaging in arts experiences, they practiced the basics of VTS pedagogy, integrated it with clinical teaching, and shared feedback.

Our intervention derived from three hypotheses: (1) providing a break in repetitive clinical teaching and consequent burnout could facilitate master teaching; (2) clinical teachers could find practical use for VTS tools and insights; and (3) works of art could emulate conditions for clinical learning by provoking an experience of uncertainty (similar to situations requiring clinical reasoning) within a context of psychological safety (fundamentally different from the dynamics of the clinic). These hypotheses arose from our experiences in teaching reasoning skills to students and in training teachers; we found commonality in helping teachers and students learn to be "comfortable being uncomfortable." Distinct from most arts interventions in medical education, we explored a "teach the teachers" approach: how might arts-teaching tools benefit faculty?

We drew directly from the Visual Thinking Strategies teaching protocol yet tailored the training to the unique concerns of clinical teachers (thus the workshops differed substantially from the "school-wide, three-year professional development model" of standard K–12 VTS implementation). The goal was to cultivate fresh eyes by having workshop participants learn to (1) facilitate "technically strict" VTS conversations and to (2) hone in on the topics of clinical observation, navigation of clinical uncertainty, and team communication. We included literature on patient safety, clinical teaching, and organizational development, making clinical connections a cornerstone of our discussion and reflection. Despite these modifications, we adamantly preserved key components of VTS training: a community of teacher practitioners, interactive encounters with carefully selected works of art, facilitation practice, coaching, feedback, and all elements of the VTS teaching method itself. In this method, teachers facilitate open-ended discussions of works of art with student groups. Rather than directing students where to look, the teacher paraphrases students' responses while identifying new vocabulary, themes, questions, and student thought patterns. Prompting students to distinguish fact from inference and to continue searching (even after findings are identified), the teacher nourishes students in actively looking, listening, voicing uncertainties, and benefiting from differences in opinions.

Our innovation rolled out over four stages: (1) planning, (2) recruitment, (3) implementation, and (4) assessment. In planning, we began by asking: "How can we most effectively apply the tools of the visual arts to enhance learning among medical students and residents and promote professional growth among faculty?" More specific questions then emerged: "How can we harness VTS to improve clinical reasoning and help learners work better amidst uncertainty?

How can we tap into knowledge across disciplines to help learners integrate the differences and strengths of others to form more effective teams?" These questions drove our subsequent needs assessment and further shaped the program design and funding applications.

Our next step was to engage a professional learning community. In addition to internal programmatic discussions, we offered two introductory talks designed to pique interest, to demonstrate the credibility of research in medical humanities and arts education, and to get people actively discussing the arts. We invited faculty, administrators, and students. We requested their lively participation and solicited their feedback. Data from these surveys were essential to securing an in-house grant for educational pilots. Using a 0–5 scale (in which 0=strongly disagree and 5=strongly agree), nineteen faculty and chief residents attending one seminar scored the workshop 4.82 for "relevant to my work as teacher," 4.73 for "facilitators were effective in communicating the goals and teaching the content," and 4.64 for "I would like more sessions to build on this one." The feedback further helped us customize the workshops.

At the implementation stage, each workshop engaged participants in practicing VTS pedagogy, exchanging feedback, and reflecting on teaching challenges. All participants committed to experimenting with VTS between sessions and to reporting back about their experiences. The sessions were organized into these three themes, emphasizing the intertwined nature of skill sets in observation, critical thinking, navigation of ambiguity, and team communication:

- The art of observation. What does it mean to look and see? What are known principles of clinical observation?[2] How do we see others? How do we make meaning? How can our visual capacities help us get at truth? Where might they interfere with truth?
- The art of ambiguity. Interacting with art as a means to gain comfort and skill in ambiguity, participants reflected on the challenges and opportunities of ambiguity, ending with pedagogical strategies[3] and literature on management of clinical uncertainty
- The art of teamwork. Identifying key concepts on team performance, participants explored them in VTS experiences and reflected upon their translation into clinical practice, teaching, and assessment of teams.

We collected feedback throughout the series. Participants voiced desire for practice in new approaches, structures for feedback, and reflection, so we changed the design of the second two sessions to include more opportunities for faculty to practice VTS teaching with one another. The assessments impressed us with the high quality of participation throughout the series, indicating that a major outcome was rigorous engagement, reflection, and dialogue. Participants further reported curricular experimentations, such as an arts-based module (four sessions) for fourth-year students on team communication skills. Chief residents reported paying more attention to their choice of language when facilitating discussions of complex cases in morning reports, based on the VTS questions. Two participants used VTS in a grand rounds presentation on compassion fatigue as part of physician wellness following the 2013 Boston Marathon bombing. These experiments suggest that the Art Practicum nourished personal and programmatic renewal.

What does it mean to cultivate fresh eyes? Fresh eyes are about curiosity, more than visual skills. Curiosity leads us through uncertainty's discomforts and drives responsible decision making. The visual arts provided the kind of new context needed for such fresh eyes, allowing BUSM faculty to see, and re-see, long-standing pedagogical issues affecting quality of care and patient safety. At the same time, the VTS techniques provided concrete tools for addressing challenges in observation, ambiguity, and teamwork with deliberate teaching and practice.

NOTES

We extend our thanks to Dabney Hailey, who contributed to the design of the teamwork workshop, as well as to Joel Katz, MD, and to the Boston University School of Medicine's Office of Development and Diversity.

1. Philip Yenawine, *Visual Thinking Strategies: Using Art to Deepen Learning across School Disciplines* (Cambridge, MA: Harvard Education Press, 2013).

2. J. Donald Boudreau, Eric J. Cassell, and Abraham Fuks, "Preparing Medical Students to Become Skilled at Clinical Observation," *Medical Teacher* 30 (2008): 857–62.

3. Dale Guenter, Nancy Fowler, and Linda Lee, "Clinical Uncertainty: Helping Our Learners," *Canadian Family Physician* 57 (2011): 120–22.

Soup vs. Art

MONICA KIDD, LARA NIXON, AND TOM ROSENAL

It started, as they say, with a happy accident. Monica's short attention span had gotten the best of her, forcing her to pip off from the conference she was attending in Toronto. Walking back to her hotel on Queen Street West, she passed the Edward Day Gallery, paused, and stepped into that big white space.

If buildings can have hangovers, this one had one. It was the morning after the Sobey Art Award ceremony, which had taken place at the neighboring Museum of Contemporary Canadian Art, where attendees, wearing skinny jeans and dark glasses, spilled over into Edward Day. Monica knows this because she had considered going but—seeing the crowds and in late stages of her pregnancy—decided in favor of knitting Christmas presents in her room at the Gladstone Hotel.

As the gallery (metaphorically) savored its coffee and plate of bacon, Monica made her way into a small back room and found the painting she had come looking for. There hung *Sticky,* a middle-aged woman, larger than life, naked, kneeling in front of a bed, and covered with sticky notes.[1] Visible only from the back, her face was completely obscured. She leaned in a particular way, slightly to the side, suggesting she was preparing to rise, or fall, or was struggling under the weight of something.

Perhaps the answer lay in what was written on the sticky notes: "poor," "fat," "unloved," and the like. Dozens of sticky notes printed in a deliberate hand covered her back and head, almost like a cloak of feathers. The insults were dizzying. The cruelty of the words on the notes, plus the sad, filtered light in the woman's room brought Monica to tears.

It didn't take long for a scheme to take root. Monica wondered what kind of medical conversations could take place around an image such as this. She snapped a clandestine photo with her phone and sent it to her friend and colleague Lara Nixon, who was equally moved by it. Monica and Lara quickly brought in Tom Rosenal, chair of a new committee tasked with increasing medical humanities offerings at the University of Calgary, and the ideas (and questions) started flying. Could we rent the painting and truck it out to Calgary? Would the artist (Margaret Sutherland of Kingston, Ontario) be interested in attending? Where would we hang it? Whom would we invite to the conversation? Would anyone come? What would we talk about? How would we go about leading such a conversation? How would we know if the conversation—assuming we could pull it off—meant anything to anyone? And who would pay for it?

Acres of digital trees were slaughtered in answering these questions, but, one by one, the questions were put to rest. Yes, we could rent it, and yes, the artist would be delighted to attend. We would bring it out for a humanities symposium we were planning in a few months' time (this was November, and the symposium was scheduled for March). We would hang her (we quickly started referring to the painting, with some affection, as "she" and "her") in the medical school's Bacs Learning Resource Centre, where she would share a space with anatomical models and software for demonstrating anatomy and pathology. During the day, *Sticky* would be both visible and supervised; at night, she would move into the vault in the undergraduate medical education (UME) office. The university gave us a certificate of insurance. And Bruce Wright, the associate dean of UME, cut us a check and warned us that "this had better be good."

Once we put the logistics to bed, it became a matter of figuring out exactly what we were up to. Like a game of intellectual spin the bottle, each time we faced a new pedagogical challenge, we spun the bottle and let it come to rest on another colleague: Roberta Jackson (English), Ian Mitchell (Pediatrics), Glenda Bendiak (Pediatrics/Medical Education), Laurie Pereles (Family Medicine), Lisa Hughes (Classics), and of course, the artist Margaret Sutherland. Finally we assembled our team and designed a one-hour workshop we called "Sticky Questions." We'd situate the painting on an easel at the front of the room, covered dramatically (we hoped) with a drape. We would start with a mini-lecture from Lisa on how to "read" a painting. Then we would do the reveal, give people a few minutes with the painting (with a stack of sticky notes on which they would write down questions the painting raised for them), and have them break into small groups to discuss their collective questions. After a few minutes back in large group, Maggie would do a question-and-answer session. Ethics approval arrived the day before the workshop.

Lara opened the workshop, and at first we were a little disappointed: there were a lot of empty chairs in the auditorium. But almost as soon as the bed sheet was pulled off of our friend *Sticky,* we could see that something magical was happening. Workshop participants, at first reserved and polite, slowly started crowding in to get a closer look at the painting. Standing at the back of the room, Tom saw a wonderful parallel: the woman in the painting appeared to be on something of a pedestal, and she was flanked by rows upon rows of the backs of viewers. The small groups were abuzz, and when Maggie shared the backstory of the painting and her relationship with her subject, we had to cut off questions in the interest of time.

We've since rolled out the workshop in other contexts, and the enthusiastic response is the same. Is it the painting itself or the act of collective reflection that so moves people? It's hard to say for sure, but there is a text that we think can shed some light on this question. In comedian Lily Tomlin's one-woman Broadway show *The Search for Signs of Intelligent Life in the Universe,* "street philosopher" Trudy struggles to explain the human pursuit of art to the "space chums" in her mind.[2] She shows them a can of Campbell's tomato soup and Andy Warhol's painting of a can of Campbell's tomato soup. "This is soup," she tells them, "and this is art."[3] She shuffles the two behind her back, reveals them, and asks them which is which. They get it wrong—and continue to get it wrong throughout the play until the very end, when they've decided to leave Earth. In a letter of farewell, they tell Trudy they finally followed her advice to go see a play, and had had the very human experience of goose bumps: "Yeah, to see a group of strangers sitting together in the dark, laughing and crying about the same things . . . that just knocked 'em out. They said, 'Trudy, the play was soup . . . the audience . . . art.'"[4]

Sticky, in our opinion, is far from soup—so much so that one of us now has her hanging in her home. But to us, watching a group of medical people stop and let the image of a vulnerable woman guide their reflection on what it means to do the work they do was art.

NOTES

1. Margaret Sutherland, Calgary, Alberta, "*Sticky,* Oil on linen, 40" x 60" ©2012, Private Collection," accessed June 5, 2015, http://maggiethered.com/images/Sticky.htm.
2. Jane Wagner, *The Search for Signs of Intelligent Life in the Universe* (New York: Harper & Row, 1987).
3. Ibid., 29.
4. Ibid., 212.

Exploring Art and Clinical Experience with Doctors in the Early Years of Postgraduate Training

KELLY THRESHER, SAMANTHA SCALLAN,
JONATHAN LOUIS SMITH, CHRISTOPHER OWEN,
LYNDSEY BOREHAM, AND PIPPA GARDINER

This innovative teaching session was undertaken with Foundation Year 2 (FY2) trainees while on a four-month attachment in primary care. These are UK trainees in the second year of broad-based medical training prior to focusing on specialist medical training. The teaching session was aimed at encouraging the trainees to step outside the primary care consulting room and to look at their clinical experiences through a different lens. We wanted to offer trainees the opportunity to reinterpret their clinical experiences through reflective writing, using a medical-related work of art as the stimulus.

In the autumn of 2011, five foundation trainees undertaking their four-month placements in primary care, their tutor (KT)* and a researcher (SS) visited the Wellcome Collection in London for an off-site education session. During the visit, the trainees were encouraged to browse the exhibitions to seek out ones that resonated with a clinical encounter or experience and to discuss what they saw during the visit. After the visit, we asked them to write a reflective account, linking an exhibit and a clinical encounter.

At the time of visiting the Wellcome Collection, two major exhibition rooms contained exhibits representative of a range of art genres and interpretations. For the most part, the group stayed in just one of the rooms, "Medicine Now." This permanent exhibition presents a range of ideas about science and medicine, reflecting a range of perspectives.[1]

In the week following the visit, the trainees wrote their reflective accounts linked to exhibits from "Medicine Now." They each linked their choices to a recent clinical encounter and wrote about the memories recalled and the impact

---

* The initials refer to an author of this essay.

it had had on them as clinicians. The trainees wrote narratives of some considerable length, structured under headings to explore and "unpack" their thinking. Their accounts were reviewed by KT and SS, who considered them for common topics and themes, which concerned attitudes and assumptions about disease, how their views and beliefs as doctors may be shaped by their worldview, and appreciation of the nature of evidence-based practice.

The sculpture *I Can Not Help the Way I Feel* prompted two trainees to reflect on clinical cases linked to obesity. For one trainee, it brought to mind social perceptions of obesity and the trainee's own assumptions about obese patients. This led to considering how clinical judgment may be shaped by feelings within. "I found the piece stimulated me to think about obese patients in a different way," the trainee said. "Although obesity is the root cause of many health problems, I realized I was just seeing an overweight patient and not the patient as a person. The piece helped me to reflect on this as the sculpture depicts an obese person without a head/face."

For the second trainee, it brought to mind a difficult consultation with an obese patient. In the course of the consultation, the interpersonal dynamic between the patient and doctor noticeably changed and was interpreted to indicate that the patient had become offended by the approach to advising on weight loss. In this case, an emotional reaction to the sculpture prompted reflection on attitudes toward the patient and whether the trainee's body language in particular had unintentionally conveyed inner feelings during the consultation. "I did not take probably enough chance to explore his expectations and struggles regarding his weight before I jumped in with my opinions," the trainee said.

At the follow-up focus group, the trainees reported that they did not have clear expectations of the day and found it a very different learning experience compared to their usual, more formal educational sessions. They liked having the freedom and time to consider the exhibits and felt this session was relevant to them as doctors even though it was not overly "medical." In general, the trainees felt there was too much choice of reflective subject matter, which made picking one item to write about quite difficult. Knowing they had to pick something to write about shaped the way they looked at the exhibits: they viewed pieces while also recalling clinical encounters. This was thought to help contextualize reflection and their reactions, as well as provide scope for new connections—by being "surprised" by exhibits and by seeing the familiar in unfamiliar ways. The trainees valued having time to undertake the visit, and, although not a "traditional" educational session, its relevance to their learning was apparent and resonant.

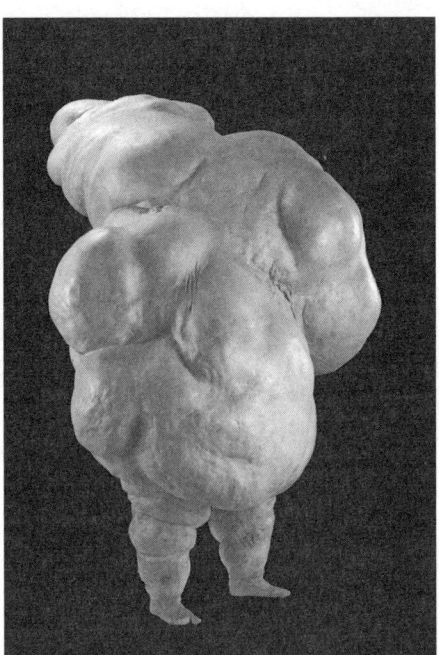

John Isaacs, *I Can Not Help the Way
I Feel,* 2003. Courtesy of Wellcome
Library, London.

The challenge for educators remains: How can we enable trainees to develop
and demonstrate depth to their learning in a world of training that speaks
of competencies, standards, and outcomes? How can space be provided for
trainees to develop and express their attitudes toward their evolving professional identity—of being a doctor and understanding the complexity of clinical
practice? The reflective writing of our group collectively demonstrated engagement with themes commensurate with deeper levels of learning: the feelings,
assumptions, beliefs, and values of practice, all of which are recognized as part
of learning and are required by the training curriculum they follow. From the
perspective of the trainees, the strength of this session was that it was not a
specific, structured learning event; rather, it offered participants freedom to
construct their reflections on clinical practice as suited them. There was also
opportunity for this learning to be shared with others in the postsession small-
group discussion. The session has become a regular part of the educational
curriculum for foundation trainees who spend time in primary care. We are
now exploring how we can further include art to facilitate reflective learning
with other learner groups.

NOTE

The authors wish to acknowledge and thank Dr. Lucy Dennison and all participating FY2 trainees who contributed to developing this innovation during the period of time they spent with us in Southampton, UK.

1. See www.wellcomecollection.org.

Visual Representations of
Personal Philosophies of Nursing

Use of Art and Reflection

JOANNE K. OLSON, OLIVE YONGE, AND SYLVIA BARTON

It was our good fortune to take part in a Faculty Learning Community (FLC) in the Faculty of Nursing at the University of Alberta during the 2012–2013 academic year. An FLC is a form of professional development that brings together faculty members with similar interests for ongoing discussions about a topic of their choice for about eight sessions over an academic year. We opted to promote each other's deeper learning about "integrating arts and humanities into teaching and learning." We co-constructed knowledge both from literature and from each other. We asked deep questions, discussed, debated, and ultimately challenged each other to use our knowledge about the effectiveness of incorporating the arts into teaching in various ways in the courses we were teaching.

I (JKO)* was teaching a graduate-level nursing course designed to promote inquiry into nursing knowledge and examine the contributions of art, philosophy, history, and science to the nursing discipline. Three of the course objectives were (1) to enhance awareness and understanding of the nature and development of nursing knowledge, (2) to explore beliefs about nursing, and (3) to examine how beliefs about the nursing profession influence practice.

Most of the thirteen graduate students were at an early stage in their master of nursing program. Some had years of nursing experience, while others had only recently graduated from their undergraduate programs. Most students were from Canada, but several came from other countries. Their nursing experience varied widely. Some had worked in emergency rooms, community health, and such areas as geriatrics and pediatrics. While many of our class

*The initials refer to an author of this essay.

discussions focused on "others'" ideas about what nursing is and how the key concepts related to nursing practice are defined, it seemed that one of the best ways to help students grasp the importance of these philosophical discussions was to examine their own nursing practices. This included inquiring into the assumptions and values that informed each student's approach to nursing, and the concepts that were most integral to their own practice.

I considered having the students write a paper about their thoughts and ideas, but there were already several written assignments in the course. Therefore, with the encouragement of my colleagues, I decided to try using art and reflection to entice students to access and express their personal nursing philosophies. Nursing literature provided us with examples of how others had used art to promote learning in nursing curricula. Whitman and Rose's[1] work with undergraduate students was especially useful in guiding this graduate-level learning experience. Ewing and Hayden-Miles[2] and Frei, Alvarez, and Alexander[3] also provided us with helpful insights into using art and reflection as we developed our approach.

Students were invited to express their personal philosophy of nursing using a selected art form in an optional assignment. They were then asked to share their creations with each other along with special guest faculty members (OY, SB). The students were invited to create an image or other representation that expressed their personal philosophies of nursing. Art forms could include drawings, paintings, a collage of images, poetry, music, or other representational forms. Students were invited to first write their own brief philosophies of nursing, if that was helpful to them, as part of their creative process. However, the students were told that their written statements would not be submitted or shared as part of this assignment; only their artistic creations would be shared and considered by their fellow students. There was no evaluation attached to this activity; the activity was merely designed to promote creative reflection, students' insights, and sharing. Students were told that there was no right or wrong way to express their own personal philosophies of nursing and informed that this "assignment" was optional. The students were each given five to seven minutes to share their artistic representation with peers and faculty guests. I shared that I (JO) would be participating in the activity along with the students by producing my own art product.

Twelve of the thirteen students elected to participate in this optional "assignment." The artistic products were varied, and their personal philosophies of nursing were depicted in collages, drawings, poems, photographs, a collection of symbols, and freshly baked chocolate chip cookies. The students shared their artwork with the class and each verbally described how it represented his or her personal philosophy of nursing. The students that participated reported that the exercise was challenging but satisfying. It helped them gain new insights into their personal philosophies of nursing and promoted more engaged discussion when considering authors' philosophies and perceptions of nursing.

For us, the outcomes of this experiment confirmed the importance of tapping into students' own creative reflection through various artistic modes, beyond writing skills, even in a graduate course. This invitation to use art to communicate a personal nursing philosophy resulted in creative products and insights that would have been only partly revealed in the more traditional written assignments. We have been encouraged by this experience and look forward to future opportunities to explore further incorporation of the arts and the humanities, and of reflection, into graduate nursing courses.

After the course was completed, I received an e-mail from one very excited student (used with permission):

> Hello Dr. Olson, I hope that you're doing well. There has been interesting activity that came out of your assignment in NURS 502 about visually representing our nursing philosophy. Upon encouragement by my supervisors, I submitted an abstract for a poster presentation, and it has been accepted. I shall be presenting a poster about my personal philosophy of nursing at a national conference! I thought you would be interested in this, since it had been the first time you had tried this assignment. Thank you for presenting the opportunity to articulate our ideas.

NOTES

1. Brenda L. Whitman and Wanda J. Rose, "Using Art to Express a Personal Philosophy of Nursing," *Nurse Educator* 28 (2003): 166–69.
2. Bonnie Ewing and Marie Hayden-Miles, "Narrative Pedagogy and Art Interpretation," *Journal of Nursing Education* 50 (2011): 211–15.
3. Judith Frei, Sarah E. Alvarez, and Michelle B. Alexander, "Ways of Seeing: Using the Visual Arts in Nursing Education," *Journal of Nursing Education* 49 (2010): 672–76.

Moral Imagination

The Use of Visual and Written Texts to Create Circles of Empathy and Understanding

LARA NIXON, TOM ROSENAL, LAURIE PERELES,
AND ROBERTA JACKSON

To encourage sensitivity to patients' lived experiences and promote self-reflection, we introduced the use of photos of people of differing ages and ethnicities as reflective triggers in a writing exercise we developed to invoke moral imagination. Moral imagination may be defined as the ability to translate moral principles to new challenges—a (cognitive) bridge that overcomes the gap between moral theories or common-sense morality and practical decision making or everyday behavior.[1] We have used this easily replicated approach to create a safe, interactive space for learning. By inviting medical students, residents, and practicing physicians to create a story about another person, we hoped to stimulate awareness of their own thoughts, values, and feelings, while also enhancing their appreciation for the lived experience of another person.[2]

We compiled a diverse array of photos that we selected from free-access websites and appropriately attributed. In groups of six to eight, participants were invited to choose a picture, reflect on the experience of the person in the image, and write about it in any format they chose. Participants were given ten to fifteen minutes to construct the story. Then each participant read his or her story to the group. In the next five minutes, the group gave feedback to the reader on what responses the story evoked in them. A facilitator monitored the time and endeavored to create a supportive and safe environment for readers. Although the stories were not directly autobiographical, there was an understanding that they would not be shared outside the group without consent. Writers did not have to share their stories if they did not feel comfortable doing so.

The facilitators judged that the creative thought revealed in the participants' stories demonstrated both curiosity and empathy toward those in the pictures. Participants used prose and poetry to create rich, descriptive narratives in a very brief amount of time. The three writing samples presented below are from participants who experienced this exercise at family medicine conferences in Canada and consented to have their writing excerpted here.

The example below is titled "Portrait of a Young Man."

The first day of school. A new country, a new language
A new school, a new class. No one I know
Probably no one who understands, no one who cares.
I'm scared. What if they don't like me?
My clothes are not right, I don't look like them.
I think I'm bigger than everyone else.
And I'm fatter. I don't know how to act. I don't fit in.
They don't know what war is like.
I can shoot a gun. My dad is dead.
My mom has to work [and] my little sister is sick.
They're counting on me.
It's time to . . . go . . . in . . .

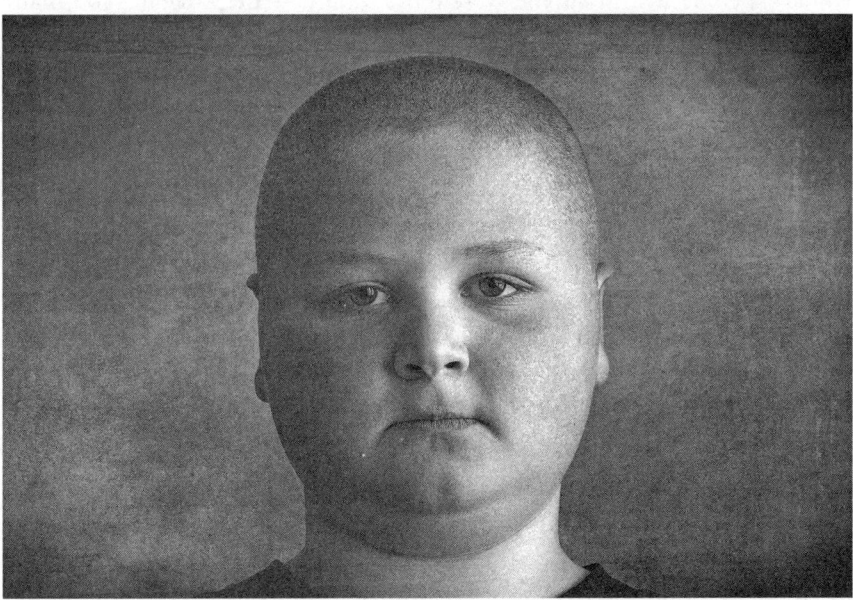

Glen Bledsoe, *Portrait of a Young Man,* 2003. Courtesy of Glen Bledsoe.

Our second example, untitled, is a portrait of an elderly woman who appears to be in her nineties. There is a tentative smile on her face, but her eyes reveal confusion.

I wish I could find my teeth. It should be easy. The young ladies who run this place seem to know where everything is—I mean, they know when it's time to eat, when I should sleep, when I need to wash. I don't have to think about anything. Maybe that's why I can't find my things.

I was married once. I think. I say that because sometimes a nice woman comes by and tells me she's my granddaughter. That means I must have had some children. And since you can't have children out of wedlock, well, ... when she comes, I can't seem to find the proper words to tell her how grateful I am for her presence. So I give her my best smile. The one into which I put all my love, and all my happiness, and try to tell her with my eyes that I'll miss her when she goes away. But you can't smile like that without any teeth. I wonder if she'll show up today.

Our third example, also untitled, is of an elderly man wearing a cap of plaid wool pulled low on his forehead so that it obscures his eyes: "I am comfortable being alone, it is easier than the messy complexity of life with people who love you, people who want to change you, people who think you are more than you are, people who wish you were more than you are. Love has too many expectations. Loneliness is comfortable. Predictable. I just want to get by."

Evoking different perspectives and empathy in a creative, collaborative, safe space facilitates learning and reflection about oneself and others, an essential component in doctor-patient relationships.[3] We found this to be especially true when group members all wrote about the same photograph. The unstructured sharing of writing encouraged empathy and understanding among the participants and appeared to promote deeper reflection than a question-and-answer session led by a facilitator. Rather than forcing a response to "the (imagined) standards of an (imagined) professor," our approach encouraged participants "to take control of their own education."[4] Reflection was also promoted by authentically inviting participants to make their own meaning and share only what they were comfortable with in the micro-context of the session, in keeping with approaches suggested by Boud and Walker.[5]

This exercise can be easily incorporated into courses that include empathy and dealing with ambiguity and empathy as learning objectives. With respect to ambiguity, we have observed that some participants express discomfort with speculating on the lived experience of the person in the photograph. There seemed to be some fear of "getting it wrong." A discomfort with the possibility of stereotyping the subject in the photographs arose and provided an opportunity to discuss ambiguity in medicine and the daily need to assess others on limited or nonverbal information and alter our impressions as more information becomes available. When multiple group members wrote about the same photograph, ambiguity became explicit and provided opportunity to navigate personal assumptions and ambiguity together.

As a group-based exercise, an additional degree of safety is afforded to the participants as they write about what they imagine another person is experiencing, rather than writing directly about themselves. Little equipment or preparation is required, and the exercise can be completed in a short period. Images could be chosen to address areas of known local concern (for example, photos of individuals who look like members of particular marginalized populations). This would increase the chance of addressing potentially sensitive issues, while challenging personal assumptions. The technique is also somewhat independent of the initial stimulus for the narrative. Rather than photos, one can use brief videos, first lines spoken by a patient in a physician's office, and other narratives. Such choices might overcome language challenges (as at a bilingual conference) or other sensory challenges of participants. While some participants may outline only sketched talking points, when invited to share their reflection most will narrate much more detailed versions of their stories. Using both imaginal and creative skills, participants experience what it is like to be a narrator while contributing to the collective construction of new understandings. In addition to enhanced appreciation of different perspectives, successful exercises will also foster camaraderie and group bonding

NOTES

1. Patricia H. Werhane, "Moral Imagination and the Search for Ethical Decision-Making in Management," *Business Ethics Quarterly* (1998): 75–98.
2. Mark Weisberg and Jacalyn Duffin, "Evoking the Moral Imagination: Using Stories to Teach Ethics and Professionalism to Nursing, Medical, and Law Students," *Journal of Medical Humanities* 16 (1995): 247–63.
3. David Boud and David Walker, "Promoting Reflection in Professional Courses: The Challenge of Context," *Studies in Higher Education* 23 (1998): 191–206.
4. Weisberg and Duffin, "Evoking the Moral Imagination," 251.
5. Boud and Walker, "Promoting Reflection in Professional Courses."

Reflective Doodling—
A Method of Visual Learning

M. MICHIKO MARUYAMA

What did I learn today? Let's see. Rubbing temples and closing eyes. It was a long day. I woke up early so that I could print today's lecture notes and review the learning objectives before two full hours of PBL, problem-based learning. OK, memory, what is the differential diagnosis for the PBL patient—a young adult male with a two-week history of intermittent epigastric pain and a one-day history of nausea and vomiting with bright red blood and clots? What a long list of differential diagnoses! During PBL, we looked at images taken from an esophagogastroduodenoscopy. Oh, that reminds me, I have to read about Barrett's esophagus and management of esophagitis and peptic ulcer disease before Friday. I will add that to tomorrow's Battle Plan. Battle Plans—what a great way to stay organized! They tell me where to be and when and what I need to do. OK, concentrate. Close eyes, rubbing temples. Visualizing. After PBL, we had a lecture on the physiology of gastric secretion. I can recall discussing five main types of gastric cells—surface mucous, parietal, chief, endocrine, and G cells—we talked about proton pump inhibitors, the function of mucous, regulation of acid secretion, H. Pylori, and the list goes on.

Such a busy day and I have learned so much! Reflecting, Reflecting, Reflecting, but I am not reflective writing in the traditional sense because truthfully I am not much of a writer. Instead, I draw—but look at the time! It is getting so late. I don't have time to draw a detailed picture, but I can squeeze in a doodle or a quick sketch. Let's see, how to turn everything that I learned, from morning to night, into one single image? How does everything connect? The main topics discussed today were the physiology of gastric secretions and peptic ulcer disease. There was a diagram on the top left-hand corner of our lecture notes showing a section of the upper gastrointestinal mucosa, which was covered by a layer of mucus. The surface mucous cells release bicarbonate into the mucus, which neutralizes incoming protons. The layer of mucus is relatively impermeable to pepsin, an enzyme that breaks down proteins into peptides, thus acting like a protective blanket for the underlying mucosa.

OK, imagination, time to transform what I learned into a Daily Doodle. Doodling happy mucous cells lying under a blob of content mucus that is hugging the mucosa with angry pepsins trying unsuccessfully to get through. Some of the pepsins are sad because they cannot play with the surface epithelium, creating craters (ulcers) that they can fill with gastric acid or use to grow their flagellated pets, H. Pylori. Setting timer for thirty minutes and go! Color, color, color, and done! Another doodle to add to the pile and soon I will have all four years of medical school in pictorial form. Many memories captured in color, each a result of my daily visual reflection on what I learned.

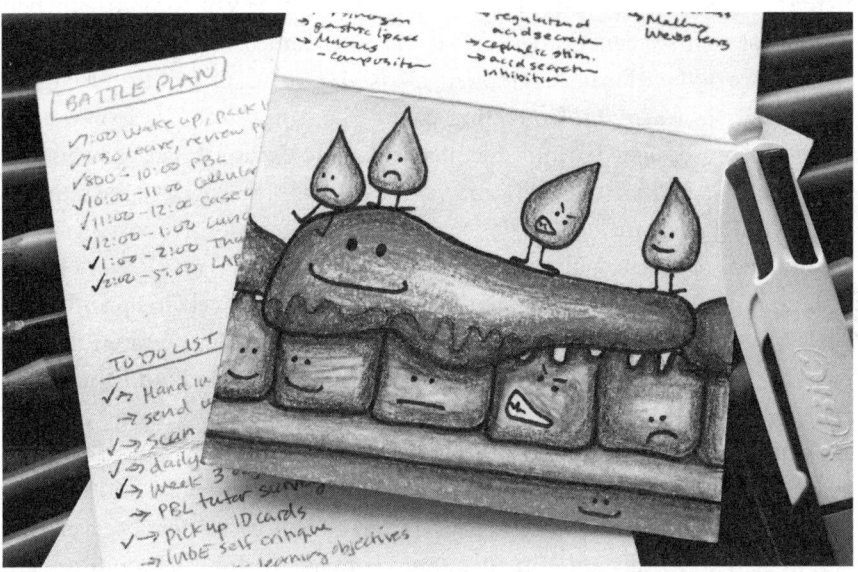

M. Michiko Maruyama, *Reflective Doodling,* 2011. Courtesy of M. Michiko Maruyama.

Drawing (on) Life Experience

Reading and Creating Comics as a Reflective Practice in Medical Education

SHELLEY WALL

In the fall of 2012, the Faculty of Medicine at the University of Toronto launched an illustrator-in-residence program to complement its existing medical humanities elective options for undergraduate medical students. One of the program's first initiatives was the introduction of the "Drawing (on) Life Experience" seminar series, designed to introduce participants to the use of visual narrative as a tool for observation, reflection, and communication. Specifically, the seminar focuses on "graphic medicine"[1]—that is, the study and creation of comics within the domains of illness, health care, and medical education.

Graphic medicine is a rich and growing field. As Michael Green and Kimberly Myers declared in 2010 in their groundbreaking article, "graphic stories have an important role in patient care, medical education, and the social critique of the medical profession."[2] The combination of words and pictures can often communicate the complexities or contradictions in a situation more powerfully and economically than words alone. Reading comics—and learning to create them—about illness and health care not only cultivates observational and interpretive skills but also encourages empathy within the multifaceted, lived experience of individual patients, their support networks, and health-care providers.

Over the past year and a half, as illustrator in residence within the Faculty of Medicine, I have developed and continue to lead this seminar series. I am also a medical illustrator and assistant professor in the Biomedical Communications program at the University of Toronto, where we research and teach all aspects of visual communication within science and medicine. My interest in graphic medicine arises from two sources, which quickly merge into a single stream. The first is professional: medical illustration is a form of visual storytelling; it combines image and text, research and experience, time and space, language and line, and so forth, to convey complex messages, and so the affinity with comics seems obvious, although not simple. The second source of my interest is personal and arose when it seemed that the only medium flexible enough to convey my individual experience with illness, caregiving, and the health-care system was the graphic novel. In the same way that comics bring together image and text, drama and reflection, and humor and pathos, the study of comics seems to permit the symbiosis of academic and personal, and of theory and raw experience. It is this combination of observation/analysis and expression/creation that I strive to build into the graphic medicine seminar.

"Drawing (on) Life Experience" is a series of five ninety-minute, weekly seminars. To date, it has been offered to undergraduate medical students across all years of study, and, as of 2014, to students in all allied health professional programs. Enrollment is capped at ten to allow for intimate and informal conversation. Each session consists, in more or less equal parts, of a guided discussion of preassigned readings and a hands-on creative exercise. In the first half of the session, participants interpret and discuss the experiences of patients, caregivers, and health-care professionals, as depicted in published examples of graphic medicine, and analyze the roles and interaction of images, words, and layout. In the hands-on exercise, participants are encouraged to make use of the language of graphic medicine to reflect on their own experiences—as medical students, future health-care providers, patients, or family caregivers. In this way, the sessions are designed both to foster empathy toward patients and families and to give students an opportunity to think critically and creatively about their own relationship to illness and the culture of biomedicine.

At our first meeting, I introduce the group to the emerging canon of graphic medicine, emphasizing the range of stories, narrative approaches, points of view, and illustrative styles. We review the anatomy of comics (panels, gutters, speech balloons, thought bubbles, emanata, and so on) using excerpts from Abel and Madden's *Drawing Words and Writing Pictures*,[3] to ensure that the class has a common vocabulary. As an exercise, participants design a simple avatar for themselves. This exercise—like all the exercises in the series—is not about "being able to draw," a frequent concern of students; it is, rather, about storytelling, about symbolic thinking, and about identifying key attributes that participants associate with themselves or think others might associate with them. After each short, guided drawing exercise, participants are invited to share their work with the group, and we discuss the process and results. Ground rules introduced during this first meeting serve to structure the space of our encounters. I invite participants to share only as much of their personal experience as they are comfortable revealing, and I ask that they not identify others (patients, staff, or students) in their work.

In the second session, we continue the exploration of how comics work, including the use of visual space, pacing, transitions, and focalization. Layout and panel structure (for example, regular or irregular panel sizes, regimented or scattered disposition on the page) convey meaning in themselves; pacing and transitions likewise inflect the reader's experience of a graphic narrative; and focalization—the use of characters as "lenses" through which to experience a story—can profoundly affect the emotional valence of a narrative. Abel and Madden define a taxonomy of transitions that provides a useful starting point. After the discussion, participants are asked to think of an experience in their training that posed an ethical dilemma, or that they found troubling, and to tell the story of this experience in a three-panel visual narrative. We look at these comics, and then participants are asked to tell the same story a second time, using completely different panel-to-panel transitions. This exercise has worked beautifully to demonstrate how changing the mode of telling can alter the meaning or focus of a story. Limiting the comic to three panels not only means that the exercise can be completed within the time frame of the seminar but also helps participants structure their story into a beginning, middle, and end.

With an understanding of comics' "anatomy and physiology" in place, we look more closely at content. The readings in these later sessions feature clinical encounters represented from the points of view of a physician, a patient, and a family caregiver, and excerpts from graphic novels on themes such as cancer, aging, and mental health. The exercises completed in these weeks build toward the final project, a one- to two-page autobiographical comic that is completed outside of class time, as students continue to explore the possibilities of the comics form through open-ended writing and drawing prompts.

The course thus moves from thinking about how comics make meaning through structure, style, and word/image combination, to a consideration of how these specific visual narrative modes inflect stories of illness and health care and capture the multiple layers of seemingly straightforward situations. At each stage, participants analyze examples of the form, practice applying these visual narrative strategies to moments in their own lives, and talk about their experiences with their peers.

In the final week, participants present their own comics; together we read and discuss them and move into a larger debriefing conversation about the seminar series. Some of the final comics have been playful (for instance, harmless but embarrassing rookie mistakes made on the ward); others have been powerfully raw (for instance, the death of a patient, or a participant's own journey through life-threatening illness). Whatever direction the comics have taken, I have found participants to be open and generous with one another in their responses, and fruitful conversations have arisen at both ends of the tragicomic spectrum.

Participants have responded very positively to the seminars to date. An informal survey completed at the end of the series has elicited comments such as these: "an amazing experience that I will remember and hopefully incorporate as I continue my training in medicine"; "a different way to cope and be mindful of things around you"; "a wonderful introduction to the art of viewing medicine from a unique perspective"; and "I really liked having time in my week to devote to thinking in a different way." Such comments capture the expanded perspective and reflective tools that graphic medicine can impart.

NOTES

1. Ian Williams, "Graphic Medicine: Comics as Medical Narrative," *Medical Humanities* 38 (2012): 21–27.
2. Michael J. Green and Kimberly R. Myers, "Graphic Medicine: Use of Comics in Medical Education and Patient Care," *British Medical Journal* 340 (2010): 574.
3. Jessica Abel and Matt Madden, *Drawing Words and Writing Pictures* (New York: First Second Books, 2008).

A Reflective Practice Curriculum for Team-Based Humanistic Patient/Relationship-Centered Care and Ethical Decision Making

HEDY S. WALD, PAUL GEORGE, AND JULIE SCOTT TAYLOR

Interprofessional education (IPE) curricula initiatives are proliferating within health professions education, given the importance of training in team-based practice for provision of safer and improved patient– and relationship-centered care (PRCC) in a rapidly changing health-care context. Health professions educators are thus challenged to foster interprofessional (IP) collaborative practice core competencies, as set forth by the IP Education Collaborative in 2011, including Values/Ethics for IP Practice, Roles/Responsibilities for Collaborative Practice (role clarification), IP Communication (including conflict management), and IP Teamwork and Team-Based Care. Reflective practice for informed flexibility and practical wisdom with narrative competence can promote effective IP teamwork. It can also deepen learning from experience and enhance IPE through development of self, other, and situational awareness, mindful presence, and emotional insight; recognition of everyday practice dilemmas; challenging one's assumptions; and appreciating multiple perspectives, leading to transformative and/or confirmatory learning.[1] Further, critically reflective practitioners' skills, including dispositional mindfulness, contribute to an IP team's recognition, management, and/or resolution of ethical dilemmas that can arise in patient care.

Few examples of IP education curricula that include formally structured techniques for promoting reflection to foster humanistic interprofessionalism (including team-based ethical decision making) have been reported. Since 2008, colleagues at Alpert Medical School of Brown University, University of Rhode Island Colleges of Pharmacy and Nursing, and Rhode Island College of Nursing collaborated on an IP curriculum for a team-based, PRCC experience using problem-based clinical cases with standardized patients involving second-year medical students, fourth-year nursing students, and fifth-year pharmacy students, with two required IPE sessions within the academic year (November, April). A written, structured curriculum evaluation for trainees' facilitated self-, professional, and IP reflection; it revealed trainees' increased confidence within IP practice, clarified their own profession's role within the team, promoted deeper understanding, appreciation, and respect for each profession's roles and responsibilities, and taught teamwork collaboration skills, including communication skills, appreciating multiple perspectives, and task delegation to improve patient care. Learners appreciated learning from "live" standardized patients within IPE, highlighting the potentially formative role of simulated clinical experience for emerging professional and IP identities.

Given this encouraging feedback, we designed an "advanced" IPE module fostering reflective and narrative competencies[2] for more effective teamwork within ethical decision making. The advanced IP ethics curriculum module innovation includes (a) an ethics decision-making paper case with a health literacy component, (b) a new student/faculty ethics module guide titled "IP Approach to Ethical Decision-Making," and (c) the newly devised "REFLECT-IDEA"[3] conceptual framework for guiding critical reflection for ethical decision making (reflection before, in, on, and for Action [RBIOFA], with appreciation to Frank Wagner of the Toronto Central CCAC and University of Toronto Joint Centre for Bioethics for permission to adapt the "IDEA" framework and IPE ethics case). A structured framework for team-based critical reflection, including reflection-inviting questions on case-specific topics, helps guide small-group, team-based, and large-group ethical decision making, and faculty-guided student debrief.

We incorporated reflection on common ethical dilemmas encountered in clinical environments and the role of IP team process in negotiating and managing such dilemmas. Overarching objectives included development of reflective practice with incorporation of narrative medicine within an IP context to appreciate stories of patients, patients' families, and team members for humane and effective medical practice.[4] The ethics case included the following learning objectives:

1. To gain awareness of ethical dilemmas, knowledge of ethical principles, and development of ethical mindfulness to guide PRCC
2. To experience narrative competency-fostered cultural sensitivity/humility with awareness of cultural context
3. To learn about each other's discipline-specific roles/responsibilities
4. To develop a shared approach for IP ethical decision making with observing

and practicing effective team communication, problem-solving skills, and overall ethical IP collaboration

5. To use reflective practice skills to address potential barriers to ethical practice—including challenging assumptions, potential biases, and/or power differentials
6. To use reflective practice skills to assess individual and team performance and incorporate feedback for future practice improvement
7. To improve perceived self-efficacy for IP experiential learning.

Students from medicine, nursing, pharmacy (same schools as in 2008–12), social work (RI College School of Social Work), and physical therapy (University of RI School of Physical Therapy) participated in the spring 2013 advanced IPE curriculum. The curriculum included three components: (1) an icebreaker activity for small IP groups, (2) an IP team-based standardized patient clinical case, and (3) an "advanced" IPE ethics curriculum module. IP faculty and fourth-year medical students (who facilitated the ethics curriculum module) received faculty development instruction. A guide to reflective practice in IP education was provided for students and faculty prior to the session. The following features are incorporated into a Team-Based Competencies Skills Grid for RBIOFA to facilitate student self-assessment and faculty/standardized patient debriefing and assessments of teamwork competencies for the IP problem-based clinical cases:

1. Team members explaining and/or clarifying their roles on the team
2. Adaptive leadership supporting team effectiveness (clarifying roles/responsibilities, delegating tasks, receiving assigned tasks, facilitating discussion and problem-solving as relevant)
3. Collaborating with mutual support and respect to develop a care plan
4. Attending to pertinent elements in patients' or team members' narratives (identifying needs/ preferences, dilemmas, etc., as relevant)
5. Communicating effectively (for example, exchanging information, eliciting opinions, managing and communicating emotionally sensitive information with patients, exploring differences, negotiating, and resolving team conflict)
6. Giving and responding to feedback
7. Attending to additional components of patient-centered care (such as provision of culturally sensitive care, shared decision making with patient/ family, assessment of patient satisfaction)
8. Considering potential consequences of actions
9. Achieving defined goals.

We have found that grid use with multisource feedback (from faculty, standardized patients, and self-assessment of teamwork competencies) scaffolds effective IP teamwork skills development.

Faculty development sessions have been integral to the success of our module. Involving fourth-year medical students as small-group facilitators for the IP ethics curriculum module was also a successful innovation. The development of a reflective practitioner is integral to effective IP teamwork, helping to promote ethical IP collaboration-in-practice (relationships within team and with patients/families). Given inherent differences in knowledge frameworks and practices and the often complex nature of ethical decision making, it is important to enhance the capacity of IP team reflective learning and practice to promote ethical decision-making processes for patients and their families, across members of the IP team for humanistic patient- and relationship-centered care.

While this intervention is feasible and well received within our institution, we are interested in its generalizability within other institutional settings, as well as its educational impact beyond a standardized patient paradigm. We plan to evaluate students' perceived self-efficacy for IP team-based competencies and for IP ethics awareness and decision making. Faculty's perceived self-efficacy for facilitating IPE for clinical cases and for learning about ethics awareness and decision making will also be evaluated. This innovative curriculum may represent a path forward in fostering reflective and narrative competencies for more effective, humanistic IP teamwork for ethical decision making in emerging health-care professionals.

Dr. Wald is grateful for support from a Gold Humanism Foundation Harvard-Macy Scholar Award, a Brown University Pre-doctoral Training Grant #D56HP20688, and Robert Wood Johnson/Tufts Health Plan PIN 6 grant.

NOTES

1. Hedy S. Wald et al., "Fostering and Evaluating Reflective Capacity in Medical Education: Developing the REFLECT Rubric for Assessing Reflective Writing," *Academic Medicine* 87 (2012): 41–50.
2. Rita Charon, *Narrative Medicine: Honoring the Stories of Illness* (New York: Oxford Univ. Press, 2006).
3. K. W. Anstey and F. Wagner, "Community Healthcare Ethics," in *The Cambridge Textbook of Bioethics,* ed. Peter A. Singer and Adrian M. Viens (New York: Cambridge Univ. Press, 2008).
4. Charon, *Narrative Medicine.*

Inspired by Visual Art

Exploring Practice through Collage Making

KAREN GOLD AND INGRID COLOGNA

The visual arts provide a powerful method for reflecting on professional practice by promoting empathy, embracing ambiguity and complexity, and acknowledging the link between the personal and professional. In this piece, we discuss a unique arts-based reflective process involving collage making. Constructed from fragments of images and text, collage draws our attention to the relationship between disparate elements and suggests new possibilities for making meaning. Through the use of already existing materials, collage allows us to make something new from "bits and pieces"; it is a means of deconstruction and reconstruction. Kathleen Vaughan describes collage as a "borderlands epistemology," as it accommodates different texts and visuals in a single work and values multiple meanings.[1]

Part of a three-year reflective practice project with social work and counseling students on hospital internships, we experimented with collage making to create opportunities for reflection on practicum learning. In particular, we were inspired by the work of contemporary Toronto artist Barbara Astman, whose photo-based art explores issues of identity, relationships, and "random particulars from her own life." Astman's "Daily Collage" project struck us as an accessible and evocative method for exploring practice experiences. Relying on very few images and using decidedly low-tech materials—a moleskin journal, a pair of scissors, and a glue stick—her collages employ a "minimalist" aesthetic to construct loosely defined narratives of everyday life.

In 2009, Astman decided to make one collage every day from the morning newspaper. The practice was appealing: choosing, isolating, cutting, gluing; the negative shapes in the edges trimmed away; the surprising juxtapositions

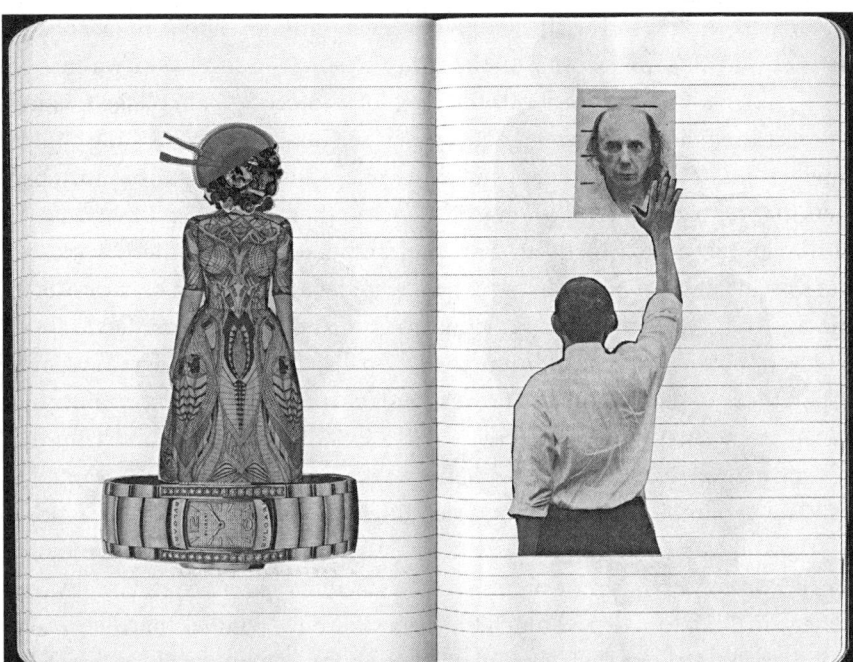

Barbara Astman, *Collage #5* (from "The Daily Collage Series"), 2011. Courtesy of Barbara Astman and the Corkin Gallery.

of the bits tossed aside; and then the letting go and moving on with the rest of the day, with the energies of the collage left to waft like sparks from a fire.

We began the project by discussing visual art as a method of reflective practice and the connections between collage making and professional social work practice. When Astman attended one of our reflective practice groups as a guest presenter, she discussed the process of the daily collage project and highlighted practice-related themes, such as self-awareness, and the implications of self-disclosure. Mindful of the influence of self-censorship on the creative process, Astman encouraged students to be aware of their own critical inner voices and value the role of intuition and serendipity in their art making. We gave our students a take-home assignment. We asked them to create a series of three to five collages depicting (1) a relationship with a patient/client; (2) an element of their practice that they are struggling with; or (3) a recurring theme in their work with patients/clients, such as depression, chronic illness, or loss.

Participants were instructed to bring their collages back to the next session and be prepared to share and discuss their work. When we met a month later, we invited students to write silently for a few minutes about their collages before discussing their work with the group. During the discussion, we encouraged students to reflect on both the content and process of collage making. In describing their collages, students described depicting challenging clinical interactions, the impact of personal experiences on professional identity, barriers to listening, and the meaning of silence in therapeutic conversations. We also encouraged participants to share their responses to each other's work and, in particular, how the images or text resonated with their own experience. By moving back and forth from individual to group reflection, we aimed to create a sense of community. In addition, the group discussion normalized students' experiences in the therapeutic process with clients, in which uncertainty and expectation often threaten to create narratives of inadequacy and failure as a beginning social worker. As audience to each other's stories, we wanted to validate the unfolding dramas and rich interactions of day-to-day practice.

The collage making served as a tangible way to acknowledge the moving, and deeply personal, nature of our work. As facilitators, we were struck by how collage making functioned much like Rita Charon's "parallel chart," in which students write about their experience caring for patients.[2] Like the parallel chart, the collages allowed students to use images and words to express what they could not say in clinical records but needed to document somewhere.

There are many ways to extend this exercise and deepen the reflective processes. These could include inviting peer responses to collages using writing or art, creating writing exercises related to the themes identified in the collages, and writing in different voices to promote greater awareness of multiple perspectives (for example, in the voice of the patient, a family member, or another practitioner). While students often recognized the therapeutic value of creative expression and its important role in practitioner self-care, it is equally important to situate the purpose of these activities in terms of professional skill development. As facilitators, we tried to be explicit about the role of arts-based reflection in enhancing our ability to listen and attend to the stories of others—in other words, to better prepare us for our roles as empathic witnesses and compassionate observers.

The beauty of collage making is its accessible method and its numerous possibilities. It lends itself to exploring the relational dimensions of practice through the juxtaposition of fragments of images and words. Several students commented on their initial uncertainty about the process and their surprise at the meanings that emerged. As practitioners and educators, we were continually struck by the rich and often unexpected connections that emerged from this creative process.

NOTES

The authors thank Barbara Astman for her inspiration and involvement in this project as well as the Bertha Rosenstadt Fund at the Factor-Inwentash Faculty of Social Work for its support.

1. Kathleen Vaughan, "Pieced Together: Collage as an Artist's Method for Interdisciplinary Research," *International Journal of Qualitative Methods* 4 (2008): 27–52.

2. Rita Charon, *Narrative Medicine: Honoring the Stories of Illness* (New York: Oxford Univ. Press, 2006).

Fostering Reflective Capacity in Health Professional Education Using Art and Reflective Narratives

KHALED KARKABI, HEDY S. WALD, AND ORIT COHEN CASTEL

Reflective capacity is integral to core health-care, professional-practice competencies. Reflection also has a central role in teacher education, as reflecting on teaching behaviors with critical analysis can potentially improve teaching practice. The humanities, including narratives and the visual arts, can serve as valuable avenues for fostering reflection. Reflective writing integrated with written feedback from faculty fosters health professionals' development of reflection skills. In addition to cultivating insights into the process of patient care and promoting health-care practitioner well-being, reflective writing within health professions education (for both students and faculty) can promote reflective self-assessment, a component of personal, professional, and interprofessional development.

Various arts modalities can foster reflection. An interactive exhibit of abstract photographs, for example, can be used as a catalyst for health-care professionals, patients, and families to reflect on illness in a health-care context.[1] Guided reflection in museum settings and multimedia, including use of visual methodologies in digital storytelling, is another vehicle for stimulating reflection in health professions education.

Over the last several years, we have been using a combination of visual arts and narratives in faculty development workshops to foster reflective competence and compassion in health-care providers and medical educators.[2] We have also found these combined modalities (written narratives on paintings) to be useful for stimulating medical students' reflection on their own experience with patients as well as examining their emotions and actions. Recently, we embarked on designing a novel faculty development program to enhance reflection and deliberately selected abstract art—in contrast to our prior and more popular work with figurative paintings. We used abstract paintings because we believed they could facilitate viewers' connection with the self and with their own inner world, thus engaging both cognitive and affective abilities. Such an exercise would facilitate the transition to the next step: writing a reflective narrative.

Table 1. Fostering Reflection through Art and Reflective Narratives: Workshop Format

Activity Timeline	Activity Description
Introduction	Present workshop goals. Provide a brief overview of reflection, focusing on its key components and why it is needed in health professions education and practice.
Close, "arts-based" noticing	Use a projector to project images of three famous abstract paintings, varying in form and color (e.g., "Orange and Yellow" [M. Rothko]; "Full Fathom Five" [J. Pollock]; "Composition number 6" [V. Kandinsky]). Ask participants to closely observe the images. Ask participants to choose one of the paintings to focus on. Each participant was provided with a small photograph of his//her selected painting (10cm x 7cm). Participants closely observed "their" painting and let the painting "work" on them; allowing emotions to emerge spontaneously, rather than focusing on specific details they see in the painting.
Enhancing emotional awareness	Invite participants to engage in quiet, individual contemplation (several minutes). As a group, invite participants to describe emotions that emerged while observing their selected painting.
Reflective writing	Encourage participants to remain open to their emotional response, as they return their gaze to their selected painting. Invite participants to write a personal narrative describing a meaningful or challenging situation with an undergraduate medical student or a resident physician (15 minutes). Various reflective domains are encouraged allowing their emotional response to accompany the writing exercise.
Deepening reflection	Working in pairs, participants share their narratives by reading them aloud. After the narrative reflection has been read, the listener is encouraged to ask reflection-inviting questions to promote depth and breadth of reflection. Members of the participant pairs then switch roles.

The faculty development workshop aims to enhance reflective capacity in health-care professionals within the educator-learner context. At the conclusion of the workshop, participants would be able to (1) describe thoughts and emotions, breakthroughs or tensions, emerging during a specific, meaningful educational interaction with a learner; (2) identify challenges; and (3) utilize reflective writing as a strategy for addressing and managing such challenges in future educator-learner interactions.

We have thus far conducted two faculty development workshops, one within our own institution in 2011 and the other with medical educators at WONCA 2012, an international family medicine conference in Vienna. For our initial workshop, participants within our division of family medicine included family medicine physicians and residents as well as a staff psychologist (n = 26). Feedback on the workshop was positive, and participants felt that the combined use of writing and abstract art helped them engage successfully in reflection. Qualitative assessment of the WONCA workshop feedback indicated that the combined use of visual arts and written narratives was well received and participants felt that viewing abstract paintings had facilitated a valuable mood transformation, preparing them emotionally for the reflective writing exercise (see note 3 for a more detailed summary of the themes we identified).[3] Of interest to us is further study of the potential long-term impact of this faculty development workshop on the reflective capacity of health professions educators. Based on participants' experiences and feedback thus far, we may speculate on achieved impact on personal and professional development and on reflective learning and practice within teaching. The application of skilled reflective process for more meaningful and effective educator-learner interactions and, ultimately, for improved patient care is a potentially valuable future area of inquiry.

NOTES

1. Hedy S. Wald, Diana Rico Norman, and Joel Walker, "Reflection through the Arts: Focus on Photography to Foster Reflection in a Health Care Context. Living Beyond—An Interactive Photographic Exhibit," *Reflective Practice* 11 (2010): 545–63.
2. Khaled Karkabi and Orit Cohen Castel, "Suffering and Compassion in Paintings: The Gift of Art," *The Israel Medical Association Journal* (2007): 419–23.
3. Khaled Karkabi, Hedy S. Wald, and Orit Cohen Castel, "The Use of Abstract Paintings and Narratives to Foster Reflective Capacity in Medical Educators: A Multinational Faculty Development Workshop," *Medical Humanities* 40 (2014): 44–48. A portion of this article has been used in this chapter.

"Not So Funny"

Prompting Reflection through Single-Panel Cartoons

NEVILLE CHIAVAROLI AND STEVE TRUMBLE

The humanities are frequently used by medical educators not only to promote reflection but also to challenge beliefs and preconceptions. This capacity to unsettle can also be a useful way of prompting students to reflect on important professional issues. A relatively underutilized material for this purpose is the single-panel cartoon.

Humor has been shown to assist learning, partly by promoting student engagement.[1] Green and Myers have shown how sequential cartoons, or "graphic stories," can be profitably used in the education of students, patients, and practitioners.[2] However, the single-panel cartoon, usually found in newspapers and magazines, is different from the drawings in graphic novels. While graphic novels use sequential images and text to tell a story, the single-panel cartoon offers more of an immediate social commentary than a narrative. Its point goes beyond the humor and is usually implied, nuanced, or even obscured. But this makes the medium particularly appropriate for reflective and critical purposes.

The use of cartoons for educational purposes came to us through an appreciation of their potential to spur critical thought and a wariness of trying to teach serious professional issues through didactic approaches. We saw elsewhere in the curriculum the benefits of using a problem-based learning approach to promote active, contextual, and engaged learning. We felt that something from "left field" might better challenge students to pause and reflect on professionalism, rather than assume the reflex cognitive attitude of passive receptivity in an area so crucially dependent on analytical and critical thought. We therefore decided to introduce the use of cartoons in the first week of our MD course to stimulate thought and prompt discussion of a complex professional concept: what makes a good doctor.

The medical profession is a frequent target of cartoonists, and suitable cartoons exist in abundance. In our experience, the effective use of such cartoons for educational purposes requires three steps: (1) judicious selection, (2) strategic consideration of the teaching opportunity, and (3) facilitated discussion.

We illustrate this process through the following three examples of cartoons, which we have used to prompt reflection about what it means to be a "good doctor." Due to limitations of space, only Cartoon 2 is reproduced here; the other cartoons can be accessed online.

Cartoon 1: A doctor enters the room where a patient is waiting to be seen.

- Caption: *"Ah, Mr. Bromley. Nice to put a face on a disease."*
- Source: Mike Twohy, www.cartoonbank.com (search for image "TCB-38483")
- Purpose: To introduce the notion of patients "being seen" by the doctor
- Teaching opportunity: Making the patient feel at ease and valued, considering the person as distinct from his other disease, refraining from unguarded and unprofessional remarks
- Facilitated discussion: How would the doctor's remark make you feel? How important is small talk between doctor and patient in creating rapport and trust? Based on this initial interaction, what judgments is Mr. Bromley likely to make about the doctor?

Cartoon 2: A doctor attempts to convince a patient that he empathizes with her spiritual suffering.

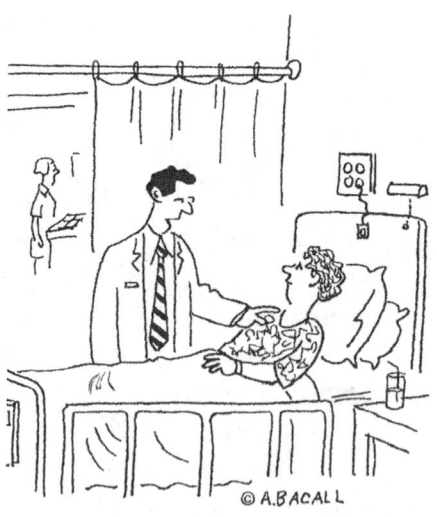

"Of course I'm listening to your expression of spiritual suffering. Don't you see me making eye contact, striking an open posture, leaning towards you and nodding empathetically?"

- Caption: *"Of course I'm listening to your expression of spiritual suffering. Don't you see me making eye contact, striking an open posture, leaning towards you and nodding empathetically?"*
- Source: Aaron Bacall, www.cartoonstock.com *(search for image "aba0445")*
- Purpose: To introduce the notion of genuine empathy and its expression
- Teaching opportunity: Understanding what empathy is and isn't, reflecting on ways of conveying empathy, understanding what makes empathy authentic

- Facilitated discussion: What is the cartoonist suggesting about this doctor's bedside manner? What underlying behavior by professionals might the cartoonist be alluding to? Is it possible to be empathic yet insincere?

Cartoon 3: A doctor gesticulates while his patient attempts to guess his meaning, as if they were playing charades.

- Caption: *"Hop? Jig? Dance? You're a dancer? Sounds like? Prancer? Cancer? Cancer? I got cancer!"*
- Source: John O'Brien, *www.cartoonbank.com (search for* image "TCB-43786")
- Purpose: To prompt reflection about how health professionals may avoid talking about difficult issues
- Teaching opportunity: Communicating bad news to patients, reflecting on what might prevent health professionals from communicating effectively and caringly, helping students better deal with their own emotions during difficult conversations
- Facilitated discussion: Why is the doctor in the cartoon behaving this way? Why does the patient keep guessing? What behavior by professionals is the cartoonist alluding to?

On first glance, the above cartoons are whimsical and even a tad absurd. But this does not mean they are trivializing serious topics—quite the opposite. Like all caricature and satire, cartoons identify a key aspect of an issue and exaggerate it for comic effect. The interpretive challenge—and the resulting teaching dividend—starts with discovering what themes the cartoonists are identifying, and magnifying, in the cartoons.

Thus, the third cartoon alludes to the tendency of some practitioners to prevaricate about bad news—to resort to tone, facial expression, euphemism, or jargon to convey the serious nature of a diagnosis without genuinely confronting the emotional challenge of communicating clearly. How such communication ought to be achieved is not for the cartoon to convey; it is simply commenting on the potential insensitivity of a notorious, and possibly typical, way of communicating.

However engaging the humor may be, the educational value of such cartoons is in the shock of recognition that comes when the cartoon's message hits home. It is at that moment that the students are rendered most "teachable"—far more teachable, in our experience, than from a didactic lecture on the topic. However, we have also found that, left to their own devices, students usually fail to appreciate and appropriately reflect on the point, choosing instead to focus on the superficial humor or absurd aspects of the cartoon or dismiss the deeper message because of its superficially trivial form. This is where we have come to see expert, guided facilitation as essential. The tutor models and facilitates the interpretive skill required to understand the underlying seriousness of the cartoon's message. That message may well be contentious, but the importance of the issue, the need to go deeper and reflect on its implications and its application to clinical practice, is reinforced by sound facilitation skills.

Well-chosen cartoons can illuminate perspectives that otherwise remain concealed and can do so humorously, succinctly, and often provocatively. Like much in the medical humanities, they can serve to jolt us into recognizing something we may have neglected to think about, or preferred not to; to unsettle us long enough to learn; to make us "laugh for five seconds and think for 10 minutes."[3] As medical educators, we have the opportunity to "draw out"—according to the Latin etymology of *educate*—the understanding relevant to the realistic analogues of the situations depicted in the cartoons.

NOTES

1. John B. Ziegler, "Use of Humour in Medical Teaching," *Medical Teacher* 20 (1998): 341–48.
2. Michael J. Green and Kimberly R. Myers, "Graphic Medicine: Use of Comics in Medical Education and Patient Care," *British Medical Journal* 340 (2010): 574–77.
3. Attributed to William Davis, U.S. author and cardiologist.

PART 3

Performance and Reflection— Theater, Music, and Film

Dramatizing Reflective Writing

MARTIN KOHN

"WE DON'T DO 'CHEESE'"

There I was, getting ready for the regular Friday noon session that provides feedback to course directors on that week's problem-based learning case and seminars. I was only a few months into my directorship of the Foundations of Medicine seminar (aka Medical Humanities) and had just witnessed, a few days prior, our first attempt at dramatizing student reflective writing. I was fairly confident that the student feedback (based on facilitators' polling of students immediately prior to our noon meeting) would be good, but, I was humbled by just how positive the response was. Interestingly, more than one student responded that they expected the play to be "cheesy." But, nearly unanimously, they reported how powerfully the dramatic vignette affected them. Hence, my faux huff response to the other course directors: "We don't do cheese!"

Why was this creative venture successful? I believe that the success was due to our collaboration with a professional playwright and top-tier actors, the Cleveland Clinic's culture of innovation, and our students' comfort with writing.

AESTHETIC STENOGRAPHER

Nearly twenty years ago, my work in medical humanities took a turn toward the arts—in particular, dramatic arts. While codirectors of the Center for Literature and Medicine, Carol Donley and I began collaboration with a Cleveland-based professional theater company. Through our work with Great Lakes Theater, I met Eric Coble, one of our nation's leading young playwrights, and continued that relationship with him at Cleveland Clinic Lerner College of Medicine (CCLCM) in our reflective writing project. Eric, as playwright in residence at

CCLCM, likened his initial work with us to that of an "aesthetic stenographer."
In addition to spending time in our Tuesday morning sessions, he had conversations with students and, most importantly, had access to their de-identified
reflective writing. For his dramatic vignettes, he looked for repeated threads
that he could weave together into thematic links, searched for strong images
that would provide drama when spoken, and, only when necessary—because
he relied primarily on verbatim content—added some "connective tissue" of
his own.[1] The results, when given voice and embodied by professional actors,
have had a significant metareflective impact on many of our students (and
faculty) in terms of professional identity formation, social justice, vulnerability,
and uncertainty—the themes our writing prompts are designed to uncover.

BLOW IT UP!

Our reflective writing project has grown through Cleveland Clinic's embrace
of innovation, a stance toward experimentation that extends to the curriculum
of CCLCM as well. When I suggested that the first two years of the medical
humanities curriculum be changed significantly, the associate dean's response
was to "blow it up!" And although not all of our experiments have turned out
as well as the one described here, the Cleveland Clinic's nonpunitive approach
toward innovation creates space for the creative energy of artists.

WILLING TO BE VULNERABLE

Students in the CCLCM five-year medical school track (CCLCM is one of three
medical school tracks within Case Western Reserve School of Medicine) are
part of a unique system that includes two research-based summer blocks, a
full research year, and an electronic portfolio competency-based assessment
system. They receive no grades and take no tests (other than the USMLE), and
the Cleveland Clinic subsidizes their tuition at Case Western Reserve University. Four of the nine competencies in particular pertain to work we provide
in the medical humanities: professionalism, health-care systems, personal
growth, and reflective practice. Students spend a significant amount of time
and effort training for and producing narratives for their formative and summative portfolio submissions. They learn how to provide evidence that they
are meeting the yearly standards for their competencies and are unabashedly
self-critical in the process. That is why they are able, as part of this reflective
writing exercise, to share their vulnerabilities—first with themselves as they
engage in the writing, then electronically with their small-group preceptors,
and finally face-to-face with members of their discussion groups.

What the dramatic vignette provides is the metareflective whole-class experience of dramatic art. As one student put it, "When we came together and watched a dramatization of our experiences, I saw my words melded with those of my classmates into something more than just words. As the actor, portraying a cadaver, rose and began to speak I felt the power of a living moral community. The act of awakening opened up a dialogue: with the person inside the body, with the unspoken thoughts and feelings of my classmates, and with my own inner fears and vulnerabilities."[2]

CONTINUITIES AND CONCERNS

Now into our third year of this venture, we've created similar opportunities during year three in the curriculum (our students' first full clinical year); and, beginning with the class of 2015, we plan to provide graduating students with copies of their first-year dramatic vignettes during their two-week capstone block. We also anticipate that our literary arts magazine, *Stethos,* will continue to print selected essays from our students. During our first year, we had the opportunity to present two of the dramatic vignettes as part of the Cleveland Play House's FusionFest, a well-attended, community-based production that provides the public with an inside view of medical education. The discussion after the public performance was as robust and revealing as the ones in class.

One of our concerns is playwright fatigue due to similar responses to prompts. This can be remedied by changing prompts or playwrights. The other concern is that we've heard students talk of writing toward the drama, vying for extensive coverage in it, and thereby possibly undermining the primary purpose of the assignment.

NOTES

1. Martin Kohn et al., "Multiple Exposures—Reflective Writing in the First Year of Medical School," *Virtual Mentor* 13, no. 7 (2011): 471–74.
2. Ibid.

SUGGESTED RESOURCES

1. Mann, Karen, Jill Gordon, and Anna MacLeod. "Reflection and Reflective Practice in Health Professions Education: A Systematic Review." *Advances in Health Sciences Education* 14.4 (2009): 595–621.
2. Shapiro, Johanna, Deborah Kasman, and Audrey Shafer. "Words and Wards: A Model of Reflective Writing and Its Uses in Medical Education." *Journal of Medical Humanities* 27, no. 4 (2006): 231–44.

Acts of Reflection

Combining Medical Readers' Theater and Reflective Writing

CAROL SCHILLING AND SUSAN ARJMAND

Todd Savitt has conceptualized medical readers' theater as public performances of script-in-hand readings of plays about medicine. Savitt's project calls for health professionals and students to perform these minimally staged readings in community settings to generate open discussions about timely "social and ethical issues in medicine."[1] While we agree that such public discussions are valuable, we have adapted Savitt's project for a medical school humanities seminar for another purpose. We wanted to offer students the experience of reading the words of a character aloud in class and reflecting on the experience of taking on the role of another. Our own experiences as performers led us to anticipate that inhabiting a character, even briefly, would give students insight into the embodied experience of another. What do we mean by "inhabiting a character"? An unusually loquacious student in our class found out when she played the role of Imelda, the title character in Savitt's dramatization of Richard Selzer's unsettling short story about treating a young surgical patient. Our student had to remain silent while her colleagues read the parts of the surgeon and his medical student. In response to playing the silent patient, our student said with exasperation, "I hated hearing what they were saying about me and not being able to speak. All I had to do was lie there! It was so frustrating." We hoped that these dramatizations would bring such difficult truths to the surface.

Plays, like other works of fiction, encourage reflection about the characters' experiences and the moral dimensions of human encounters. However, neither silently reading a literary work (whether drama, poem, or prose) nor listening to someone performing it matches the experience of speaking the words of a character in the presence of listeners. We asked students to experiment with ways of delivering lines and discussed the possible consequences of various deliveries. Through speaking, listening, and self-reflection, students became alert to how the pitch, speed, volume, timbre, and affect of their voices, along with their body language, can profoundly influence the way others perceive them. We welcomed the dilemmas arising from the ambiguity of language, discrepant interpretations, and the uncertainties implicit in human relationships. Our goal was not a finished performance but rather open-ended reflection.

Our five-week course met two consecutive hours a week as a humanities elective in the Northwestern University Feinberg School of Medicine undergraduate program. The class of nine second-year students read three scripts: two short scripts from Savitt's anthology, "Ambulance" and "Imelda," and the play *Wit* by Margaret Edson. During the first two weeks, we read from and discussed Savitt's short dramatizations. The third week, we focused on the script for *Wit*. In the fourth week, students viewed the film version of *Wit* (2001), and read and discussed selected scenes in class.[2] For our fifth session, groups of students chose scenes from the three plays to perform, script in hand. Our discussions focused on the decisions the groups grappled with as they prepared their scenes, the experience of playing the characters, and, for the audience, the experience of witnessing the reading. Prior to each class, students e-mailed us a short, written reflection on one or more lines from the play that they could identify with or that they found puzzling. In addition to giving students an opportunity to slow down their reading and reflect, written responses also encouraged them to read attentively and increased the likelihood that they would participate in the discussions. Reading the students' responses in advance helped us identify scenes to read in class and questions to ask. Our students appreciated the first two scripts because they dramatized experiences the students easily identified with: being the least-experienced member of a medical team and navigating relationships and responsibilities within hospital hierarchies. However, they found *Wit* most compelling because of the dissatisfying communication and interactions between almost all members of the medical staff and a dying patient. In the remainder of this essay, we focus on Edson's play to illustrate our activities and outcomes.

When asked to write about a moment in *Wit,* many students wrote about one of two aspects: (1) the character of Jason, a brash resident, or (2) the question that vexes the dying protagonist Vivian—"How are you feeling today?" Jason, who "really mastered the technical side of medicine" while being "completely oblivious to Vivian's unspoken needs," as one student put it, appalled them. Close to their own clinical encounters with patients, students quickly generated a long list of Jason's offences: his callous pelvic exam, his blatant disregard for her DNR order, his expressed delight in the intellectual challenge of researching cancer while ignoring its effects on his dying patient, his description of clinical manners and compassion as "crap," his clueless response when he takes his patient's expression of fear as a sign of mental deterioration, and his perfunctory grasp of taking a patient history via a series of staccato questions that ignore his patient's intelligence, reflective pauses, and fear. Seeing Jason as a foil for the kind of doctor they hoped to become, students pledged to provide, as one wrote, a "listening ear for the patient's worries and fears."

However, reading the medical history scene aloud, with students taking the parts of Jason and Vivian, added a palpable sense of unease about both delivering and listening to Jason's oblivious, matter-of-fact, clipped manner of speech. "I really don't want to be that person" is the best way we can summarize the students' responses. We wanted, though, to move beyond self-congratulation for deploring Jason's lack of empathy and to explore the character more fully. We asked students in what ways Jason (and Dr. Kelekian, Jason's role model) were admirable. We also asked them to rewrite Jason's interrogation in ways that would be more considerate of his patient's fears. The students read their newly scripted interviews in turn, and authors and listeners commented on the language and delivery. The acts of writing, revising, performing, speaking, and listening layered reflection upon reflection and complicated the students' original responses to Jason. They left the class session with their own internalized scripts for conducting more empathic interviews. During the second class on *Wit,* we watched and discussed other selected scenes. One scene dramatized Vivian's perspective as a patient during grand rounds, when the residents and senior physician speak over Vivian as she lay on her back, barely acknowledging her as they poke her belly. We showed this scene with the sound turned off and asked students to write (as they watched) an interior monologue of what Vivian was thinking while subjected to this treatment. They read their monologues, a series of sensitive understandings of what it must feel like to be this objectified patient. One imagined Vivian mentally chastising the resident for touching her warm belly with cold hands.

Asked what they thought of writing about the plays before class, students revealed that the process of writing reflectively challenged them to try to identify with a character and made them aware of their emotional responses. However, students felt they actually changed their views of certain characters when reading the plays aloud. After hearing *Wit* read in class, students observed that vocalizing words made the characters seem more realistic. One student noted that performing "forced [me] to relate to, and think about the characters in a way that reading to yourself doesn't." Another concluded that reading aloud made her "realize the power of words and of delivery." The students discovered an increased awareness of the way that emotion, body language, vocal inflection, and mood affect physicians' encounters with patients. As one student optimistically wrote, "I will use these insights to understand patients better and to accept them."

When asked whether there is a difference between feeling an emotion and acting one out in character, several students wrote that acting increased their awareness of emotions. As one student discovered, "I think that often emotions are locked inside. . . . To act an emotion, one has to be consciously aware of it to bring it to the forefront of one's attention, and determine the best way to express it." Students concluded that physicians must be aware of the importance of emotions, words, and tone of voice. Otherwise, they believed, unacknowledged biases could surface, affecting physicians' interactions with patients. Reflecting on a class discussion about the perplexing question of whether revealing a true emotion is always the best clinical choice, one student worried that a physician might sound "fake" if he or she concealed genuine feelings.

Empathy involves adopting the vantage point of the "Other" and examining one's own assumptions, biases, and beliefs. Certainly medical readers' theater helps students imagine being another. The writing exercises shared during class also contributed to students' understanding of characters and their responses to them. "Hearing everyone's insights," a student observed, "made me step outside my perspective of the reading." We believe that stepping into a character and outside one's self in a medical readers' class encourages such transformative acts of reflection.

NOTES

We thank our students in Northwestern University Feinberg School of Medicine for their kind permission to quote from their writing.

1. Todd Savitt, ed., *Medical Readers' Theater: A Guide and Scripts* (Iowa City: Univ. of Iowa Press, 2002), xvi.
2. Margaret Edson, *Wit: A Play* (New York: Faber and Faber, 1993); *Wit*, directed by Mike Nichols (HBO, 2001), DVD.

Developing Personal Artistry

Physicians and Artists Explore the Art of Health-Care Communication Excellence

IRENE MCGHEE, KATE ECCLES, AND ANGELA ELSTER

Patient communication is an art as much as a science. Sooner or later each physician must delve into the murky, "unscientific" world of human relationships to fully understand his or her capacity for connection and leadership. This is not easy territory. Increasing subspecialization and intense focus on evidence-based practice encourages narrow silos of scientific expertise. While fundamental to building intellectual discernment and rigor, this does little to prepare us for the complex human dynamics that characterize the real world of medicine. High-pressure situations in which patient and physician confront powerful emotions are the norm in many subspecialties. Making instantaneous high-stakes decisions while collaborating within complex, multidisciplinary teams is the norm, particularly in fields like emergency medicine, anesthesiology, surgery, and nursing.

How to help specialists in training gain exposure to humanistic ways of thinking was the basis of a joint learning project by Sunnybrook Health Sciences Centre, University of Toronto, and the Royal Conservatory of Music's Learning through the Arts program (LTTA). Anesthesiology residents came to the new TELUS Centre for Performance and Learning at Toronto's Royal Conservatory for an arts-based, experiential elective module called "Context, Collaboration, and Communication," designed to deliver seven outcomes detailed in the Can-MEDS Physician Competency Framework (medical expert, communicator, collaborator, manager, health advocate, scholar, and professional).

In her role as chief creative director of LTTA, Kate Eccles, and leading arts and education expert Angela Elster conceived the initial approach using playback theater, an improvisational theater technique developed by artistic directors Jonathan Fox and Jo Salas. Specially trained LTTA artist-educator

Heather Dick, a theater director and expert in improv, was the lead facilitator. All worked closely with Dr. Irene McGhee, Sunnybrook anesthesiology resident coordinator, who ensured content met medical and scientific learning outcomes rooted in the realities of the specialty.

Prior to the workshops, Dr. McGhee developed scenarios from real-life experiences that had been related to her by previous residents. The residents' anonymity was preserved, but all the details of very stressful or upsetting operating room situations (such as challenging clinical or communication problems, interpersonal team conflicts, adverse events, errors) assured abundant material. Participants—using one of the provided scenarios or sharing one from their own experience—were asked to write, on the right side of a piece of paper, the actual dialogue and precise sequence of events that took place as they remembered it. On the left side, they recorded thoughts and feelings they'd had but didn't express.

Heather, Kate, and Irene collected the scenarios and created "movie scripts" out of them—short professional "plays" for residents to star in, playing themselves, with Dr. McGhee and LTTA actors as supporting characters. Scenarios focused on such challenges as communicating with patients whose first language is not English, hostile or anxious patients in a pre-op interview, angry and belligerent surgeons, and high-anxiety resident colleagues. Students reenacted these situations in front of an audience of peers and then replayed the action, stopping whenever they wished to discuss what was taking place. The scene was then repeated with other students able to stop the action and step into one of the roles, experimenting with what could have happened if one or other person had acted differently. Audience members could also step onto the stage like a Greek chorus to represent the "left column"—responses arising from our better judgment or intuition but that we ignore, hide, or don't express.

Playback theater is a highly effective mechanism for learning. Because each scenario represents a unique moment in time—an "ecosystem" of individuals, patients, families, and specialists—there is no correct outcome. The scenarios devolve into real-time improvisations in which students come to better understand how thoughts, feelings, words, and body language quickly forge a path to particular responses in others and create dynamic outcomes. In our case, students could discuss their learning in real time under the expert guidance and supervision of Dr. McGhee. These discussions concerned their performance as physicians, but learners also benefited from the related experience of actors who daily inhabit a landscape populated by improvisation, the need for essential, instantly clear communication, and the ability to work daily in multifaceted, ever-changing ensemble settings.

On the second day, students broke into smaller improvisation groups led by actors and writers, allowing them to practice improvising scenarios from scratch. One student would play the anesthesiologist, having no idea what was going to happen. Another student, playing the patient, was given a cue card outlining what the scenario would be. For example, one cue card read, "You have been in a serious accident, are badly hurt, and need an immediate operation. You saw the movie *Awake* and fear that you'll be able to feel the pain of the operation but won't be able to communicate that you are not actually asleep. When the anesthesiologist approaches to conduct the pre-op interview, you are beginning to panic, asking a lot of questions in rapid succession and starting to breathe very heavily."

Students took turns trying different approaches to playing the roles, followed by group discussions about what the emerging excellent anesthesiologist could glean professionally from standing in the shoes of the person on the other side of the dialogue. The two-day event was recorded by a professional multimedia artist who, at the conclusion of the workshops, created an edited DVD that students could use for personal reference and submit as part of their CanMEDS[1] portfolio. While many residents expressed how useful the workshop was as a one-time event for learning about the multiple roles and abilities of effective physicians, the challenge of including it as an ongoing approach to learning about CanMEDS competencies was funding. No one could figure out how this kind of learning could fit within budgets, and so, as of right now, we have not repeated the workshop.

Anesthesiologists are the patient's primary caregiver through a critical period. Until they have an up close and personal experience with illness themselves, many medical professionals can not appreciate how vulnerable patients may feel in the moments before induction. For the anesthesiologist, the ability to readily engage and connect at this time is essential. Beyond the serious responsibility of managing a patient's life functions during surgery, anesthesiologists have an integral role in ensuring optimal team performance. In their work, they are dependent on surgical and nursing personnel, machines, drugs, and very sophisticated equipment to practice safely. This necessitates close liaisons with many team members at once. It is absolutely vital that they learn to communicate effectively, develop situational awareness, speak up about concerns, and listen actively, and continually work at forging positive connections with others to facilitate safe surgery, collaborative accountability, and patient-focused, high-quality care.

In this workshop, we discussed the many challenges anesthesiologists face as physicians, as well as the challenges patients may experience when navigating the health-care system. By helping residents to increase their awareness of these challenges and providing them with an opportunity to work toward developing key interpersonal communication and collaboration skills using LTTA methods, it is hoped that these CanMEDs competencies remain a touchstone and are realized in the professional lives of residents.

NOTE

1. Royal College of Physicians and Surgeons of Canada, CanMEDS Physician Competency Framework, http://www.royalcollege.ca/portal/page/portal/rc/canmeds, accessed Dec. 16, 2015.

Theater in the Theater

The Cancer Tales Experience in Four Acts

TREVOR THOMPSON AND WILL GOODISON

PROLOGUE

Keeping the reflection fresh is a matter of presentation, of making it real and relevant. Clinical situations give rise to the most poignant opportunities, but in our work with students in the early years at Bristol (UK) we face a particular challenge—they don't yet have much clinical exposure. Philosopher Donald Schön distinguishes reflection-in-action from reflection-on-action, to which we would have to add reflection-before-action. In our search for ways to make reflection fresh, we have for the last seven years been bringing theater to the lecture theater, using extracts from the play *Cancer Tales: True Stories* by Nell Dunn.[1] In this essay, I am joined by Dr. Will Goodison, one of our recent graduates, who, as a student, directed several stagings of the play.

ACT I: THINKING "AS IF"

I remember it like yesterday, Tennessee Williams's *A Streetcar Named Desire* at the Lyric Theater, Belfast, Northern Ireland, one of those early indelible initiations into art that works. Viscerally engaged, narratively convinced, I was right there with Blanche DuBois as she unraveled in the Louisiana heat. This is what theater at its best can do: take us by the scruff of the neck and haul us into a foreign territory of the imagination. So touched, we see the world differently, with more awareness of life's complexities, with more potential for compassion. Gretchen Case and Daniel Brauner introduce the idea of "thinking as if." Aware that I can never truly leave my own perspective behind (or want to), I can at least think "as if" I were "the other person."[2] For audiences of nearly three hundred, we have not found a better way of engaging hearts and minds than through the medium of live theater. This is not a novelty but the latest in a long tradition within medical education.

Every lecturer should consider the performative aspects of their craft. Teaching, like medicine, is both art and science, and the art of teaching is how we engage the enthusiasm and imagination of the student, to inspire as well as to inform. Handily, we are provided with various accoutrements for this worthy task, including actual theaters. The lecture theater is like any other theater, with a stage, lighting, and raked seating, otherwise impractical spaces designed to focus the attention on an unfolding drama. The idea of the "operating theater" first stemmed from public demonstrations of anatomical dissections in front of a paying audience in the 1300s.

There are various ways in which theater lends value. Through theater we see behind the social mask to the agonies and ecstasies of the inner life, without leaving anybody emotionally exposed (except perhaps the audience). The play delivers a condensed and considered narrative that is so often missed, suppressed, or drowned in the noise of fast-paced, real-world clinical encounter.

ACT II: OUT OF OUR HEADS

Tucked within the early years at our medical school is a short module, "Medical Humanities and Whole Person Care," in which we unabashedly champion the art of clinical medicine, including such nuances as creating rapport, engendering trust, and dispensing hope. We also describe the arts in medicine, including medical themes in history, literature, and philosophy. In turning these notions into curriculum activity, we draw on students' creative capacities, in a program of "compulsory creativity."[3]

Bringing the art of medicine to life in the lecture theater setting has been a particular challenge. In 2005 we came across *Cancer Tales: True Stories* by Nell Dunn and recommend this play to any teacher seeking to engage the undivided attention of a large audience. *Cancer Tales* was written by Dunn as a way of making sense of her father's passing. She decided to be "more friendly with death,"[4] spending many long hours talking with cancer patients in the waiting rooms of London's Royal Marsden Hospital and in interviews with their health professional careers. Her research resulted in the creation of five interwoven narratives that portray seven women's experiences of disease, loss, death, and restoration. Not surprisingly, health professionals are treated realistically in *Cancer Tales*—the play shows examples of both exemplary and cack-handed care. All of these highly personal stories offer diverse starting points for engaged, thought-provoking discussion.

In busy curricula, it is possible (though not artistically ideal) to enact a single story, or selection of stories, rather than the entire *Cancer Tales* script. In our curriculum, we present two of the stories unabridged, including the story of Rebecca, a young woman diagnosed with leukemia, and her mother, Mary, as a performance lasting around twenty minutes. Mary describes the difficulty she has watching her daughter suffer. At one point, building on a multilayered narrative, Rebecca asserts, "I am alive now, not dying, living."[5] A bit later, when it becomes clear that Rebecca is dying, Mary appreciates the direct, caring approach of Rebecca's doctor: "He was so straight he was wonderful he was clear then you know what to do you have the truth and you've got to deal with it."[6]

ACT III: ROUTES TO REFLECTION

Because of the play's rawness, students are warned that the stories may be upsetting, particularly for those who have family members experiencing cancer or other serious illness. Because medical students in the UK enter medical school right out of high school, they are younger than in North America. We have had feedback from tutors that the play can be overwhelming and capable of rendering ensuing group work unfeasible. However, we feel that it is a good thing to rehearse such discomfort in the early years and to challenge the idea that such emotional reactions should be buried.

In the seven consecutive years we have staged *Cancer Tales,* the standard of performance has been extraordinary, at times as good as any professional company. This essay does not tackle the educational benefits of theater for performers, but since medicine itself is a type of theater—with roles, scripts, props, and improvisation—the parallels are convincing. Each year a student director casts the play and makes his or her mark on how it is staged. We fund professional lighting, and the play is performed without scripts and with the use of basic props and costume.

We have experimented with various ways of aiding reflection in the small-group seminars that follow the performance. It is normal to get caught in the narrative sweep and to miss the many themes as they dash by. To remedy this, we have produced a short document that prompts discussion on four topics: "Cancer Narratives," "Care-giver Narratives," "Therapeutic Relationships," and "The Doctor's Story." We provide salient verbatim quotations from the text for reference.

We invite a senior oncologist to join the students in discussion immediately after the play. *Cancer Tales* does not give voice to the doctor's story and so the students can find out from the clinician if the play seems realistic and how the oncologist would have dealt with the issues that arise. It is also important for students to learn how cancer care has evolved in the UK since the play was first published in 2002—for instance with the emergence of oncology nurse specialists in clinic settings. We have also asked students to role-play aspects of the drama that we don't see on stage—like two doctors talking about one of the characters.

ACT IV: THEATER IS BRILLIANT!

Of our 2013 cohort, asked to rate the *Cancer Tales* session either "brilliant," "pretty good," "OK," "not great," or "atrocious," 75 percent rated it as "brilliant" (n = 210, response rate 84 percent). By comparison, our next most highly rated element, a creative and interactive lecture, received a "Brilliant" rating of 28 percent. It is fair to say that *Cancer Tales* is highly popular. But why? For this essay, each of our students was asked to return feedback on the use of "theater in the theater" and to share one particular episode that hit home from the *Cancer Tales* experience.

Students frequently opined that theater "brought issues to life" in a way not possible in the normal lecture. Many considered the value of visualizing situations rather than hearing them reported, even when the speakers were reporting their own experience (we make regular use of such testimonials). The play "really emphasized the kind of deep emotions I will have to deal with during my training and when I qualify," one student said. "I would have been horrified if this had happened to me and felt very uncomfortable just watching," noted another.

Students found themselves reflecting on aspects that are often invisible in the clinical encounter. "The play really made me consider the complexity of people's lives," a student said. "Often on the surface people project a certain exterior and you have no idea what is really happening." The mother-daughter relationship was particularly impactful. Said one audience member: "So moving . . . the daughter had an acceptance, and it seems much harder to witness someone dying than to be the one that dies."

The play caused the students to reflect on how they would practice in the future in terms of privacy ("the lack of patient privacy really struck me as something I want to alter about my future practice"), the use of language ("a throw-away comment can have such a profound effect on people"), disclosure ("if the patient wants to know all the details you shouldn't hide them from them"), and physical empathy ("coming down to patients' eye level, these simple things are skills that can't really be taught").

EPILOGUE

Although efficient for capturing the attention of a large group of students, staging a play is resource intensive compared to showing a film or a film clip, where the educator can remain in command of content and the remote control. However, the immediacy, unpredictability, and novelty of theater wins the day. A key to success is handing the whole thing over to the student community, trusting in their creative and emotional intelligence to give and receive these unforgettable stories.

NOTES

1. Nell Dunn, *Cancer Tales: True Stories* (Oxford: Amber Lane Press, 2002).
2. Gretchen A. Case and Daniel J. Brauner, "Perspective: The Doctor as Performer: A Proposal for Change Based on a Performance Studies Paradigm," *Academic Medicine* 85 (2010): 159–63.
3. Trevor Thompson, Catherine Lamont-Robinson, and Louise Younie, "'Compulsory Creativity': Rationales, Recipes, and Results in the Placement of Mandatory Creative Endeavour in a Medical Undergraduate Curriculum," *Medical Education Online* 15 (Nov. 2010), www.ncbi.nlm.nih.gov/pmc/articles/PMC3037267.
4. Monica Desai and Adrian Gonzalez, "Theatre: Cancer Tales," *British Medical Journal* 326, no. 7399 (2003): 1151.
5. Ibid., 75.
6. Ibid., 87.

Fostering Reflection-in-Action through a Performance Arts Workshop

JULIE CHEN, LYNN YAU, NANCY LOO,
ANDERSON TSANG, AND L. C. CHAN

In September 2013, a new Medical Humanities curriculum was launched as part of the core medical program at the University of Hong Kong (HKU). Drawing on the fine arts, performance arts, literature, history, and the social sciences through interactive lectures and experiential workshops, the first-year class of 210 undergraduate medical students explored three themes: "What is meant by the medical humanities?" "The person behind the white coat," and "The history of medicine in Hong Kong."

Performance arts, such as drama, have been used successfully in other settings to explore themes relevant to medical practice and to build skills transferable to clinical work.[1] In addition, we introduced the concept of "reflection-in-action,"[2] in which students demonstrated how their thinking was reframed while they were doing a task in response to an unexpected or unsettling idea or outcome. This concurrent action and reflection on the issues raised in the workshop helped students to consolidate concepts, challenge assumptions, and develop self-understanding. Here is an example of a performance arts workshop that specifically addressed issues related to "the person behind the white coat" as an educational opportunity to foster student reflection-in-action.

We partnered with the Absolutely Fabulous Theater Connection (AFTEC), a community organization with expertise in drama education, to design a three-hour performance arts workshop, which was held five times, with forty-two students per session. The workshops were led by two AFTEC artist-educators who were skilled in drama and music and assisted by one HKU medical faculty member. Each workshop had three parts. It started with a series of professionally designed theater games that aimed to break the ice and simultaneously introduce the role of emotional intelligence in the practice of medicine. For example, in the exercise "emotional mirror," students paired up and mirrored each other's facial expressions and body movements for approximately ten minutes, with each partner getting a chance to lead and follow. They changed their expressions and actions according to mood cues from live piano music. Another game demonstrated how changing the tone, volume, and expression of the voice could carry powerful emotions. In a two-person dialogue, students said, "Hey, you," "Who, me?" "Yes, you," varying their voices and expressions each time.

This was followed by smaller groups of five to six students who reviewed a dramatic script and then selected one of the scenes to read and perform in front of the class. The short story "Imelda," written by surgeon Richard Selzer,[3] was adapted into a script with four key scenes by Dr. Vicki Ooi, AFTEC's artistic director. "Imelda" was selected for the rich entry-points it provided for discussion about medical error, professional/unprofessional attitudes and behaviors, and what defines humanism in medicine. The plot charts the journey of Dr. Franciscus, a haughty surgeon who performs cleft lip surgery on a young patient who dies on the operating table from anesthesia complications. The surgeon later returns to the morgue to finish the operation on the dead girl.

The last part of the workshop required students to reconsider their understanding of the scene from "Imelda" using new insights they identified from the dramatic reading of the script. They were then invited to either rewrite or extend the scene in an imaginary way, performing the scene in a way that addressed one of the issues that resonated in the scene (for example, the nature of the doctor-patient relationship, ethical dilemmas, or professionalism). In both situations, students had to incorporate their understanding of the role emotions play for any of the characters. Guiding questions were included in each key scene to assist with critical reflexivity. Prompts and questions included: "Describe any character's feelings and your own feelings as you watch the performance," "What did you understand from the performance that applies to you as a medical student and future doctor?" and "Discuss any ethical issues you may have with Dr. Franciscus performing surgery on Imelda's body." After the performance of the selected scene, students on stage led a discussion with the "audience" based on the questions. Feedback obtained from students and facilitators indicated that the performance arts workshop had a positive impact.

Illustrative student feedback (used with permission) follows:

"It would be important in terms of learning to be a benevolent, ethical doctor and managing emotions. Drama portrays life to some extent and gives people an experience even though they are not actually in it. It helps doctors look into their profession and themselves. Music on the other hand is a medium to clear one's mind, and can act as a refuge for doctors under great pressure."—Ngan Chiu Kei Kenneth, first-year medical student

"I learned to look for patients' body language, voice quality and emotions to identify what they need most. I think it is very important as it helps us to identify our role as a doctor and also to observe and listen carefully to the surroundings."—Sun Wai Chuen, first-year medical student

Feedback from facilitators included the following:

"For students who did not know or were not interested in music, music was more challenging to interpret and comprehend. In one of the workshops, I spoke of my godson's funeral—he died of leukemia—and played the song he composed before his untimely death. That personal gesture encouraged the students to share similar life stories and became a start of endearing them to music. My son is a doctor with long working hours and few holidays. It's painful watching him drag his tired self home. Doctors deal with life and death, and every decision is crucial. I told the doctors that they are the ones who walk the final journey with patients. They are the ones who are in need of rest and relief. The Medical Humanities programme asks of them to understand their own feelings. They must learn to express their emotions before learning to cure patients."—Nancy Loo, workshop facilitator

And also:

"For AFTEC, the performing arts workshops were stimulating because we experienced how the arts can positively contribute to those with a science background for the betterment of their medical journey. In addition, we were intrigued as to how we could bridge a gap between the arts and the sciences by distilling the best of both fields for teaching and learning. I was fascinated with the transformation of learning mindsets both for ourselves and the students to be more open and inclusive given that the pre-university education system locally is generally termed as "Confucian" or conservative. I think the MH programme is crucial in nurturing a culture of doctoring feelingly and meaningfully in young medical students during their medical studies and beyond."—Lynn Yau, workshop facilitator

"The practice of medicine is perhaps the most humanistic profession of all. Doctors and health care professionals absorb the sufferings and miseries of patients;

and at the same time share their joy and hope throughout the course of illnesses. It is all too easy to shrink from patients' sentiments and to treat them as a case of disease, in an attempt to isolate oneself from the burden. We believe helping medical students to be better equipped in facing the psychological challenges ahead should be part and parcel of a comprehensive medical education. In this regard performing arts and music prove to be an effective mirror for students to reflect on their emotional reaction and subconscious behavior in simulated patient encounters."—Anderson Tsang, workshop facilitator

A fundamental aim of undergraduate medical education is to nurture students to become competent, reflective practitioners. We found that the performing arts are a wonderful medium to encourage students to share their feelings in a safe environment and to be introspective and reflective—traits that will contribute to their development as humanistic doctors. Besides encouraging students to get in touch with their own emotional lives and to reflect on their own comfort with emotions, the performance workshop was uniquely suitable for fostering the skill of reflection-in-action, a skill required in all clinical situations.

NOTES

1. Ewan James Jeffrey, Jen Goddard, and David Jeffrey, "Performance and Palliative Care: A Drama Module for Medical Students," *Medical Humanities* 38 (2012): 110–14.
2. Donald A. Schön, *The Reflective Practitioner: How Professionals Think in Action* (New York: Basic Books, 1983).
3. Richard Selzer, *Letters to a Young Doctor* (New York: Simon and Schuster, 1982).

"And So the Story Grows"

The Object Exercise

NANCY MCNAUGHTON AND KERRY KNICKLE

"The twine reminded me of my grandfather's home in the country. I remembered the smells of the attic . . . that lovely musty old smell . . . and then I remembered washing my grandmother's back in the bath as a young girl . . . she needed my help . . . her hands were so crippled from arthritis . . . and I was reminded of what a wonderful outlook she had about life . . . and how much she loved me. . . ." This reflection by one of the authors is inspired by a roll of twine, one of an assortment of objects placed on a table as part of an evocative object exercise. It was the twine that "spoke to her," evoking emotion and stimulating her memory.

Sunwolf, Lawrence Frey, and Lisa Keränen claim that the "sharing of stories between tellers and listeners provides a symbolic framework offering myriad connections between story, self, other and experience."[1] Transformational theory suggests that emotion and affect are as important for learning as formal abstract reasoning, and that by engaging the affective dimension of storytelling we have "an opportunity, for establishing a dialogue with those unconscious aspects of ourselves seeking expression through various images, feelings, and behaviors within the learning setting."[2] For health professional educators, this means actively creating opportunities for learners to experience and reflect on not only what they are learning but how they feel about what they are learning. In this essay we describe the "object exercise," a learning activity we developed for health professional learners and practitioners to reflect on affective dimensions of learning. The central goals of the workshop are to actively learn about how emotion and affect impact listening and storytelling and to gain understanding about how trust, connection, and empathy shape our communicative processes.

A Bible, spectacles, a bone fragment, a coil of twine, sharks' teeth, a black-and-white photograph, postcards, and a faded blood donor card sit on a draped table at the front of the room. These "evocative objects"[3] were chosen for their texture, color, shape, implied history, and symbolic and aesthetic value. The object exercise is a reflective undertaking, highlighting the integral connection between emotion and communication. Participants actively engage in storytelling and listening in partnership as they experience the nature and quality of empathic exchange.

As described by Sherry Turkle, "We are on less familiar ground when we consider objects as companions to our emotional lives or as provocations to thought." She notes that evocative objects underscore the "inseparability of thought and feeling in our relationship to things. We think with the objects we love; we love the objects we think with."[4] The "object exercise" reinforces Turkle's suggestion that objects bring together intellect and emotion and connect daily life to practice. In this exercise, learners across professional disciplines, skill levels, and cultures have the opportunity to call up unique emotional memories and to share their stories. This is a reciprocal collaboration in which themes of connection, empathy, emotion, and communication are explored and discussed.

To begin the exercise, participants are asked to "drink in" the objects on the table and choose one object that evokes a memory or story. They then return to their seats and work in pairs. There are two consecutive five-minute interactions in which each person engages with their partner as a storyteller and also as a listener. Consider the story that was introduced at the beginning of this essay. As the storyteller's partner listened, she was affected by the teller's description of her grandmother's outlook on life, which in turn reminded her of her time growing up in Italy and missing her family at home. This prompted a series of inquiries and tellings:

> Listener: Was she able to cook with her hands so crippled?
>
> Storyteller: No, she couldn't cook but she could play piano. I remember my friends would stop playing so they could come and talk to her when she was at the piano. As a nine-year-old that drove me crazy. I wanted my friends to come play with me.
>
> Listener: She must have been a lovely person. My own grandmother loved music as well. I haven't been able to see her in over a year.
>
> Storyteller: I envy that you can still visit her. My grandmother passed away when I was eleven, and I often wished I had appreciated her the way my friends did.

After ten minutes of sharing reflections and asking questions of each other in pairs, the whole group reconvenes. Participants are asked to reflect on their experiences, first as storyteller: "As the storyteller, how did your object inspire your story? What was the first thing you wanted to tell?" Next the participants are asked to reflect on their experiences as listener: "What did you hear? What stood out to you? How did the story affect you? Images? Feelings? Memories? What was the first thing you wanted to ask? Why?" Finally participants revisit their experience as the storyteller: "How did the listener affect you and the story you told? Did your story change in unexpected ways? If so, how?" The exercise concludes with a facilitated discussion.

Participants have shared how surprised they are at the intensity of the empathic listening they experience and the emotional memories they recall when sharing memories evoked by their selected object. The group reflects on how trust and honesty is dependent on the sense of safety that may develop in varying degrees in each partnership. The group considers what it is it about the quality of an interaction that invites us to share more and why we may be less inclined to share in other instances. We see that "story sharing is a dynamic process in which stories are transformed in the telling, and, then, further transformed in the receiving period. . . . When we listen to a teller we hear our own story."[5]

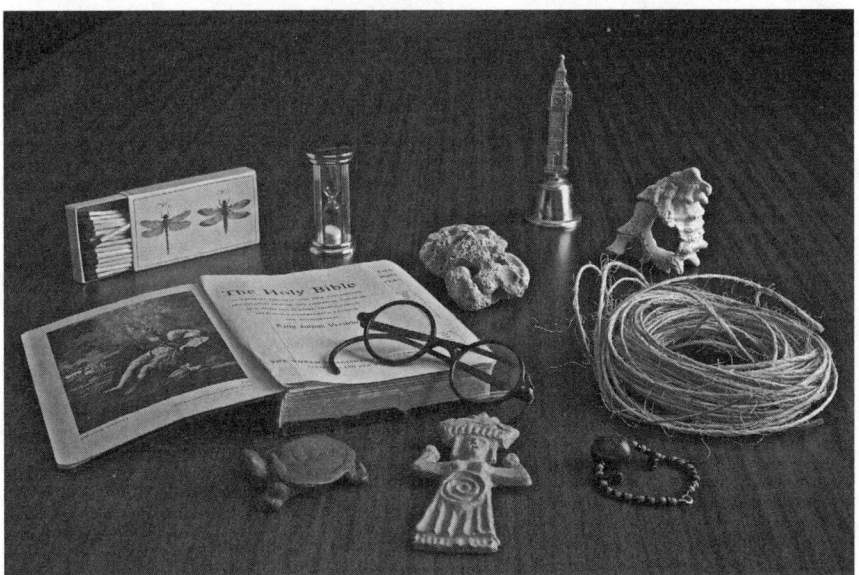

Cameron MacLennan, *Memory,* 2013. Courtesy of Cameron MacLennan Collection, Standardized Patient Program, Faculty of Medicine, University of Toronto.

For the past five years we have presented this workshop locally and internationally for professionals and learners both inside and outside of health care. It was formally presented during the second Creating Spaces symposium meeting in Banff, Alberta, in 2011.

This exercise highlights the relational power of story as a co-creation that can inspire recollection and reflection in rich and unexpected ways. The storyteller and listener are directly affected and effected by the connection that develops between them during the exchange. It has utility across the health-care continuum and can be applied beyond health professions to explore the art and practice of focused, empathic communication. The exercise offers a potent means for transforming emotional memory into knowledge and cultivating awareness of another's experience. It also allows learners to explore empathic communication and actively engage as storytellers and listeners within the context of the patient/clinician exchange or in conversation with family, friends, colleagues, or strangers.

Despite different circumstances and backgrounds, people can come together through shared connection. Just as emotion influences communication, communication influences emotion. Evocative objects can transform the empathic communication between storyteller and listener and can inspire new relational possibilities through mutual narrative experience.

NOTES

1. Sunwolf, Lawrence R. Frey, and Lisa Keränen, "Rx Story Prescriptions: Healing Effects of Storytelling and Storylistening in the Practice of Medicine," in *Narratives, Health, and Healing: Communication Theory, Research, and Practice,* ed. Lynn M. Harter, Phyllis M. Japp, and Christina S. Beck (Mahwah, NJ: Lawrence Erlbaum, 2005), 240.
2. John M. Dirkx, "Engaging Emotions in Adult Learning: A Jungian Perspective on Emotion and Transformative Learning," *New Directions for Adult and Continuing Education* 109 (Spring 2006): 22.
3. Sherry Turkle, *Evocative Objects: Things We Think With* (Cambridge, MA: MIT Press, 2011).
4. Ibid., 5.
5. Sunwolf, Frey, and Keränen, "Rx Story Prescriptions," 241.

The Use of Musical Autobiographies in Shaping Professional Identity

AMY CLEMENTS-CORTES

In music therapy, music is the primary therapeutic tool used in the client-therapist relationship to work toward clinical goals and objectives. To be an effective music therapist, it is essential not only to be a highly skilled musician who continually develops his or her craft but also to have an intimate relationship with music and the role it plays in one's life. The importance of music in one's life contributes to the development of who we are as therapists and is a significant factor in shaping the professional identity of student music therapists as they begin their practical placements. This narrative outlines a musical autobiography assignment I have given my class, and a reflection on this assignment by a student.

Why did I create this assignment? Music therapists may actively engage older adults and those in palliative care in writing songs and creating musical autobiographies and "legacy" projects to further the life review and facilitate grieving processes. In the undergraduate creative improvisation class at the University of Windsor, music therapy students learn multiple ways of implementing improvisational techniques through a variety of mediums, including music, art, dance, and drama. Students complete this course either before their clinical placements or alongside their first practical placements as they began learning about who they are as therapists. I designed this assignment to help them access the importance of music in their lives as an avenue for developing a reflective practice and facilitating the initial steps in building a professional identity.

What is a musical autobiography? A musical autobiography involves a written narrative that is accompanied by musical examples that highlight important stories in one's life. By adding music to one's stories, the stories become more animated, dramatic, emotional, and engaging. For this specific musical auto-biography assignment, there were three major components: audio, visual, and written. The audio component involved creating a recording of selections of special music, sounds, voices, and freely composed music, such as a song that helped portray the student's life story. The visual component involved a range of options, including creating a mural or collage, which may have included photos to accompany selected audio examples or may have incorporated video samples or PowerPoint presentations with visual images that advanced the autobiography. The written component included a four-thousand-word narrative documenting the stories with in-depth reflection referencing major milestones and the reasons for the selections of music.

Students were encouraged to use the entire term to prepare this assignment to ensure they had adequate time to reflect and truly facilitate a comprehensive analysis. As a starting point, it was suggested that the students begin by collecting details about their music-listening and music-making experiences at different stages in their lives and creating a music chart or narrative that described the ways that music influenced them during these stages. The students were also encouraged to reflect on significant events, experiences, music mentors, and favorite music that influenced or inspired them.

Stage two involved students making the recording of sounds and music that they associated with various events, periods, people, relationships, or feelings from their past, starting with their earliest memories and proceeding chronologically to the present. Stage three involved students experimenting with visually artistic ways to enhance the musical selections while demonstrating personal expression. Students had an opportunity to share significant aspects and highlights of their autobiographies with the class. They were graded in four areas: (1) audio collection—presence of thought and reflection in the arrangement and appropriate length of selections; (2) visual representation—scope of reflection, creativity, presence of effort, and personal expression; (3) quality—the caliber of work and appearance; and (4) written narrative—depth of reflection, scope of review, elaboration of ideas, presence of thought and effort, narrative flow, and grammar.

The following student reflection bears on the value of the assignment in relation to the student's professional identity formation as a future music therapist:

> I had the chance to create my own musical autobiography in this class. At first, I was very intimidated: I did not know where to start, and, frankly, I wasn't sure exactly what place music has had throughout my life. However, as a future music therapist, I saw the potential benefit of such a musical reflection.

Choosing how to describe the impact music has had on my life isn't easy, because life isn't linear or categorical: it is eclectic and filled with highs and lows, turns and bumps—a journey. And this journey takes many forms, sometimes as a friendship and sometimes as an excursion in a foreign culture. It is also the passage between important milestones in our life. My musical autobiography was housed in a backpack, which contained travelogues (or travel diaries) describing journeys I have taken. I numbered these chronologically and included pictures and objects relevant to the story being told. Musical selections were also included in the written narrative. Taking the time to reflect on the place of music in my life has made me realize how omnipresent music is and how diverse the ways are in which we associate music with different parts of our life. I have also come to appreciate the therapeutic benefit of this exercise.

In terms of my own music therapy career, this process helped me assess the different experiences I have had, not only with music but also with other life experiences that have helped me to become a good therapist. Being able to document, reflect on, and assess your past—what you have experienced, accomplished and learned—is an essential skill for music therapists. I strongly believe in the importance of reflecting and evaluating, because it contributes to the improvement of the services I will provide. I also included my ambitions related to my music therapy career. Reflecting about my long-term goals prompted me to research graduate programs in fields related to music therapy. It also revitalized my true passion for the profession.

Having general guidelines and opportunities to use a range of media stimulates the creativity of my students. It allows individuals to represent their lives in ways that are most meaningful to them. I sincerely believe that a simple reflective paper would have not been as beneficial as the musical autobiography project. The creative process that my students experienced through this exercise has helped me to identify a variety of themes, including those related to professional identity formation; person– and relationship-centered care; social justice assumptions about class, race, ability, power, gender, diversity, and equity; interdisciplinary and interprofessional exchange and learning; community building; and changing cultures of health-care education. I have used my own stories and accompanying musical selections to discuss these issues. Further, this process helped me understand how music has shaped my life and affects the type of therapist I am becoming. I think that all music therapists can benefit from creating their own musical autobiographies. It helps us see our own experiences, values, and beliefs, all of which impact our practice.

NOTE

It has been an honor and privilege for me, as the professor in this class, to facilitate this exercise and learn about my students and their musical and personal experiences. I thank them all for sharing their stories with me. I am reassured that I am helping to introduce the benefits of reflective practice to a new health professional group—music therapists.

"Parallel Narrative" in a Close Reading of the Film The Savages

MAURA SPIEGEL

First-year medical students enrolled in a narrative medicine selective at Columbia University College of Physicians and Surgeons are required to watch the film *The Savages* (2007). A primary objective in using film with medical students is to offer them strategies for accessing their own experience through the mediation of films. I propose the term *parallel narrative* to describe the experience we all share of drawing connections to our own lives—to events or emotions—that are aroused or awakened by a movie. This idea of parallel narrative has met with a mixed response, gaining traction in discussion of some films more than others, and I was hoping to find a way to break through in the final class. I experienced a eureka moment when it occurred to me that the students could get closer to their own experiences when our discussion got closer to the film—that is, when we read it closely. Let me walk you through that process.

I began the class with a little preamble, telling them about my parallel narrative while I was rewatching *The Savages* in preparation for class. What repeated in my mind was, "Oh dear, you [the students] will not identify with these characters," a brother and sister who are unable to complete things, to commit to relationships, and who, approaching midlife, are still grappling with their abusive and abandoning father. "I worried," I continued, "that these characters would merely get on your nerves. You'd see them as losers and reject them. Maybe they'd call on parts of yourselves that you can't afford to think about right now."

I kept talking with such transparency because I could see that I had aroused their genuine interest. I was describing how they, the medical students, had taken up residence in my imagination, how I was seeing the film through their eyes, or my projection of what they might see in the film. In telling them about my parallel narrative, I demonstrated that parallel narrative was not merely a literary-analytical term but a recognizable part of what occurs when we watch a film. The proposition: noticing one's own thoughts can be useful, can reveal something that is occupying or preoccupying one's mind. Once identified, the thoughts can be considered on their merits or challenged in some way. These are not foreign ideas to most adults, but sometimes such familiar notions come into focus in a new way. A tangible drop in resistance was perceptible in the room, as it seemed they were considering that introspection might—in some instances—be an asset instead of a threat to their functioning. In prior weeks, we had had fruitful discussions about the vicissitudes of sympathy— how complex and contingent it can be. After writing to the prompt for five minutes, they shared experiences in which something internal had interfered with their capacity to care for or about a person in their lives. I felt this was a theme especially pertinent to this film, both because I'd worried that their sympathy for the main characters might be troubled and because the characters themselves have difficulty feeling for and caring for one another.

Turning to the film, we began with the scene in which Jon (actor Philip Seymour-Hoffman) receives a phone call during class, informing him that his father is dying. After he folds his cell phone, he stands looking dazed when a student asks him, "What is the difference between plot and narrative?" Focusing on a small moment—one we agreed was understated by the camera work and the quiet of the room—engaged my students immediately. They noted that the student had no idea what Jon was undergoing in that moment and that the scene effectively revealed how a distance can open up suddenly between people. Another commented that the student's question pointed to a distinction between the plot of the father's life, now coming to an end, and the narrative of his life, which was far from over.

We turned then to an earlier scene, the surreal slow-motion sequence of the oldsters in Sun City, Arizona, dancing to "I Don't Want to Play in Your Yard." They were right on it, noting that this introduces the theme of the denial of death and sets up an opposition between a euphemistic approach to death and the tough-minded acknowledgment of decay and mortality the film will later explore. They observed how Wendy (actor Laura Linney) and Jon represent two sides of this issue. One student recalled that the nursing home was called a "rehabilitation center," and this led to further discussion of the use of euphemism in death's proximity. Another student reminded us of Jon's explosion outside the upscale nursing home, where he avers that such places prey on family members' guilt and denial while doing nothing significant for the patient. Agreement with that point of view led to a discussion of what physicians do for the family of the dying person. The discussion had veered far from the idea of parallel narrative, but the students were enjoying the close reading—taking pleasure in articulating what was happening in the film. It seemed to me that they were experiencing the value of such articulation, of giving language to their experience.

From here we looked at the scene in which Wendy picks her father up at the hospital to begin their journey to Buffalo, New York. I asked the students to recount what we already knew about Wendy's character before this point in the film. They noted that she writes her grant letter while on the job and shovels office supplies into her purse; she lies about her PAP smear to Larry (actor Peter Friedman), her married boyfriend, and reaches out to Larry's dog during sex; she pockets the Percocet she finds in the recently deceased Doris's medicine cabinet. So before the travel scene with her father begins, we have plenty of evidence of Wendy's neediness and of how she resorts to lying, stealing, and manipulating in an effort to fill the void.

Returning to the clip, I asked the students several questions: "Why does Wendy take the suspenders and baseball cap off her father? What did you see in the interaction in which the nurse provides Wendy with a small mountain of medications and pile of diapers for her father? What feelings is Wendy having? And what are we as viewers feeling for and about her? How does the film manage our feelings toward the characters? How does humor figure in? Did you feel the film was sometimes critical of the characters? What thoughts did they have when Lenny was yelling that he needed the bathroom? How did they feel about how Wendy handled it?" I was fascinated that many of the students were critical of how long it took Wendy to get up from her seat and to realize that her father's pants had fallen down. Here the discussion turned to the challenges of traveling with an ill person, of caring for someone who is irascible, and of feeling inadequate to a task. I asked them if they had stories from their own experience that interfaced with this scene. Many of them nodded significantly.

Next we looked at "Movie Night," when Jon and Wendy screen *The Jazz Singer* at the nursing home. The students again were quick to the draw:

- Lenny believes he is seeing himself and his family in the film when he says, "See, there she is, there's my mother." (Here I resisted drawing attention to Lenny's parallel narrative.)
- From Lenny's reaction, we learn that he was beaten by *his* father. (Later in the film, we see that Lenny repeated this behavior with his son Jon.)
- We take in the affront to the African American staff when Al Jolson applies his blackface makeup. Wendy and Jon slink out of the nursing home after the screening, mortified that the film has offended the staff.

We then discussed other points where racial issues are raised in the film: Lenny's subtle racism in not being able to distinguish between his two male aids; Wendy's assumption that Jimmy is Jamaican, when he is in fact Nigerian. And we discussed the real-world fact that white patients living in nursing homes are often cared for by persons of color. The film sought to acknowledge this fact and some of the ways it is problematic. We agreed that it doesn't solve any of the issues raised but simply offers an acknowledgment that these are subjects that belong in the discussion.

Finally, we discussed the scene near the end when Jon watches the rehearsal of Wendy's play. What did the students make of Jon's tears? Why does seeing a representation of one's own story move one to tears? The answers to these two questions were, I believe, known in an intuitive way to all of the students, but they did not resent being asked to give language to those intuitions. I asked each of them which moment in that scene they had found most moving. The students responded warmly, earnestly. Coming to the end of the film, there was a feeling of accomplishment in the room—that we'd done something together. I quickly gave them a writing prompt: "Write about a time you needed support and got it from a family member." Their written reflections felt more open than in the past—more immediate and charged—and they even included an increased use of detail, following our attention to detail in the film.

SUGGESTED RESOURCE

1. Heiserman, Arthur, and Maura Spiegel. "Narrative Permeability: Crossing the Dissociative Barrier In and Out of Films." *Literature and Medicine* 25 (2006): 463–74.

A Red Nose, Floppy Hat, and the Arts

The Trainers' Workshop

PAUL DAKIN

A big red nose and floppy hat may seem odd additions to a trainers' workshop, but these unexpected tools were provided at our annual "Away Day." As educators in postgraduate general practice, we look forward to escaping the bustle of North London for the stately Tudor pile of Cambridge University's continuing education center. But to be sent out of the room with a nose and hat and then asked to perform with a fellow trainer in front of thirty colleagues—well, that's far removed from consulting room or lecture hall! Two clowns, one a doctor, had been asked to provide input for the day. Starting with a variety of awareness exercises, such as mirroring the movements of a partner, they encouraged us to enter a state of mindfulness by walking us continuously around the room without interaction, much like so many smoke particles in Brownian motion. Splitting into pairs, with no script or preparation, and wearing only the accoutrements of a clown to mark our transformation, we acted and played, silently sensing one another's mood and reacting without conscious thought—a process that subverted the filter of rationality we rely upon when dealing with patients and professionals.

On reflection, this rather peculiar set of exercises may not actually be so far removed from everyday practice. Through training and practice we become expert in reading and responding to the moods of our patients. We become proficient in training others how to observe subliminal cues in body language and paraverbals. We teach the importance of attending to our "gut feeling," the inward detection of so many subtle signs and indicators that we find them hard to categorize and put into words. Theater-based activities such as these can help promote self-awareness and provide us with ideas on how to teach more effectively. For example, perhaps we might better make use of the actors we employ in our standardized role-play scenarios. Instead of just asking them to adopt the role of patient from whom trainees bounce their consultation skills, they could teach us the acting techniques they learned at drama school. This might help our trainees better connect with patients, informed by sources of genuine emotion and internalized memories that would allow their consultation script to write itself with care and connection.

We have also introduced the consideration of poetry into our trainers' workshop. Precisely chosen words and crafted rhythms can slip past our conscious defenses, inspiring new insights, understanding, and awareness. We have enjoyed workshops with the now nonagenarian doctor-poet Dannie Abse, who, when reading from his published collections, mesmerizes fellow medics with the significance of his frequently recurring motif—"white coat/purple coat"—reminding us that we are both physicians and magicians in the eyes of our patients and in the power of our pronouncements. And we have tried to write our own poetry, presenting it to one another—an uncomfortable process for colleagues of a strictly scientific persuasion.

The use of books such as *Middlemarch* to explore professional identity is commonplace and valuable, along with graphic novels (or "comics" to the unpretentious) that have the capacity to thrill a student, provoke a postgraduate, and disturb a trainer into further consideration of what it is that makes us tick. Images of artwork such as Hodler's "The Disillusioned One" or Munch's "The Scream" trigger a discussion of emotional communication, body language, and interest in what was conveyed from the mind of the artist.

Film is often a "secret weapon" that confronts our complacency. All of us enjoy watching a picture story unfold (and what is better than sitting in front of the screen as an excuse for work or education?), but movies like *Wit* (2001) or *The Doctor* (1991) strike at the foundation of our professionalism, forcing us to consider whether we would have behaved in the same way and what inner and personal resources we have to fall back on should we encounter times of illness, anxiety, and stress. *The Third Man* (1949), set in the safe remoteness of postwar Vienna, lulls us with its zither tones until we are made to feel uncomfortable by the fallen ethics of a doctor complicit in the sale of black-market penicillin. Surely in this day and age with our heightened sense of ethical awareness we could never find ourselves in such a compromised position?

To protect against these various awareness-promoting activities and reflections from becoming an entirely solitary affair, our trainers' workshops are subdivided into small groups of four or five; these meetings, held regularly, are considered to be the most important and protected component of the afternoon. The aim, ostensibly, is to discuss with our peers the difficulties we have in training our individual registrars, postgraduate doctors specializing in general practice. But of course in the process, we are actually revealing, sharing, communicating, and reflecting upon our own performance as educators. We consider issues of personality, workload, work/life balance, stress, recovery, burnout, joy, and despair—all inspired by the astute questions from trusted and sympathetic colleagues whose pressures and resources mirror our own and who keep us safe without words of criticism, nor its equally dangerous opposite, complicity. So powerful are these reflective interactions that a colleague on the point of retiring told me recently that what he will miss most on leaving general practice will be his visits to the workshop—"my support group."

Performative Reflection

A Theater Elective Directed to Promoting Relational-Responsive Awareness among Medical Students

MICHELE FLEIGER, ALIM NAGJI, AND
PAMELA BRETT-MACLEAN

The contributions of theater in medical education have been described in various ways, including providing a means of enhancing empathic understanding of patients' stories. This was a guiding objective of a six-session "Understanding the Patient's Story" special studies module that was piloted five years ago at the University of Alberta. Conceived by Alim Nagji (as a first-year medical student), the elective has grown and evolved based on an ongoing collaboration between the Department of Drama and the Arts & Humanities in Health & Medicine (AHHM) program in the Faculty of Medicine & Dentistry. The expertise of theater artists at the University of Alberta has been integral to the success of the elective. Initially realized with the facilitation of Michael Kennard, actor, director, and inspiring teacher in physical theater, this longitudinal theater-based experience has been devised and facilitated by artist-educator Michele Fleiger since its inception in 2010. Pamela Brett-MacLean, in her role as director of the AHHM program, helped to conceptualize and continues to substantively contribute to the evolution of the class, which is currently offered as a formal undergraduate elective. Student leads assist in coordinating the scheduling of sessions and modeling understanding of the developmental process of the elective (given their experience as participants in the previous year). Alim remained involved in the class during his time as a senior medical student and resident at the University of Alberta.

As we have been engaged in the process, we have become acutely aware that, as a physical art, theater provides a powerful means of reflecting on embodied and tacit knowledge. Structures of engagement grounded in theatrical principles provide a means of prompting and helping medical students to reflect on their intellectual, physical, and emotional responses to various clinically relevant scenarios. By constructing imaginative realities that demand an open attentiveness to the here and now, theater serves to enhance the potential for expanded awareness, insight, and empathic responsiveness. Recalling Bakhtin's work—which offers a conception of development that is explicitly relational and dialogical, one in which we are always in the process of "becoming"[1]—we introduce theater exercises that encourage students to reflect on stories of "persons-in-relation" and help them to expand and deepen their interpretive and responsive capabilities. Following a developmental arc and flow, iterative, scaffolded theater exercises encourage the participants to develop an awareness of, and open and alert responsiveness to, the relational possibilities that arise moment by moment in everyday experiences with patients, families, and colleagues.

Six two-hour sessions are scheduled over the course of three months. The first three sessions introduce participatory elements (group building and improvisational exercises) and collaborative reflection, which lead to role-plays and forum theater exercises in the last three sessions. These early sessions are directed to enhancing awareness of self, and self in relation to others, as well as acknowledging assumptions. When we introduce role-play exercises—a structure of engagement that is both familiar and perceived to be directly connected to medical practice—we begin with "silent scenes" to highlight the applicability of what the students have learned in previous sessions. For example, students are encouraged to consider the influence of different aspects of the physical environment and behavioral cues on the relational responses they may consider. Later, verbal role-plays involve students taking on the roles of the doctor, patient, and witness, with students improvising in relation to various prompts. All exercises are followed by open-ended reflective sharing by the actors involved and by any observers. The final session includes an adapted forum theater exercise that provides the students with an opportunity to employ what they have learned in mindfully redirecting various problematic scenarios. This is followed by a closing group celebration.

When students are invited to, or spontaneously share reflections about what they are learning, we have been impressed by their keen insights into the multifaceted and contextual aspects of clinical care and by the responsive possibilities that exist for them as caring professionals. In 2012, recognizing the developmental potentials (personal and professional) of the elective, we renamed it "Performative Reflection: A Theatre-based Elective in Medicine." We believe this shift has worked to foster a deeper inquiry into and understanding of relational encounters in health care and also has helped to support the developmental growth of our students. Just as we invite the students to reflect on what they are learning, we also continuously reflect on the sessions (highlights, lowlights, and other surprises), to ensure the integrity of process. We regularly collect and read written feedback from the students and consider modifications to introduce the following session.

Maintaining the integrity of the pedagogical trajectory is always a balancing act. Typically, during the early sessions students articulate a desire to move more quickly into role-play. Most of our students are unfamiliar with improvisational theater exercises, and there are always a few who misinterpret the intent of our early formative explorations, believing these to be unrelated to learning how to communicate with and care for patients. We have learned, however, that without these foundational experiences the students' role-playing will reflect a narrow range of responses informed by assumed projections and restricted insight and awareness, which will limit the emergence of new understandings. As an example, we introduced the following role-play exercise in the fourth session of the elective. Students were encouraged to offer partial statements or phrases that could be expected as part of an opening gambit in a clinical encounter. These phrases functioned as triggers for an imaginative response. Students were divided into doctors and patients. Students playing a patient randomly selected an index card and completed the phrase with information that suggested something about their condition or presenting concern. They then entered the imagined clinical space of the encounter. Following this, the doctor entered the scene and, after greeting the patient, began to explore and develop a shared understanding of the patient's concerns, hopes, or expectations for the appointment.

In theater it is crucial to maintain the integrity of an authentic imagined space, so the students are encouraged to stay with the reality they create. In one memorable session, a student playing the patient completed the phrase "I don't want . . ." with the response "to go on. I just want to kill myself." There was some nervous laughter, but this dissipated fairly quickly as a number of the students asserted the potentiality of the statement in a clinical context. As the scene unfolded the response of the doctor moved everyone to a deeper appreciation of the potential for responding authentically and empathically to a challenging, highly charged patient encounter. The doctor's response resonated with the group. The doctor imaginatively conveyed a depth of understanding and formed a reassuring and caring connection with the patient. We paused the scenario, and when we invited students to reflect on what had taken place, a story was shared.

The student who had played the doctor related a story of how a former partner had made light of a friend's cry for help and the friend's subsequent suicide two weeks later. As a community of learners, we shared a contemplative moment of silence. A collaborative, reflective discussion ensued that supported the value of making meaning of difficult experiences and, in particular, doing so in the context of a supportive community. The students touched on how we live, act, and respond to others through our own personal narratives, and they emphasized the value of being aware of the personal frames of understanding through which we contextualize our encounters. These insights occurred given the students' willingness to invest in the imaginative reality created and the continuously emerging, developmental opportunities that are found in the context of a collaborative learning involving clinician learners and an artist-educator.

Fred Newman and Lois Holzman propose that development is continuously emergent, involving movement "from fixed mental states and identities to relational possibilities with others."[2] Development involves a shift from knowing to learning. How we engage with others, the life-world and structures in which we are immersed, displays our relationally responsive understandings. We are continuing to explore ways in which improvisational structures of theater-based engagement can foster a heightened understanding of relational processes and can also help promote the development of a sense of community among our learners. We offer medical students a stage on which to try out and reflect on their relationally responsive understandings; over the past five years, almost two hundred students have completed the elective. With respect to the next step in our evolution, an ongoing question is how we might incorporate performative reflection within the core curriculum. We look to our graduates and faculty for their inspiration!

NOTES

1. Mikhail M. Bakhtin, *The Dialogic Imagination: Four Essays,* ed. Michael Holquist, trans. Caryl Emerson and Michael Holquist (Austin, TX: Univ. of Texas Press, 1981).
2. Fred Newman and Lois Holzman, *The End of Knowing: A New Developmental Way of Learning* (London: Routledge, 1997), 131.

The Challenges of Effective Student Reflection in a Predoctoral Dental Communication Simulation Course

MARK SCARBECZ AND MARCIA S. SEEBERG

Communication skills are associated with practice success in dentistry. The Commission on Dental Accreditation expects dental graduates to be competent in their use of communication skills to effectively address patient needs. Surveys of dentists in the United States show that general dentists, and especially younger dentists, underutilize their communication skills. In 2011, the University of Tennessee College of Dentistry developed a simulation course titled Patient-Centered Dentistry (PCD) aimed at helping students develop effective relationship and communication skills. In this essay, we describe the role of student reflection in the course.

In the course, following preparation sessions using a team-based learning format,[1] third-year student-dentists interacted with standardized patients in clinical scenarios. A standardized patient is a person trained to portray a patient for the practice of communication and examination skills of a health-care provider. Each simulation scenario in PCD has an associated set of behavioral and communication competencies; students are observed in real time and assessed by the course directors, clinical dental faculty, and the standardized patient. There were six scenarios, ranging from "Initial Interview with a Patient" to "Delivering Bad News to Patients;" due to time constraints, each student participated in two different scenarios.

The underlying foundation for PCD is patient-centered care—care that embodies the qualities of empathy, unconditional positive regard, and congruence, or genuineness. Patient-centered care is associated with patient satisfaction and improved health outcomes.[2] Reflection may be defined as a set of "intellectual and affective activities in which individuals engage to explore their experiences in order to lead to new understandings and appreciations."[3] In PCD, students are offered several structured opportunities to reflect on their performance in the scenarios.

Immediately after completing the scenario, the course director asked the students to verbally reflect on their performance, relative to the simulation competencies and how they could improve. Feedback was provided by faculty observers and the standardized patient. The sessions were video-recorded, stored on a password-protected website, and made available to students. The opportunity to review their recorded performance allowed students to more accurately assess and reflect on their own performance. Students were also given their completed competency checklists to refer to when completing their reflection assignments.

Team debriefing presentations to their classmates offered another reflection opportunity. Students were preassigned to teams and participated in the same simulation. Teams were expected to show samples of video from their simulations, illustrating examples of best practices and areas that needed improvement, and to list concrete suggestions for communicating with patients in specific clinical situations. The team presentation allowed students who did not participate in a given simulation to learn from their classmates' experiences.

The final required reflection component was a written paper that was graded. Students were asked to consider what they did well during their simulation, how they could improve, and how they could apply the lessons learned to their clinical practice. Students were expected to base their reflection on the simulation competencies as well as on instructor feedback and to use critical thinking skills to constructively critique their performance.

Despite substantial variation in performance, many students thought they did "OK" immediately following their simulations. Students may overestimate their competence for two reasons. First, we required students to multitask: perform in their simulation, attend to the standardized patient and the competencies, and assess their own performance—all in real time. This may hinder accurate self-reflection. Second, because most dental students have an established record of academic success, the "Lake Wobegon" effect may lead many students to already think of themselves as "above average" communicators. For students who were able to critically assess their performance, the initial reflection provided the opportunity to "save face" and discuss the competencies they missed in a nonthreatening environment.

The inability of many students to accurately reflect on their performance immediately after a simulation demonstrated the value of allowing students to review their videos and reflect upon their experience, both individually and as team members. Student surveys confirm this. Using a 1–5 scale, where 1 = "Not at all useful" and 5 = "Extremely useful," the majority of students rated the following activities at three or greater: "preparing and presenting the team presentations" (66 percent), "watching their own video" (91 percent) and "[written] reflection assignment after the simulation" (60 percent).

The students' individual written reflections were more thoughtful than their postsimulation verbal reflections. Students had the time to review their video and instructor feedback, and our questions (hopefully) stimulated students to think critically about their communication skills. However, although it was a graded assignment, we observed wide variation in the quality of the written reflections. We judged the team-based reflection to be a more valuable experience for the students than the written reflection for several reasons. First, students appreciated that their fellow students had a range of strengths and weaknesses, some of which were similar to their own. This commonality of experience may have helped to foster our students' awareness of their own emerging professional identity and their commitment to patient-centered care. Second, all students in a team were in the same boat, having participated in the same simulation. Whereas solitary reflection may be subject to many common cognitive biases, the team reflection may have led students to honestly discuss their strengths and weaknesses with one another in a nonthreatening environment. Third, one of the primary goals of team-based learning is for students to learn from each other. Team-based reflection may have helped the students to appreciate the many different approaches for effective patient-centered communication—that students could be successful in different ways. Fourth, students enjoyed the presentations; 80 percent of the class rated watching the team presentations at 3 or higher in usefulness. We believe team-based reflection provides an innovative and unique approach to reflection in health science education.

We found applying reliable and valid standards for grading reflection assignments to be a challenge. We dealt with this issue by developing very specific objectives for the assignments. Students' reflections were expected to discuss behavioral competencies, specific ways to improve performance, and how to apply patient-centered care to clinical dental practice. However, we did not use a specific grading rubric to ascertain whether a student met these objectives. We used a small number of grading categories (good, fair, poor) and relied on our judgment and intuitive sense of whether the objectives had been met. Our experience suggests that considerable reflective capacity is required from course directors in crafting objectives and evaluating assignments and that some level of subjectivity is inherent to the process of grading student reflections.

We have also wondered if some form of remediation may be beneficial for students who continue to struggle with patient communication during their clinical years of dental school. What form that remediation may take and how to fit remediation into an already overcrowded dental curriculum are unresolved issues.

Last, we do not know if students have applied the lessons from PCD to actual patient care during their clinical (third and fourth) years of dental school. Anecdotal feedback from students who completed the PCD course has generally been positive. Their enthusiastic descriptions of how they use communication skills while treating patients in the College of Dentistry suggest that many students have internalized the lessons of the course. We hope that the benefits of the course continue to extend to students beyond graduation and into their clinical practices.

NOTES

1. Larry K. Michaelsen, Dean X. Parmelee, Kathryn K. McMahon, and Ruth E. Levine, eds., *Team-based Learning for Health Professions Education: A Guide to Using Small Groups for Improving Learning* (Sterling, VA: Stylus Publishing LCC, 2008).
2. Christophe Bedos and Christine Loignon, "Patient-Centred Approaches: New Models for New Challenges," *Journal of the Canadian Dental Association* 77 (2011): b88, www.jcda.ca/article/b88.
3. David Boud, Rosemary Keogh, and David Walker, eds., *Reflection: Turning Experience into Learning* (Oxon, UK: Routledge, 1985), 3.

Music as Metaphor to Teach Transformation in Nursing Education

OLIVE YONGE, JOANNE K. OLSON, AND SYLVIA BARTON

As educators, we seek to create meaningful and lasting educational experiences that provoke new insights and ways of thinking about our profession. *Creativity, imagination,* and *inspiration* are merely educational buzzwords unless students can experience them firsthand. This essay describes the use of music in the classroom as a metaphor for transformation—yet another tiresome cant in our profession, but one we wish to reclaim for its original sense of lasting and profound change. *Transformation* is an easy word to bandy about, yet a difficult concept to convey in a seminar. This recognition, together with the desire to engage our students on a more affective and reflective level, drove us to jettison words, and worlds, together in a graduate course focusing on leadership.

Music is a core human experience. Few of us will never experience live music or fail to appreciate its significance as nonverbal communication, even if we are not always trolling for implicit messages. To our good fortune, we are acquainted with a highly accomplished violin and piano duo, Grace Miazga and Samantha Semler (the latter composed a work performed by the Edmonton symphony), both game enough to perform in a highly unconventional setting. The students were informed that our class would be held in a public area around a grand piano.

Recognizing that music and other arts-based teaching activities can help students gain a fresh perspective of classroom concepts, the guiding aim of the session was to provide our students with an experience that would help them to rethink the meaning of leadership through a different modality. Prior to the class, students were provided with a reading list, learning objectives, and study questions designed to guide them in reflecting on what they were learning. The specific learning objectives guiding the session were (1) to reflect on the concepts of leadership and transformation through music, (2) to consider how the arts can be integrated with nursing education, (3) to appreciate the talent that exists in our own midst, and (4) to enjoy learning in different ways.

The students were asked to consider several questions:

- What evidence is there that the arts, in this case music, lead to transformational learning?
- How will you integrate this musical performance as part of the course content?
- What are the risks and benefits of drawing from the arts for learning in other domains?
- What is the value of having a live performance versus a DVD?
- What is the role of metaphor when learning?[1]

Grace and Samantha started the class by playing "Amazing Grace." After playing the melody once, they improvised over the song's chords for several minutes. This illustrated how foundational knowledge (or in this case, the harmonic pattern) supplies building blocks for the exploration of new opportunities and perspectives—an object lesson in transformative practice. The students responded with nods, and some commented on the beauty of the piece. One student was moved to tears.

The two selections that followed were original compositions. The second was based on dissonance, chosen to reflect the tension of dealing with new knowledge and the energy of two entities impelling each other forward. The last piece provided a study in resolution, engagement, and celebration; Samantha continuously swept her hands over the entire keyboard, every note played to the delight of everyone present. After each selection, we asked the students how the music affected them and what insights they were formulating as they listened.

A professor from the Faculty of Medicine & Dentistry, who took part as a guest observer, remarked that discord resolving to harmony reminded her to be respectful of the parents of children with HIV she cared for and to listen carefully to their words. Just as the violin and the piano worked together to create a musical relationship, so too must doctors work with their patients. This inspired a few students to comment on potential links between music and their own clinical experiences. Afterward the mood was subdued. It was only the second of thirteen class sessions, and we wondered if we had managed only to bewilder the entire class.

It turned out to be the tipping point of the course—the point when teachers know they have won the students' trust and everyone feels the learning environment is safe. The seminars blossomed like a rose as the students employed other art-based strategies to explore issues related to nursing. "My favorite class," wrote one student in her final course evaluation, "was when the musicians came . . . I realized that my passion is nursing. In some ways, nursing enables me to speak [like music] because it is through nursing that I am able to express myself." The experience proved transformative in other ways, no less pleasing. More than one student inquired afterward, "Where do I get tickets to the symphony?"

The authors would like to acknowledge Grace Miazga and Samantha Semler for their musical performance and helping to develop this idea. This creative work was supported by Dr. Yonge's Vargo Teaching Chair.

NOTE

1. Alexander M. Clark et al., "What Football Teaches Us about Researching Complex Health Interventions," *British Medical Journal* 345 (2012): e8316, http://dx.doi.org/10.1136/bmj.e8316; Brenda L. Whitman and Wanda J. Rose, "Using Art to Express a Personal Philosophy of Nursing," *Nurse Educator* 28 (2003): 166–69.

Body Language

MAREN BATALDEN, CHRISTINA PHAM, RACHAEL BEDARD,
AND ELIZABETH GAUFBERG

As a physician, I work with bodies. Other people's bodies. I think about them. I read about them. I talk about them. I feel them. I listen to them. I smell them. I look at them—with my naked eyes and with the aid of all kinds of sophisticated X-ray vision. My own body, ironically, I usually ignore. My training and the relentless pace of work have actually honed my skills in ignoring my body. I learn to keep going even though I am tired; I learn to eat lunch while standing in the elevator or walking between meetings; I learn to limit my fluid intake so I can avoid wasting time in the bathroom; I pay no heed to stiff muscles or nagging nausea. Most of the time, I take my body for granted. I regard it as a trustworthy, reliable vehicle for carrying around my all-important head.

Occasionally, a reflective practice session wakes me up to my body and its power. For the last few years, our residency programs at the Cambridge Health Alliance have successfully recruited young doctors who practice and teach yoga. Without too much fanfare, we have been able to turn the space and time previously known as "noon conference" into a "now and then" yoga class. We dim the lights, push aside the tables and chairs, take off our shoes and socks, and sit down. Before my eyes, the psychiatry intern I am supervising on the wards becomes my teacher. Her voice is calm, steady, encouraging. *Feel the breath as it enters your nose. Notice the temperature of the air as it passes through your nostrils. Let your abdomen expand with your breath* ... We reach up, we bend low, we stretch and twist, we hold postures and maintain balance. Over the course of thirty minutes, I feel my center of gravity shifting from my head to my body. After the session, I feel good—more relaxed, more patient, more open, kinder somehow. I see a glimpse of what might be possible if I came to work with my whole self—mind *and* body.

A second reflective noontime session invites my body in a different way. An internal medicine resident with an avocation for Indian folk dance teaches a Bhangra class. Again, we move the tables and chairs to open the floor. He connects his iPod to speakers and the bold rhythm of the music transforms the space. The movements are gymnastic—leaping and turning, knees bouncing, arms pumping. We are breathless and sweaty by the end of the hour and full of joy. The opportunity to play together physically (with an accompanying soundtrack!) simultaneously binds us to one another and frees us from our usual professional restraint. We put our white coats back on and return to the wards somehow changed—happier, more resilient, incrementally more aware of the difference between health and the absence of disease, a little more inclined to connect to our patients as human beings.

In a third reflective noontime session, we engage our bodies yet again. As before, a resident steps in to teach. With her husband as co-facilitator, she leads a ballroom dance workshop. As we practice partnering with one another in dance exercises, we think explicitly about applying these lessons to the partnerships we build with patients. We close our eyes, place our palms against the palms of a partner, and move around the room, taking turns playing the role of follower and leader. Complexity increases as we hold each other in different ways, practice turns, learn new step patterns, and add rhythm.

The wisdom that emerges from the conversation that follows feels profound. What does doctoring have to learn from dancing? We observe that partnering—in dance and in doctoring—is governed by etiquette. As a dancer dances for his or her partner, so too the doctor doctors for his or her patient. In both dancing and doctoring, respect for the partner is paramount, and the partner's pleasure and comfort is always a fundamental goal. The first step in both dancing and doctoring, we notice, is to establish a solid connection. In dancing, partners establish the connection by achieving a careful balance between push and pull forces of hands and bodies. In doctoring, the connection is constructed with words, with the spaces between words, and with eye contact, posture, and gesture. Both centers of gravity come to play. Without this established base of connection, partnerships in both dance and doctoring fail.

In the best and most responsive relationships in dance and in doctoring, partners take turns playing the roles of leader and follower. They switch roles with grace and intentionality. Experienced dance partners signal major changes in direction or momentum with subtle modifications in the pressure of a hand or the proximity of a foot. Clear, succinct communication between partners on the dance floor facilitates confidence and safety and creates joy and beauty. What would health care look like if doctors and patients partnered like two people on a dance floor? What music would play? Where might doctors and patients take dancing lessons? In each of these sessions, I encounter my body. My body teaches me; it grounds and inspires me; it connects me to the meaning of my work, to my colleagues, and to patients. It makes me reflect on what harm a "dis-embodied" healer or teacher who is on autopilot can potentially inflict on others. What a delightful surprise to discover—in the midst of all of this work attending to the bodies of others—I have had my own with me all along.

PART 4

Learning from Patients and Clients

On Becoming Impolite

Learning to Make the Most of Collisions

JONATHAN BOLTON

On the wall of a social worker I visited in North Dakota was a sign: "Never waste a crisis." Crises come in different sizes; they are all potentially useful to the clinician and teacher. The kinds of small crises I will explore Schön called a "surprise," Garfinkel called a "breach" of expected norms of behavior, and Goffman called a "rupture" in how the participants are defining a social situation.[1] Instead, I will borrow Havens's term *collision,* which contains some of the meanings of the other terms but conveys better the sense of two people "stumbling against each other," which I take to be central to what we do when we work with students and patients.[2] The social worker's sign points out that meaning can, and should, be made from collisions. When we notice we have been involved in one, we should ask: What just happened? What have we just unwittingly discovered about the other person, and about ourselves, as a result of this collision? How do we make the most of a collision, without too quickly fixing it? And, how do we teach our students to notice and make use of collisions?

What is a collision? In a collision, one party is surprised, sometimes hurt; the other party may also experience discomfort or may not even notice. A collision challenges the assumption of a shared understanding and the taken-for-grantedness on which our everyday routines rely. It exposes an unacknowledged difference between the two participants to a situation. A collision might be a failure of expectation, a slight, a misunderstanding, or misattribution; one person might unintentionally kick over a stone and reveal unimagined pain, fear, or shame beneath. We might notice a collision when a patient gets angry when we ask seemingly routine questions, when a colleague picks a fight with us, when a resident goes quiet, or when a student bursts into tears.

165

Because they represent a break in the taken-for-grantedness, we often don't know what to do next. In *The Presentation of Self in Everyday Life,* Goffman describes how participants to a situation will employ tact and politeness to contain and limit the spread of the collision. We might laugh it off with a joke, apologize, or pretend we didn't notice. When we practice these defensive measures, we patch the situation back up. We don't open it up for examination, so we miss an opportunity to have a deeper understanding of the other person and ourselves.

To learn from a collision, one must first notice that one has occurred. Powerful people can be protected from learning from their collisions. For example, doctors are often protected from the consequences of their collisions when patients decide to look for another clinician rather than confront them. Teachers may not learn because students choose not to risk their grade. Vaillant describes how other people, "because of defects in genes, socialization, and maturation" have difficulty learning what society wishes to teach them, after they collide with agents of institutions, colleagues, friends, and lovers.[3]

The first thing that we notice after a collision is surprise. What we expected has not happened. It might be as small as noticing that a patient's response starts with "well, . . . " suggesting that they are about to make a dispreferred response. As linguists tell us, a *dispreferred* response to a yes/no question contains more information than a *preferred* response and might be made because the person agrees with the premise embedded in the question, out of politeness, avoidance, etc. The tiny "well" might indicate a hesitantly offered dissonant view.

After the surprise comes an emotion, possibly anger, frustration, or excitement. Cognitive therapists refer to these as "hot emotions," and they are often followed by action and reactions. We might feel the urge to flee to higher ground, to fight, to pathologize the other, to explain away the situation. How we do respond to the surprise and to these emotions influences how open we are to learning from the collision. We have to be open to hear what Schön called the "back talk" of the collision. We have to be prepared to care, to listen, to explore. This requires that we first "withstand and confirm" the collision, and keep it open for exploration.[4] This takes emotional work and, for most of us, training.

How do we encourage our trainees to first notice and then make use of collisions? Training a student to remain alive to the momentousness of a failure of expectation and to resist too quickly of engaging in "repair work" (by apology or tact)—or of too quickly criticizing the patient—is not easy. It goes against the grain of a person's upbringing. And it seems to contradict the "customer service" approach to "health-care delivery"—that is, the ethic encouraged by our institutions.

Unless the teacher or supervisor is present as the collision occurs, he or she may not know that one ever happened. The student might feel ashamed and fail to mention it or mention it only obliquely and then somehow blame the patient. The teacher must be alert to the collisions these evasions might be hiding, and be prepared to stop the forward action of the student's report, rewind it, and go through the episode frame by frame. The sort of fine-grain analysis required to unpack a collision is often difficult when the source of information about it is retrospective, thematic, and guarded. For this reason, audio- or videotaping sessions with patients allows analysis of microexchanges and provides a way in to difficult or surprising moments.

Medical students and residents are quick learners: they learn to do what they are trained to do and what they observe their teachers doing. If the attending punishes the student for allowing "a consent" to be anything more than a formality, then the student learns not to allow the patient to ask too many questions about their understanding and their fears about the procedure.

Unless the teacher models how to make use of a collision, the student may assume it is just another good idea that has no place in the actual practice. The teacher will find opportunities to model when the student is observing the teacher interact with a patient. The teacher may model the method by examining collisions as they occur in the relationship with the student. By asking in a relaxed manner, "What just happened between us?" the teacher shows the student how to withstand and examine a collision. It shows how the inhibiting urges to be polite or protective can be put aside in the service of understanding and a closer alliance.

If the teacher can encourage the student to see clinical and educational interactions as something like a game in which the doctor and patient, or teacher and student, are players, then interaction becomes a series of moves and countermoves, rather than interrogations and advice. The student is then asked to make miniprojections about the patient's next move or statement. The student gets immediate feedback as the projection is accurate or not, in which case the student may be out of empathic attunement or a collision may have occurred.[5] By paying attention to each turn and counterturn, students can be sensitized to signs of hesitation (for example, the "well, . . ." or slow agreement, crossed arms or a physical turn away from the clinician, eyes turned downward or away), or a too quick agreement, either of which may signal a gap or a difference of opinion. Then, the student is encouraged to consider whether or not to stop the process and explore what might have just happened between them.

Elvin Semrad, the famous psychiatric educator, famously said of our job as teachers, "You have to help the resident not to go dead."[6] Discouraging the residents from too quickly applying standardized solutions to standardized problems, and from being too polite in avoiding the examination of the fear, anger, disorientation, and disappointment that are contained within each collision can be one of our most important contributions to their development as alive and human physicians.

NOTES

1. Donald Schön, *Educating the Reflective Practitioner* (San Francisco, CA: John Wiley and Sons, 1987); Harold Garfinkel, *Studies in Ethnomethodology* (Englewood Cliffs, NJ: Prentice-Hall, 1967); Erving Goffman, *The Presentation of Self in Everyday Life* (Garden City, NY: Doubleday, 1959).

2. Leston Havens, "The Best Kept Secret: How to Form an Effective Alliance," *Harvard Review of Psychiatry* 12 (2004): 56–62.

3. George E. Vaillant, "The Beginning of Wisdom Is Never Calling a Patient a Borderline; or, the Clinical Management of Immature Defenses in the Treatment of Individuals with Personality Disorders," *The Journal of Psychotherapy Practice and Research* 1 (1992): 84.

4. Havens, "The Best Kept Secret."

5. Ibid.

6. Susan Rako and Harvey Mazer, *Semrad: The Heart of a Therapist* (Northvale, NJ: Jason Aronson, 1980).

Incorporating Patients' Voices in
Health Professional Education

WENDY A. HALL, SEEMA SHAH, LISA MARIE STERR,
AND SUE MACDONALD

The question of reflection in teaching is constantly revisited by those involved in the business of education. Participants come from many viewpoints. In our health education innovation, participants (patients, faculty, and students from the University of British Columbia, and a health-care provider from a community-based agency) joined together to develop a community-led interdisciplinary workshop for health science students. We subscribe to Jean Lave and Etienne Wenger's view of learning as a situated activity in which learners participate in communities of practice to master knowledge and skill.[1] To help learners become full participants in sociocultural practice that puts the patient at the center of all activities, we wanted to develop a model to bring students and patients together so that patients' voices were privileged. Patients' perspectives are vital to health-care providers' education because of their direct experience with illness. Moreover, at a time when professional collaboration is considered essential to responding to health-care complexity, we aimed to challenge students to reflect on changing the cultures of health-care education in the area of mental health. We were aware that interdisciplinary training components in mental health are limited, but interdisciplinary functioning at work is central.[2]

Our workshop centered on patients as community educators. The other team members provided support for their activities. We developed two interactive teaching approaches that elicited embodied reflection. One community educator adapted a story about depression as an unwanted companion by changing the story to a script;[3] five students were recruited from the group attending the workshop to act the scripted parts. The community educator led the play and explained the process to the students. After the reading in the first workshop (about fifteen minutes), the community educator shared insights about the play, used specific life examples, and helped students debrief about their feelings regarding challenges experienced with mental health problems in interdisciplinary patient-centered exchanges (again, about fifteen minutes). A story written by Krahn provided an opportunity to share patients' voices without putting patients in the difficult position of sharing personal narratives, which can result in feelings of threat and exposure.[4] It also created a distance from the educator leading the workshop that permitted students to be honest about their feelings and reactions to the workshop activities.

The second activity included in the workshop was a game show, "A Day in the Life." This activity, developed by the second community educator, was intended to demonstrate to students how extensively mental illness can negatively affect everyday living activities. In the activity, the focus was on dislocation, specifically in the context of the students' lives. The game involved two volunteer students recording their schedules for the preceding day, or whatever recent day was typical. As the students described an activity occurring at a particular time during the day, the second community educator drew cards like a game show host to indicate which life adjustments the students had to make due to their mental illness. If their activities were dislocated, they lost points. For example, the cards dictated that the students were unable to sleep one night, were unable to get out of bed the next morning, and had to drop two classes. We wanted students to experience the limits created by mental illness. A winner of the game was selected based on points. Following the game, the community educator led the discussion with the volunteer students and the rest of the group (thirteen students in total) about the similarity between the life adjustments in the game and in real-life experience and invited the students to share feelings elicited by the activity and their views of disciplinary contributions to the care of patients with mental illness. The length of the session was twenty-five minutes.

After we reflected on our learning from the first workshop, we offered the workshop format with both of the approaches described above on a second occasion. On the basis of students' reactions, we created more opportunities for them to reflect on-site. Students were asked to take two minutes to silently consider their thoughts and feelings following each activity. Students next moved into small interdisciplinary groups to discuss their insights about the potential effects of mental illness on one's self-worth, on practice, and on their specific role as health-care professionals. Students then moved into large groups to share their small-group insights for twenty minutes. We introduced ground rules for sharing at the beginning of the session, which included attention to confidentiality and respect.

Despite being offered in an evening format, the two workshops each attracted thirteen to fifteen students in the health sciences, including social work, nursing, occupational therapy, pharmacy, and dietetics. Students completed surveys about their experiences and some participated in follow-up interviews. Students indicated that they achieved our objectives, which were to recognize patients' expertise regarding their own illnesses and lives, to appreciate human-to-human experience (for example, empathy), and to describe the effects of stigma. We envision this as providing opportunities for full interdisciplinary dialogue that supported students in becoming reflective practitioners. The impacts are limited because the sessions were extracurricular and required students to commit an evening. Moving workshops into regular curricula, with the emphasis on the humanities, has the potential to take student reflection to another level and change the way students think about patients as the center of their practice.

NOTES

1. Jean Lave and Etienne Wenger, *Situated Learning: Legitimate Peripheral Participation* (Cambridge, MA: Cambridge Univ. Press, 1991).
2. Pippa Hall and Lynda Weaver, "Interdisciplinary Education and Teamwork: A Long and Winding Road," *Medical Education* 35 (2001): 867–75.
3. Ruth Krahn, "Unwanted Companion," in *Study in Grey: Women Writing about Depression*, ed. Wynne M. Edwards and Shirley A. Serviss (Edmonton, Alberta: Rowan Books, 1999), 40–53.
4. Ibid.

"What Ails You?"

Reflections on Compassion

ULRICH TEUCHER AND MARCEL D'EON

A timeless example of a tale of reflexivity in matters of health is the medieval romance *Parzival* by Wolfgang von Eschenbach, later refashioned into opera by Wagner, a painting by Anselm Kiefer, a ballet by John Neumeier, and many other artistic emulations. At its center is the coming-of-age story of the young apprentice knight, Parzival, who, at first, fails to ask his seriously ill king Anfortas, "What ails you?" In order to overcome his lack of reflexivity, Parzival will first have to gain life experience, win and lose some battles, fall in and out of love, and, in short, come to understand and reflect on his limitations, vulnerabilities, and own mortality. A matured Parzival will grasp the empathetic and ethical weight of asking the three crucial words not as a matter of convention but as indeed a moral commitment to solidarity based on mutual vulnerability.[1] In Neumeier's ballet, this act is symbolized by a grown-up Parzival offering his last shirt to the ailing Anfortas.

In a way, approaching reflexivity through words as well as gestures has informed how both of us have conceived teaching our Patient Narrative seminars in the College of Medicine at the University of Saskatchewan. Since their inception over three years ago, these seminars for credit have been bringing together every year a new interprofessional cohort, made up of fifty to sixty first- and second-year students, typically from pharmacy, nutrition, nursing, medicine, and general health sciences, meeting about five times a year. At each seminar, those attending divide into small interprofessional groups of four to six members, generally from different health disciplines so that students engage with as many interprofessional perspectives as possible. The main rationale and background of the Patient Narrative seminar series is made available to participants on a university website and introduced in abbreviated form for any newcomers at the beginning of each seminar meeting.

Generally, our vision for the seminars arises from the insight that young health-care students often enter their studies with unbridled idealism and heroism, wanting to work with people and help others. After a few terms of being inundated with health scientific course materials and data, many students are well on their way to perfecting symptom recognition and management and all aspects of cure—but many have lost sight of basic human care. Moreover, they may have become overwhelmed and begun to retreat from the sheer magnitude of patient suffering in their daily routines in some parts of health care. This has been referred to by the late family doctor Miriam Divinsky, and bemoaned in many personal patient accounts, as an "empathic failure."[2] In our own approach, we have taken many of our cues from Rita Charon's Narrative Medicine seminars at Columbia University, including the two-part structure of the seminars, beginning each seminar with some form of presentation (taking up the first half of each seminar), to be followed in the second half with some reflective tasks for participants. Observations and feedback are then shared by each group with the entire cohort. Our main objective is to present participants at each seminar with a sample patient's experience with illness in our health-care system that, after discussion in groups and a short question-and-answer period for the whole cohort, leads to the second part of the seminar, in which participants may reflect within their small groups on their own or others' experiences of illness.

Participants are encouraged to reflect by writing a paragraph and formulating their thoughts using the first-person "I," since writing in the first person can take reflection to a much more personal level. Many participants comment on the effectiveness of this writing task. However, we have also found that many participants do not like writing reflective accounts more than once. Instead, many appreciate and indeed prefer live patient presentations, in which they can ask questions of the presenters, exchange personal reflections in small groups, and share final short points of interest with the entire cohort. We have therefore varied the format of each seminar, providing personal accounts in different genres or presenting speakers with different health problems or disabilities.

Thus, we have been inviting, among others, a quadriplegic who faced stigmatization for giving birth to children; an aboriginal person who spoke about her experience with organ donations and different cultural perspectives regarding our health-care system; community volunteers with mental health problems (for example, schizophrenia, bipolar disorder, anxiety); and caregivers, family members, pharmacists, spiritual care providers, hospice workers, and health professionals. We have also presented slide shows of art (including sculptures, drawings, paintings, installations) by patients with such conditions as epilepsy, stroke, Alzheimer's, and cancer. In addition, we have used texts (including a poem by Patricia Blondal about her cancer diagnosis)[3], short personal accounts of persons with serious chronic illnesses,[4] and case discussions involving the spiritual care needs of people living with serious illness.

In the coming term, we hope to invite patients with other types of illnesses, organize a panel with a range of health professionals to discuss the role of empathy in health care, and feature an executive from a funeral home speaking about services and family involvement after the death of a loved one. In addition, we would like to invite a local group of volunteers who perform a self-written theatrical piece on problems of life and care with lymphedema. The presentations, small-group discussions, and debriefings with the full cohort typically have been raising a great variety of health-care–related questions and themes, including those of professional identity formation; the importance of cure versus care; person- and family-centered care; the roles of ethnicity, gender, and disability in patient care; access problems in disability; and much more. A recurring theme in the discussions and debriefings among patients and health-care providers is the fear of death and dying.

When we began the seminar series more than three years ago, we had hoped to use a lot more writing tasks to encourage reflection. However, we have come to appreciate our participants' wishes for more live patient presentations ("Bring more patients in: seeing and hearing has much greater impact than reading a document," wrote one student) and small-group verbal reflections. Our participants' direct questions to our presenters and during the small-group discussions have consistently revealed high levels of reflection. ("Initially thought group work not beneficial but interesting to see all the different perspectives," wrote another). Other results from the seminar include the benefits of reflection ("I have gotten a deeper insight into what it is like to be a patient, as I myself have little to no experience in this area") and plans for action ("I feel I have a better understanding of how to provide compassionate and empathetic care in the future").

Perhaps Patient Narrative seminars involving actual patient presentations and group discussions provide a rich embodied experience of words, gestures, hesitations, silences, and moral questions that engage our students in reflection and invite and encourage them into a type of selfless action—whether (symbolically) sharing their last shirts, developing resilience, witnessing and bearing the suffering of others, or externalizing their perceptions in language. We invite them to connect to the real-life concerns of patients so that they can ask more easily, "What ails you?"

NOTES

1. Michael Susmov Sanatani, "The Anfortas Question," *Canadian Medical Association Journal* 182 (2010): 1268, www.ncbi.nlm.nih.gov/pmc/articles/PMC2917944/.
2. Miriam Divinsky, "Stories for Life: Introduction to Narrative Medicine," *Canadian Family Physician* 53 (2007): 203–5.
3. Patricia Blondal, "Untitled," in *The Winnipeg Connection: Writing Lives at Mid-Century,* ed. Birk Sproxton (Winnipeg, Manitoba: Prairie Fire Press, 2006), 296–303.
4. Personal accounts were based on interviews by Ulrich Teucher.

Preparing the Soil

Fostering Reflection and Transformation through Narratives in Medical Education

JULIE BLASZCZAK AND ARNO K. KUMAGAI

As physicians, we practice medicine to alleviate suffering and optimize health. As educators, our responsibility to our patients and to our profession is to pass on humanistic practices to the next generation of physicians. The dilemma that presents itself is how to introduce humanism—that is, an orientation that affirms human values and human beings—into medical training when this approach is often at odds with models of medical education where "hard science" is prioritized over "softer" subject matters. The understanding of the emotional burden of illness, for instance, cannot be taught by lectures or assessed by multiple-choice exams; instead, it must be reinforced as a lifelong, dynamic learning process. Education in humanistic practice requires methods of teaching and learning that differ from the expert-novice, competency-based approaches dictated by current trends or past traditions. This type of education calls for methods that foster perspective transformation rather than just acquisition of knowledge or skills. Approaches that enhance a reflective orientation toward medicine in which the needs and interests of the patient are placed front and center are also required.

So how might one go about "preparing the soil" for this type of transformation? At our institution, we have relied on the power of stories to prompt reflection and dialogue about the experience of illness and the personal, cultural, and societal dimensions of medical practice. The educational context of these efforts is the Family Centered Experience (FCE), a required, two-year undergraduate program created at the University of Michigan Medical School in the fall of 2003. In the FCE, pairs of preclinical students are matched with a volunteer family in the community who live with serious or chronic illness. The student pairs make periodic visits to the volunteers' homes for a series of discussions on topics such as the impact of illness on the patient and his or her family, the patient-physician relationship, stigma and illness, and breaking bad news. These visits offer an opportunity for students to listen to the volunteers tell their life stories as the volunteers and their families experience and navigate illness. This stimulates a broadening of a student's vision through perspective-taking and exploration of the "at home" meanings that individuals and their families give to these experiences.[1]

After each home visit, students gather in groups of ten to twelve to share insights from their visits in a safe, confidential space with clinician educators who are trained to facilitate exploration of sensitive topics. Through these interactive discussions, the student groups (which remain the same throughout the two-year program) reflect upon common themes that connect their volunteers' experiences—how stories of individuals fit into the greater context of society and culture and how the students' previous beliefs, assumptions, and biases have been challenged by reflecting on the narratives they have heard. Small-group discussions are supplemented by readings from literature, newspapers, anthropology, and cultural studies, as well as short preparatory writing assignments designed to enhance personal reflections on a variety of themes, including stigmatization and prejudice, power relations, and disparities in health care. At the end of their first year, students work in teams to create an interpretive project—a work of creative art that expresses the students' understanding of their volunteers' illness experience. In these "acts of interpretation," students use a variety of art forms to embody their reflections and articulate their new understandings of the patients' illness experience.[2]

In this context, learning is driven by the power of stories to broaden perspectives. By engaging in intimate, face-to-face conversations with individuals who are living with a chronic condition and with their families, in the privacy of their own homes, students may achieve a level of understanding of illness and suffering that is personal, highly nuanced, and deeply human. For instance, aspiring physicians can learn from lectures that sickle cell anemia causes chronic pain and acute "crises" due to abnormal rigidity of red cells that "sickle" under hypoxic conditions. However, as they watch their volunteer with sickle cell disease limp to the kitchen, or as they listen to her describe how many days of work she has missed due to frequent hospital stays, or how she is appalled that doctors often minimize her attempts to manage her suffering as "drug-seeking behavior," the student's understanding about the extent to which the disease reaches into all facets of the patient's life is deepened and given context. Hearing of an experience of humiliation, disrespect, or injustice may trigger a sense of moral outrage, which may lead to a commitment to work for societal change. In the intimacy of storytelling, empathy is enhanced through honoring personal relationships. Imagination is critical here, because many students come to medical school from positions of privilege in terms of good health, youth, education, and socioeconomic status. Stories may act to foster students' personal concern and moral imagination toward patients and their medical care that may persist long after the relationship is over. By placing oneself in the shoes of someone whose background, identity, and worldview may be vastly different from one's own, one engages in a type of learning that goes beyond lectures and situates medicine and its practice in social, historical, and human dimensions.

The narratives of those with chronic illness reveal embodied suffering. The stories that are told are often those of strength, courage, and optimism. But they can also involve anger, sadness, loss, and the absence of cure or tidy resolutions. In a biomedical culture that frequently teaches students to look for the "right answer" or to "weed out" "irrelevant" pieces of a patient's story in order to determine a diagnosis, giving students the opportunity to listen to an entire life story and allowing them to feel and reflect upon the emotions the events in the story evoke is a forceful reminder of the overarching goals of medicine. Furthermore, instead of attributing medical "failures" to individual pathology or noncompliance, illness narratives have the power to reveal social suffering and societal neglect or violence and prompt students to reflect on more broadly encompassing solutions.

Stories may also challenge perspectives through discomfort and surprise. Encountering a different experience, a different identity, or an entirely different way of looking at the world may provoke intense questioning and critical reflection on one's own values, beliefs, and assumptions. This "cognitive disequilibrium" may in turn act as the ground upon which perspective transformation occurs.[3] When used with caution and humanistic intent, stories also may avoid becoming mere spectacles for a simple cathartic release of emotion and instead offer the opportunity to bear witness to another's struggles. This act of bearing witness involves an acknowledgment of a responsibility on the part of the listener—either to search for the cause of the suffering or for its solution, and in doing so, prompts the listener to action. In practical terms, this means that by providing medical students an opportunity to witness the determination and resilience of individuals with chronic illness as they negotiate their way through an unwieldy and often unjust health-care system, narratives offer a chance for students not only to bear witness to the patient's sense of agency but also to foster a sense of their own.

It would be the height of educational hubris to suppose that medical school can "teach" the intangible qualities one needs to be a compassionate, reflective, patient-centered physician. After all, one of the effects of medical education—especially under the influence of the hidden curriculum—is a hardening of previously idealistic, compassionate attitudes of students during training. Instead, by inviting medical students to listen to the stories of individuals who live with chronic illness, one may provide students with a curricular space in which they may use the power of stories to fashion their own style of humanistic care that is an individual expression of personal and professional perspectives and values.

NOTES

We thank H. Avant and all those involved in the Family Centered Experience Program for their commitment to teaching and learning. We would also like to recognize The Arnold P. Gold Foundation which Student Summer Fellowship.

1. Arno K. Kumagai, "A Conceptual Framework for the Use of Illness Narratives in Medical Education," *Academic Medicine* 83 (2008): 653–58.
2. Arno K. Kumagai, "Perspective: Acts of Interpretation: A Philosophical Approach to Using Creative Arts in Medical Education," *Academic Medicine* 87 (2012): 1138–44.
3. Arno K. Kumagai and Monica L. Lypson, "Beyond Cultural Competence: Critical Consciousness, Social Justice, and Multicultural Education," *Academic Medicine* 84 (2009): 782–87.

Psychoanalytic Approaches to
Opening Reflective Practice

RON RUSKIN

A BUSY GP AND AN ANXIOUS PATIENT: MARK AND DAN

Mark, a hard-working but soft-spoken thirty-eight-year-old Asian university professor, arrives for follow-up at Dan's busy hospital office one evening in mid-November. Mark presents with headaches, muscle tension, and academic performance concerns. During their visit, Dan, a general practitioner, reviews Mark's history, completes a physical, and orders lab work. Mark feels stressed by course work and dismissed by his department head, who is a "bully." Dan, who is in his forties and married with three children, listens to Mark but also feels pressured to see his last patient, with her acutely ill daughter. Dan suggests starting Mark on an anxiety-reducing medication. As he leaves the office, Mark mutters that Dan is a pill pusher who doesn't care about patients. That night, after dinner, Dan puts his children to bed, chats with his wife, reviews lab reports, e-mail, and phone messages, and then reflects on his interaction with his patient Mark.

Open versus Closed Reflective Space: Dan feels irritated by Mark's comments but, rather than dismissing Mark as hostile, begins to reflect on his own actions and how these may have triggered Mark's anger. He realizes that he focused more on Mark's biomedical concerns than on his psychosocial concerns. As a GP hospital physician, Dan's primary role is to diagnose and treat illness with caring efficiency. Yet having experienced therapy himself, he begins to consider the value of bridging the psycho-bio-medical divide and creating an opportunity for reflection to better understand patients like Mark, who present with physical symptoms not clearly attributable to a biomedical condition.

The next day Dan reviews Mark's patient file and notes his recommendations that Mark participate in yoga, meditation, exercise regimens, and psychotherapy. Mark episodically attends fitness classes but is "too busy" to do more. Dan believes that Mark expresses mixed feelings regarding their doctor-patient relationship. Mark looks forward to his visits with Dan yet expresses frustration when his problems are unrelieved. Recalling the benefits of his own earlier therapy, Dan offers an hour to explore Mark's personal history and interpersonal relationships.

A Psychoanalytic Approach to Reflective Practice: Dan questions if there may be factors influencing Mark's behavior and symptoms that are not directly conscious, due to limited self-awareness or an unconscious conflict. Dan imagines that offering space and time to reflect with Mark may help him gain access to his subjective experiences and help him critically process and understand his unconscious conflicts. In the extended session he schedules with Mark, Dan learns that Mark's parents emigrated from Asia when he was a child and worked long hours in a corner store to support their growing family. Mark was raised by an anxious, overprotective grandmother who spoke little English. His parents deprived themselves to send him to private school and university. His hardworking father was critical and abusive when Mark did not stand first in his class. Mark experienced prejudice and bullying as a minority in his early years. During their session, Dan also learns that Mark has been engaged to a young woman from his community for four years. Mark is working overtime to complete a promotions package for university tenure. If Mark succeeds, he will be assured of a professorship with reasonable income and security. If he fails, Mark will receive a reduced salary that will put his marriage and life goals on hold. With this broader understanding, Dan can now more effectively grasp and reflectively formulate his patient's problems and conflicts.

Busy physicians often fail to fully explore or openly reflect on their patient's past experience and relationships and how they influence current issues. In addition, while the patient or physician may be aware of a presenting challenge or conflict (in this case, promotion and tenure), there are other conflicts that lie behind the presenting issues, embedded in the patient's fears and wishes, relationships, and past life. These conflicts are typically not directly brought to light unless the physician is willing to take time to critically inquire and reflectively explore these issues and help the patient gain access to and become aware of underlying connections related to their presenting concerns.

One does not need to be an analyst to use psychoanalytic principles—they have moved beyond Freud's consulting room to our cultural lexicon. For our purposes, two basic psychoanalytic principles are relevant: the existence of unconscious conflict and transference. Consider how Dan applies these two principles in reflective practice.

Since childhood Mark has struggled with paternal injunctions to academically succeed amidst fears of punishment and loss of parental love. The disturbing emotions he has experienced in relation to these unconscious conflicts have deeply influenced him and his sense of self. A thoughtful man, Mark is conflicted about active self-assertion (he was repeatedly bullied in primary school). Mark also bears unconscious resentment toward his authoritative father, whom he wishes to surpass. Mark expresses his unconscious conflict through bodily symptoms for which he can ask for help, rather than speaking openly about his vulnerability, which causes him intense shame and anxiety.

Transference is the term used to refer to the unconscious repetition of early experience with a significant other transferred onto the figure of a therapist.[1] Mark transferred his unconscious hostility toward authorities—his department head and also his doctor, for seeming to rebuff his needs for support and attention. Having engaged in a reflective space in the patient-doctor relationship using psychoanalytic principles, both participants (physician and patient) may reflect more openly on Mark's issues as they discuss next steps in treatment. *Countertransference,* the unconscious transference of the clinician's early experience to the patient, is considered below.[2]

A SOCIAL WORKER AND HER CLIENT: SANDRA AND EVA

Sandra, a recent graduate social worker, is employed in an agency where she works with Eva, a separated mother of a five-year-old daughter suffering from severe juvenile rheumatoid arthritis. Sandra meets with Eva to secure community support for her child's care. Soon she finds herself speaking to Eva several times a week by phone. Sandra helps Eva grocery shop, buys gifts for her daughter, and makes home visits.

Opening a Reflective Space: Sandra feels preoccupied with Eva. She discusses this case with her supervisor, who asks Sandra to reflect on her client overinvolvement. Why buy gifts for Eva's child? Why make unnecessary home visits? Her supervisor points out that Sandra's professional role was to offer counseling and guidance for community support. When she asks "Why are you 'mothering' Eva?" Sandra is at a loss. She feels she "needs" to help Eva but knows from training that she is overstepping a professional boundary. Following her supervisory meeting, Sandra realizes what she has known since childhood but failed to integrate in reflective awareness. Her younger sister suffered childhood leukemia and was overprotected by her family. When her sister died at the age of six, Sandra experienced deep sadness and loss, complicated by the realization that she was now an only child and possessed her sister's toys. Sandra struggled with unconscious conflicts about survivor guilt, greediness, and punishment. Her decision to become a social worker included "mothering" transference to those less fortunate. Her awareness of this prompts Sandra to open a space for reflective inquiry to enhance her own self-awareness and professional growth, facilitated by supervisory contact.

REFLECTIVE SPACE INFORMED

BY PSYCHOANALYTICAL PRINCIPLES

Engel argues that how health professionals approach treating patients is influenced "by the conceptual models in which their knowledge and experience is organized."[3] He maintains that health-care providers are largely unaware of the power such models exert on their thinking and behavior. According to Engel, in the biomedical model the ideal is to determine as quickly as possible the simplest explanation, preferably the diagnosis of a single disease, with all else regarded as "complications," "overlay," or otherwise irrelevant to the doctor's task. The biopsychosocial model, in contrast, considers not only biological evidence but also the relationship between patient and physician, the larger group, his or her family, work, friends, community, and culture, and also recognizes unconscious factors that may influence these relationships.

Within a biopsychosocial model, reflective practice informed by psychoanalytic principles can benefit both patients and health-care workers. A meaningful therapeutic connection developed in the reflective space that Dan created, helping to address Mark's performance anxiety. Opening a reflective supervisory space offered Sandra insights that were critical to both her personal and professional development.

NOTES

1. Sigmund Freud, "The Dynamics of Transference," in *Papers on Technique and Other Works,* trans. James Strachey, Vol. XII of *The Standard Edition of the Complete Psychological Works of Sigmund Freud* (London: Hogarth Press, 1956), 99–108.

2. Alex Tarnopolsky, "Teaching Countertransference," *Canadian Journal of Psychoanalysis* 3 (1995): 293–313.

3. George L. Engel, "The Clinical Application of the Biopsychosocial Model," in *The Biopsychosocial Approach: Past, Present, and Future,* ed. Richard M. Frankel, Timothy E. Quill, and Susan H. McDaniel (Rochester, NY: Boydell and Brewer, 2003), 1.

Nervous Laughter and Taboo Topics

Using Humor to Teach History-Taking Skills

CLAYTON J. BAKER

Few things are less amusing than an analysis of humor. Just as trying to explain a joke drains the comedy out of it, attempting to define and quantify what is "funny" tends to reduce the very notion of humor to a dull, intellectualized subject. Nevertheless, studying humor can have valuable uses in medical education. Used effectively, humor promotes candid reflection of one's strengths and weaknesses, and it can powerfully facilitate self-awareness in students developing clinical skills such as history taking. This essay gives examples of the use of humor in teaching medical history taking, while leaving the reader to decide what is funny and what is not.

The development of history-taking skills is one of the most important goals of clinical medical education. Unlike some other fundamental, skill-based components of medical practice, such as the physical examination, history taking has not yet been significantly supplanted by advanced technologies. A medical history still must be obtained the old-fashioned way: by question and answer between doctor and patient. It is relatively straightforward to learn the rudiments of the medical history, and most students arrive with adequate communication skills to obtain a basic medical history, once they learn what one entails and get some practice at it. However, subtleties abound in history taking, and in complex cases great skill can be needed to gather and discern key facts. Certain "taboo topics" can be particularly problematic. Sexual practices, drug use, mental illness, criminal history, and personal secrets are among the sensitive subjects that both inexperienced students and anxious patients often find difficult to discuss. Sometimes, both parties are so reluctant to address an uncomfortable topic that they strike a tacit bargain to omit it from the interview, a phenomenon I call the "collusion of noncommunication."

During a successful medical interview, at least two processes occur. First, the doctor gathers clinical information from the patient in the form of a medical history. Second, a therapeutic relationship develops. When a collusion of non-communication is present, both of these processes are undermined. If relevant issues go unexamined, important diagnostic information may be omitted; if both parties become aware that full, open communication is lacking, trust may suffer. Conversely, physicians who persist in the effort to obtain sensitive information but who lack the requisite skills may also fail. An awkward, amateurish, or un-reflective approach to history taking, driven by anxiety or inexperience, may fail to obtain key historical facts, while simultaneously alienating, angering, or distressing the patient. Again, the medical history and the therapeutic relation-ship suffer. Greater sophistication of technique and reflective self-awareness can remedy these problems. Humor can be used to help teach both.

One can learn from both the wise and the unwise. Indeed, the latter often teach more vividly and memorably. However, students will often reflexively distance themselves from bad examples that are presented as cautionary tales (for example, "Can you imagine someone actually doing that?" or "Thank goodness that's not how I work"). Humor can help students past this obstacle. When a bad example is presented in a comical, even over-the-top fashion, the learning points become easier to identify and less threatening to consider, and can then be broken down in a thoughtful, systematic, and self-reflective manner. After watching the ridiculously botched attempts at communication found in certain Monty Python sketches, medical students' typical first re-sponse is laughter. In the sketch "The Man with Three Buttocks,"[1] for example, John Cleese nervously minces, squirms, and cravenly evades the entire point of the interview. After watching the sketch, we ask our chuckling students, "Why are you laughing?" They correctly point out the interviewer's gawky, defensive body language, his hesitant, stuttering speech, and the long stream of silly, befuddling euphemisms (rump, derriere, posterior, sit-upon) that he uses before finally using a more direct anatomic term ("your buttocks"). Fair enough, we concede, but do you ever do any of these things yourselves? Do any of you see yourselves in the John Cleese character?

With proper nudging and a flicker of insight, the heart of the lesson ensues. It is surprising how much self-awareness students can gain by dissecting the particulars of a goofy, forty-year-old English comedy sketch. Comparing themselves to the caricatures on the screen, students realize how clumsy and counterproductive an unskilled or evasive approach to history taking can be. For example, one student recounted the time she danced around a sensi-tive question so gingerly that the patient told her just to write it down if she couldn't bear to ask it out loud. Students see in broad relief the ineffectiveness of excessive modesty and evasiveness when discussing sensitive topics with patients. They see firsthand, in an amusing and nonthreatening way, how they do not want to appear to their patients. Once the gaffes have been identified, the discussion turns to preventing them from occurring in the clinic. Students strategize on how difficult interviews might be more effectively conducted. Practical approaches to everything from choice of words to body language are examined, working toward the goal of developing a skilled, practiced approach to broaching uncomfortable topics with patients.

Humor can also serve as a powerful tool for students to reflect on and develop self-awareness of their own personal attitudes, idiosyncrasies, and biases. In another exercise, students read aloud from the comic essayist Ian Frazier's piece, "The Frankest Interview Yet." By turns they recite portions of the narrator's over-the-top account of his sexual history, which begins: "A: I was having sex. I had had sex previously, found that I enjoyed it, and so was having it again. With a sexual partner, I screwed all over the floor. Orgasms were multiple for the both of us. I took a lover, also. Plus I had a tryst with a fellow in the shower room of the old Grand Avenue Y. I turned an empty office at work into a snuggery, and made use of it."[2]

This narrative continues for four pages, incrementally upping the shock value for comic effect as it goes. Upon completion, and temporarily ignoring the snickers and guffaws that invariably accompany its recitation, the teacher directs students to summarize the narrative, in fifty words or fewer, into a sexual history fit for inclusion in a patient's chart. Students then read aloud their condensed, chart-worthy versions, identifying the editing work they have just done and how it alters the narrative. By necessity they condense and formalize it, but in the process other things happen to the narrative: it is by turns jargonized, sanitized, depersonalized, normalized, minimized, pathologized, and so on. And almost without exception, the humor has vanished.

When students describe their reactions both to reading this narrative aloud and to hearing someone else recite it to them, they typically confess that "I couldn't help laughing." We press them: "Why? What are some of the reasons people laugh? What are the reasons you laughed while reading, or being read, this piece?" Embarrassment, anxiety, discomfort, disbelief, or simply not knowing how else to respond—students offer all these as explanations. Students then reflect on what specific portions of the narrative evoked these feelings and how they may have responded to analogous encounters with real patients. Given the intentionally humorous tone of the narrative and the fact that this is an exercise rather than an actual patient encounter, there is a "safety in fiction" here. The students perceive that the stakes are lower and the latitude is greater, allowing them to reflect freely on the best approaches to such sensitive subjects. By reading an over-the-top, humorous piece like this, students realize that such words can be said aloud, such ideas can be expressed, and that anxiety, discomfort, and the impulse to laugh can be managed.

Furthermore, laughter can be understood for what it often is: a warning sign of sorts that a potentially difficult portion of the history has been reached. The fact is, sometimes patients do tell doctors some pretty extraordinary things. Students must learn to recognize and acknowledge their reactions so they trigger not a reflexive avoidance or an offensive utterance but rather a skilled, sensitive, and effective response to the patient's story. One should note what the use of humor in addressing difficult and sensitive topics in the medical history is not. It is not meant to teach medical students to become stand-up comics on the wards. Humor must never be used to mock or deride others, especially patients, in clinical situations. One must differentiate humor from scorn, and if one is feeling something akin to scorn, one must acknowledge such a reaction and why one is feeling it and manage it with the best interest of the patient in mind. Such reflective self-awareness is vital in clinical medicine and represents an additional benefit of studying humor as it pertains to the clinical encounter.

The practice of medicine, while often humorous, is not all fun and games. Humor may be a useful adjunct to developing reflective skills, but it is an adjunct. The standard communication style for doctors should remain a professional, serious, yet empathetic one. Still, in the right setting, we can learn from the funny stuff—hopefully without taking all the fun out of it.

NOTES

1. Monty Python, "The Man with Three Buttocks," accessed June 5, 2015, www.montypython.net/scripts/man3butt.php.
2. Ian Frazier, *Coyote v. Acme* (New York: Farrar, Strauss and Giroux, 1996).

A Structure for Reflection Using Home Visits

ROBERT J. BULIK

Initially, narrative medicine focused on using literature and writing to enhance student insight and reflection on the art of medicine.[1] However, students are now being asked to write about other kinds of content, their patients, and themselves. In some cases, the texts that students produce are used to assess student learning. The challenge inherent in assessing student writing is in developing a scoring rubric that adequately captures learning in relation to the objectives of the activity.

The Family Home Visit Program was implemented at our medical school through an AAMC/Hartford geriatric education grant and was designed to take students out into the community to interact with intergenerational families;[2] a reflective essay based on conversations with the family was one of the required activities following the visit. To achieve student (author) and faculty (rater) acceptance of this graded reflective assignment, we developed a scoring rubric that incorporated two key elements: student reflection on the family visit and an articulation of implications for future practice.

The organization and structure provided in directions to students for the reflective writing assignment is that of a short story. They are told to include an introduction (feelings and thoughts prior to the home visit), character (who was present and how each person contributed to answering questions from students), setting (socioeconomic and environmental description), plot (how the history—migration/immigration of this multigenerational—family evolved over time), and conclusion (reflections on the "story").

Students who write the essays report it useful to have a structure for the writing task, and faculty who grade the essays report similar appreciation for the organization. While there is no word count or page-length requirement, students are advised that essays will be scored overall as honors, high pass, pass, or fail; in addition to grades, we have evaluated student responses and found evidence of true transformational change in thinking for some students.[3] The weighting of each of the five sections of the essay can be course-specific and can aid faculty in determining how well students completed the assignment. Based on a 100-point scale, the conclusion is awarded a maximum of 35 points, with the remaining points allocated across the other four sections of the short story form. In writing the conclusion, students are specifically directed to reflect on how this community-based experience might influence them in their eventual practice. Finally, the use of the terms *short* and *story* to describe the structure implies that the essay should be focused and organized. The following two abstracted excerpts from a student's essay, used with permission, provide an example:

> Excerpt 1—Pre-visit thoughts: Discovering the age of the family members assigned to this task filled my mind with fore-drawn conclusions based on stereotypical geriatrics. I thought to myself of the old mothball smell and long drawn-out stories that accompanied a neglected house and decidedly unkempt façade. Having met only one of my grandparents, information on the more aged population came from television or simple interactions around hospitals. What struck me the most was that all the older individuals I met needed assistance of some kind.
>
> Excerpt 2—Post-visit thoughts: Mr. and Mrs. B are not geriatric patients. They are mothers, fathers, brothers, sisters, grandparents, and most importantly friends. The lives they have led and will continue to lead are not stereotypical. In fact, I hope someday I could sit in my big chair and look a pretentious medical student in the eye and tell him that I lived a happy life.

The reader should not only observe the selection of words that this medical student chose to use, but read the excerpts aloud and hear the difference in feeling, tone and tempo between the first segment and the second. When patients are encouraged to tell their stories and not just relate their symptoms, students learn to hear patients, thus creating a caring and healing environment within the doctor-patient relationship. The patient's story assignment is discussed and debriefed in small student groups, facilitated by faculty.

I believe that we need to teach students to reflect on the doctor-patient relationship in such a way that the patient is encouraged to tell a story that situates and contextualizes an illness or disease within the immediate or extended family. In practice, when physicians take a patient's history, we are asking that individual to "teach" us something about him- or herself—in essence, to tell us a story. Storytelling, as an instructional method, is perhaps the oldest known pedagogical approach in existence. However, the sharing of information is not the only goal of encouraging a patient to tell his or her story. Storytelling, because it creates a relationship between teller and listener, strengthens comprehension; elicits psychosocial, health maintenance, or prevention concerns; recognizes the impact of socioeconomic issues; and helps the physician understand relationships within the family and within a cultural context. Similarly, while sickness and disease do not occur in isolation, neither should we assume that healing happens in seclusion.

Reflecting on the family visit through the structure of a short story encourages students to think holistically about patients throughout their professional careers. In order to appreciate, or at least understand someone else's situation, we are sometimes advised to "walk a mile in that person's shoes." When we ask our medical students to conduct a family home visit, we hope they will come to appreciate the wide diversity of people and circumstances with which they will be working as practicing physicians—we are asking them to at least recognize the different "shoe sizes" that exist in all our culturally diverse communities.

Consequently, it is not the lecture or the small group problem or case-based scenario that will sufficiently challenge existing schema to foster a change in student beliefs about categories of patients. Nor is it the oral presentation of the differential diagnosis that a student makes to a preceptor that will confront and challenge an existing stereotype. In an oral case presentation, the verbal "self" never exists long enough to be reflected upon. Rather, it is the consequence of writing that transforms private thoughts into concrete text. Instead of chasing an elusive verbal representation of a thought pattern, reflection on the explicit written text can bring about transformational learning.

NOTES

1. Rita Charon, *Narrative Medicine: Honoring the Stories of Illness* (New York: Oxford Univ. Press, 2006).
2. Jack Mezirow, "Transformative Learning: Theory to Practice," *New Directions for Adult and Continuing Education* 74 (1997): 5–12.
3. Robert E. Beach, Debra A. Newell, and James S. Goodwin, "University of Texas Medical Branch at Galveston," *Academic Medicine* 79 (2004): S177–81.

PART 5

Ethics and Professionalism

Saying What We Mean

Using Reflection to Articulate Core Values

RACHAEL BEDARD, MAREN BATALDEN, AND
ELIZABETH GAUFBERG

I believe, first and above all, in being kind. I believe that the only thing that concretely matters is how you feel and how you make other people feel. I believe that it matters whether you are kind or unkind in every interaction, and I believe that you always have the choice to be kind. Second, I believe in a profound egalitarianism. Third, I am driven by a happy curiosity that feels essential to lifelong doctoring. Finally, I believe that in addition to promoting equality and to being kind and curious, the fourth essential task of the doctor is to be critical. Good doctoring requires the explicit practice of self-reflection—bringing insight and intention to every action.

As a second-year internal medicine resident, I (RB)* wrote these lines as part of an essay about what I believed was true about my doctoring practice. Being kind, empowering patients, being curious, being critical: these are the core values that define me as a physician. That these things are important may seem self-evident, but achieving this clarity about my professional priorities had been a process and continues to be one. One of my colleagues might articulate "scientific discovery, working in teams, feeling useful" as her core values; another might speak of the pleasure in constant intellectual challenge. Working from a place of intention, rather than as a series of reactions, requires knowing your own first principles. At the Cambridge Health Alliance (CHA), we have used the following three exercises to help residents articulate and reflect on their core values.

In the 1950s, Edward R. Murrow began hosting a series on National Public

---

*The initials refer to an author of this essay.

Radio (NPR) called *This I Believe.*[1] Famous people and nonfamous people were invited to write short personal essays expressing a statement of conviction and to read those essays on the radio. The objective of this project was to encourage individuals from disparate backgrounds to explore and share what was meaningful to them in a time when Murrow and his colleagues felt the world was becoming unmoored. As a second-year resident, I wrote a "This I Believe" essay of my own, which is excerpted in the first paragraph of this piece. Writing the essay was an invigorating, challenging exercise that helped me to know myself better as a young physician, to understand my purpose, and to develop my sense of professional integrity.

We subsequently developed a workshop for other residents and faculty based on this exercise. We began by listening to the wonderful essays of a few luminaries. Martha Graham, for example, wrote, "Then, there is the cultivation of the being. It is through this that the legends of the soul's journey are retold with all their gaiety and their tragedy and the bitterness and sweetness of living." Leonard Bernstein wrote, "I believe in people . . . One human figure on the slope of a mountain can make the whole mountain disappear for me." We asked workshop participants to listen with intention and be attentive to their own responses. Did participants find these voices compelling? Did the voices resonate? Did these voices inspire participants to write essays of their own? We gave participants a blank piece of paper, an opportunity to write, and some time to talk. Some participants shared thoughts on the values that guide their own approaches to the practice of medicine. Others reflected on the essays we had heard. The "This I Believe" exercise encourages individuals to craft personal essays that they may or may not choose to share with others.

Two other initiatives, both supported by the Arnold P. Gold Foundation, offer learners the opportunity to express first principles aloud and to connect explicitly as a community around core values. "Public Narrative" is a leadership practice that Marshall Ganz of the Kennedy School of Government at Harvard University developed based on his long personal history as an activist and community organizer. The practice of public narrative involves telling a story in three parts. The first part, the "Story of Self," describes a personal challenge in which the storyteller had to make an important choice that illustrates his or her core values. In the second part, the "Story of Us," the individual connects his or her core values with the shared core values and intentions of a larger community. In the third part, the "Story of Now," the teller calls his or her listeners to take specific action in this time and place.

This structured storytelling exercise can be used to build consensus in times of change and to help people who work together bond over what calls them to the work they do. We have used it as a team-building exercise in our primary care clinics and as a leadership development tool across our health-care system. The initial challenge, crafting a Story of Self that illustrates core values in a compelling narrative, invites participants to reflect deeply on the formative experiences of their own histories. If a facilitator is successful in creating a safe environment for sharing, telling these Stories of Self can be powerful in fostering a collective sense of understanding and shared purpose among members of a group.

Finally, we encourage reflection on core values by asking incoming interns to write an oath.[2] New internal medicine, psychiatry and transitional year interns, fresh from medical school, gather for orientation during the last week of June. After several icebreakers and exercises designed to help them get to know one another, we do a two-part session in which the group creates a collective professional oath. We begin by asking them to reflect on what oaths mean: What purpose do they serve? How do they connect us to one another? We ask participants to reflect on the principal relationships in a physician's life. To whom must physicians make promises? What promises do they make? Participants then work in small groups. Their conversations are honest, open-ended, and generative. Questions they have considered have also included: How should we feel about the tensions between our responsibilities to ourselves and to our patients? Are we making promises we can't keep? What standards do we hold as professionals, and what obligations do we have as private citizens? Over the course of the week, they refine and revise a single collection of promises to craft statements that they might include in a professional oath. At our hospital, serving a socioeconomically disadvantaged patient population, final draft oaths often include a commitment about the physician's duty to care for the underserved and need to advocate for systemic change, which reflects and reinforces the idealism and deep sense of purpose that motivates the trainees who choose to learn here. Our residents share their final draft with the wider CHA community at our year-end transition party. We revisit the oath with the group at the end of their internship to ask: What was surprising? What still feels important to you? What changes would you make if you were rewriting your oath now? Which promises were hard to keep?

Oath making, sharing stories of ourselves, and crafting expressions of belief all offer opportunities to reflect on our values, to name what calls us to this work, and to confirm what grounds us. We come to know ourselves better in this process of reflection; articulating a sense of purpose that allows us to work with greater authenticity and integrity. When we challenge learners to say what they mean, they do so with passion and nuance. As faculty, we participate alongside our trainees in these exercises and find them equally clarifying and transformative.

What North Stars guide you?

NOTES

This is the second of three related essays we have authored as co-facilitators of "Food for the Soul," a Cambridge Health Alliance (CHA) Medicine Residency reflective practice seminar. Collectively these essays describe the main organizing principles and several of the exercises used in this seminar.

1. This I Believe, Inc., "This I Believe: A Public Dialogue about Belief—One Essay at a Time," accessed June 2, 2015, http://thisibelieve.org.

2. Maren Batalden and Elizabeth Gaufberg, "Professional Promises," *Journal of Graduate Medical Education* 4 (2012): 269–70.

Reflective Time Capsules

J. DONALD BOUDREAU

Let us emancipate the student and give him time and opportunity for the cultivation of his mind, so that in his pupilage he shall not be a puppet in the hands
of others, but rather a self-relying and reflecting being.

—SIR WILLIAM OSLER

In 2005, McGill's Faculty of Medicine introduced a new curricular component
titled Physicianship. It is grounded in the belief that the primary mandate of
medicine is healing, while professionalism refers to the framework and structures adopted by physicians and society to deliver healing services. Details of the
educational blueprint of this curriculum have been described elsewhere.[1] Suffice
it to say, for the purposes of this essay, that a flagship course of the curriculum
has been what we call the Physician Apprenticeship. The apprenticeship's main
objectives are to assist students in their personal transition from layperson to
physician and to provide a safe environment for reflection upon the professionalization process. Students, in groups of six, are assigned to a mentor—a
clinician affiliated with the faculty. These mentors are given the name Osler
Fellows. One of the strategies developed to foster students' reflective abilities
was the "Physicianship Portfolio." This portfolio was expected to serve both as
a trigger and a repository for critical and thoughtful written reflections. The
Osler Fellows were asked to use the portfolio entries as vehicles for in-depth
discussions within their apprenticeship groups, touching on issues pertinent
to enculturation, personal change, and the medical school experience.

The portfolio was intended to be open-ended, adaptable, and flexible. Given
that few faculty members and students had prior experience with reflective

writing, the portfolio was crafted such that it included a menu of specific rec-ommendations. A few of the recommendations were linked to key events (for example, the White Coat Ceremony, the Commemorative Service for Donors of Bodies, the beginning of clerkships). They were educationally stage-specific; that is, it was assumed that sources for personal reflections would be more linked to patient encounters in the senior than junior years. The portfolio template included mandatory and optional entries. A few of the mandatory entries were to be shared between student and Osler Fellow. Most of the mandatory entries and all of the optional entries were to be read by the Osler Fellow exclusively at the student's invitation.

I will comment on two specific portfolio entries that were well received. I label these two writing exercises "Reflective Time Capsules." A time capsule is a container that holds objects, records, or texts that speak about current is-sues and describe hopes and aspirations for the future. They are often placed in special physical places, such as the cornerstone of a new building. There is an expectation that the time capsule will eventually be cracked open in order to reveal its messages. The Physicianship Portfolio incorporated two time capsules in its blueprint.

The first was called the "Secret Personal Message." It was described to students at registration and orientation to medical school as follows: "A memo—written to yourself at the beginning of the program—that speaks to any insights, hopes or fears concerning anything at this important transition point in your life. This message should be placed in a closed envelope and remain sealed until the end of the program."

The second was called the "Dear Me" letter. Students were expected to write this letter several days before the start of the clerkship rotations, rotations in which they are accorded substantial responsibility for patient care. The instruc-tions were:

> Write a brief letter (250–500 words) addressed to "Dear Me." This pre-clerk-ship letter should address any of the following: In what aspects do I feel most prepared and/or least prepared to begin clerkships? What aspects of clerkships are most exciting and/or most worrisome to me? What features of my personality do I want to be most evident to the patients for whom I will have responsibili-ties? What kind of impression do I want to leave my clinical supervisors? What do I want to emphasize in the first rotation? What are my personal goals for the next 12 months? It may help you to think of it as an autobiographical letter similar to the one you wrote for admission to medical school, except that in this instance it is an autobiographical letter for "admission" to clerkships.

Both time capsules were to be housed in the portfolio—a binder that was provided to each student by the faculty. The expectation was that students would open their "Secret Personal Message" one month before graduation. They were not required to discuss it in the context of the Physician Apprenticeship unless they wished to do so. The "Dear Me" letter, however, was to be reviewed in a one-on-one meeting, between the student and his or her Osler Fellow, three to four months into the clerkship. We know, based on privileged feedback from several Osler Fellows, that the "Dear Me" letters were reviewed occasionally, especially when students were struggling, and that they contributed to meaningful and supportive dialogues. We believe they have the potential to be of assistance by providing an entry for recognizing unmet needs, unrealized aspirations, and gaps between expectations and reality. (Additional research is required to substantiate this claim.)

In a subsequent year, the faculty attempted to reap additional benefits from the notion of time-activated reflections. Again it asked all students at the beginning of the clerkship year to compose a "Dear Me" letter. In this iteration, however, it instructed students to anonymize a copy of their letter and to deposit it in a cardboard box, similar to a ballot box, positioned at the front of the class. Confidentiality was guaranteed. This was conducted on the last day of the Introduction to Clerkship course. We have now embarked on this exercise annually for five years. Although we do not monitor who complies and who does not, the response rate has been consistently over 98 percent. None of the letters contain names, student numbers, or other markers that might result in identification. In a sense, the sealed box acts like a collective time capsule for an entire class.

We have analyzed the student reflections documented in the "Dear Me" letters collected in this manner and have found them useful. We have generally done so at the three-month mark into the clerkship year. In 2008, three main themes emerged. Most prominent were anxieties concerning clinical work (for example, making mistakes or wrong decisions and fear of unclear expectations or being left alone). The second was a perceived need to balance the professional and personal sides of life (being afraid of being submerged by medicine, not wanting to lose one's personality, and preserving time for sleep and pleasures). Lastly, there were issues relating to performance assessments (constant evaluations, concerns about looking stupid, coping with competitive environments, and needing to impress tutors) and the impact of all these on career planning. All in all, despite the salience of anxieties, the tone of the letters was generally positive and the concluding remarks often optimistic. These letters revealed a cohort of students who were intent on trusting their basic personalities and secure in the notion that their core humanity would constitute an unfailing lifeline during clerkships. These findings were then shared with the Osler Fellows at one of their regular faculty development workshops. It was suggested that they might wish to explore some of these issues with the students in their apprenticeship groups. Although the specific reflection could not be linked to any particular individual, the themes had arisen from the class and were thus imbued with an aura of authenticity. They served as multilayered triggers for ongoing reflections. The potential of reflective time capsules was fulfilled, albeit not exactly as originally planned.

The strategy of a time-activated reflection is not a novel idea. Allan Peterkin, referring to medical students' autobiographical letters, has suggested, "I think they should tuck the letter they wrote to get into med school in their journal as an antidote to cynicism."[2] Presumably, Peterkin assumed that students would retrieve these letters at some later point in time and use them to gauge which aspects of their core values and worldviews might have evolved and which might have endured. He did not refer to a time capsule per se, but it is implied. A critical feature of a time-activated reflection is that there is a built-in time gap. During this hiatus, it is inescapable that there will be a potential for changes in perspectives. Personal commentaries, packaged in time capsules, hold promise as a strategy for catalyzing and guiding post hoc reflections. They open up avenues for insights into personal maturation and professional identity formation.

NOTES

1. J. Donald Boudreau, Sylvia R. Cruess, and Richard L. Cruess, "Physicianship: Educating for Professionalism in the Post-Flexnarian Era," *Perspectives in Biology and Medicine* 54 (2011): 89–105.
2. Allan Peterkin, "White Coat Ceremonies: Not So White (or Black)?" *Atrium: The Report of the Northwestern Medical Humanities and Bioethics Program* 9 (2011): 24–26.

An Arts-Based Approach to Ethics Education in the Health Professions

ELIZABETH ANNE KINSELLA, SHANON PHELAN,
AND SUSAN BIDINOSTI

As a professor in a faculty of health sciences, whose scholarship focuses on ethics, reflection, and reflexivity in professional life; a professor with interests in reflexivity, ethics, and identity; and an artist and researcher interested in the intersections between the arts and health-care practice—we have come, over time, to be convinced of the power of the arts as a means to engage reflection in deep and meaningful ways in health professional education.

At Western University we offer a course titled Ethics and Professional Practice in Context in the second year of an entry to practice master's program for occupational therapists. Throughout the course, which spans two terms, students engage in reflection (individual, collective, and guided) on their own values, assumptions, and ethical commitments with the aim of deepening their capacity for moral agency and ethically based decision making in professional practice. For one of the course assignments, students have asked to develop an arts-based representation of ethical practice. The project was assigned in September and due in March. It has variously been worth 20 to 40 percent of students' final grade, and in some years it has been accompanied by a two-day exhibition in which students display their work along with a brief artist's statement. The exhibit, curated by students and the course instructor, is open to professors, staff, and students in the Faculty of Health Sciences.

Students are provided with the following instructions:

> The purpose of this project is to engage in reflection on the question, what does ethical practice mean to you? Each of you will have a unique response to this question. A range of possible mediums may be used to represent one's ethical stance through artistic means. You may choose to develop a 3-dimensional model,

a piece of visual art (such as a painting, collage, pen and ink drawing); literary works of art such as a collection of poetry, a dramatic performance or script, a short story. Be creative! Have fun with this.

In addition, students were required to complete three additional assignments:

- A 750- to 1,000-word paper that makes explicit the intended meaning, significance, and/or symbolism of the work, as well as insights garnered in the process of its construction. References may be used if they extend or illuminate the intended meaning of the project; however, they are not required.
- A short (one-paragraph) artist's statement on a separate page. The artist's statement provides a brief overview of the project.
- A one-page reflection on learning, responding to the question: "What, if anything, did you learn through the 'process' of completing this project?"

Students are encouraged to work with metaphors or symbols in their creative projects as a means to deepen their reflection and are reminded that the project is not about their skills as artists but rather about working with and reflecting on ideas through the medium of the arts.

Over time, we have discussed and developed the following criteria to grade the projects: depth of critical thinking, depth of reflection, creativity, a well-explained rationale, links to personal experience, links to ethical practice, use of metaphor to foster reflection, evolution of thinking, sensitivity, originality, quality of expression, willingness to take risks, use of moral imagination (to imaginatively project oneself into the future), and respectful representation.

Analysis of the student projects over five years has been supported by a Social Science and Humanities Research Council Grant. Findings have illuminated how an arts-based approach contributes to student reflection, self-awareness, and the learning process. Students' work represented an array of themes related to ethical practice that illustrate their personal reflections. Prevalent themes included ethics as care, ethics as negotiating complexity, ethics as seeking balance, ethics as ways of seeing, ethics as a living thing, ethics as a journey, and ethics as professional responsibility. Interestingly, more than half of the students used symbols of the body in relation to ethical practice (that is, a human figure, hands and arms, heart, faces, gut, eyes, and brain) in the form of images and written text. Additionally, students identified diverse outcomes in their written reflections on learning, including becoming aware of values and beliefs, discovering creativity, valuing reflection, acknowledging complexity, and imagining praxis. A number of themes and representative quotes (below), used with permission, arose from students' written reflections related to the process of engaging with the arts-based project.

Depth of Reflection: "Creating a piece of art about what ethical practice means to me forced me to think about ethics on a much deeper level than I would have in just writing another essay or reflection. . . . Despite my original misgivings, I am now quite grateful that we had the opportunity to do a project like this."

Critical Thinking: "The project makes you think more critically and deeply about the subject and is a good exercise to reflect on professional practice."

Self-Knowledge: "Although some ethical decisions may be part of a tacit process, I've learned that self-evaluation and critical appraisal is not only important but necessary in professional practice. This learning experience has been truly self-revealing."

Personal Insights: "By creating this artwork and writing about how it relates to my practice, I have developed insights into the process behind my decision-making. Ultimately, I feel this experience has helped me understand and realize the underlying basis for decisions I have made in the past and future, which will allow me to become a more self-reflective practitioner."

Making Connections: "Each morning and night my eyes are drawn to this sculpture. Not only because I think it is attractive, but also because of the meaning and symbolism I have now attached to this . . . each day I am aware of my personal notion of ethics and my ethical abilities in relation to . . . practice. I am also aware that ethics is a part of everyday activities and that my actions . . . no matter how seemingly insignificant, will always impact others in health care."

Transformative: "I began to feel as though I had stepped out of my comfort zone, challenged my prior thoughts and opinions, and discovered new ways to see and think about the world."

Challenging Boundaries: "This project has taught me that I am capable of doing things that make me slightly uncomfortable. . . . Now I have more confidence [so] that when I face things that are unfamiliar to me, I will be able to attempt them; and if the result is not exactly what I had hoped for, I can learn from the experience and build upon it in the future."

Recognizing Diversity: "I have also come to find that every individual is different in regards to their values, morals and most importantly their ethical reasoning. But that you will learn and grow from understanding a different perspective."

Imagining Others' Perspective: "When I was reflecting, I found that a lot of the times, I was immersing myself in the client's situation so that I may gain a better understanding of their experience as well as their needs and wants. . . .

I found that by letting my imagination run and deeply reflecting it has helped me gain at least some understanding of the [client's] experience."

Ways of Knowing: "What I have learned from this process is that just as much learning can be achieved from an artistic assignment as can be achieved from a research-based academic assignment. In fact, the learning I have done here is more transferable to practice than what I learned from writing a research-based paper."

Memorable: "Without contest I feel that I am more likely to remember what I have learned in doing this project than what I have learned from the hundreds of journal articles I have read in writing other assignments. . . . I now have a visual image ingrained in my mind of what ethical practice means to me and it is something I will never forget."

Resistance: "Initially . . . I was skeptical. I thought it seemed rather ridiculous to convey through art what could just as easily be conveyed through essay or reflection form. I found it quite difficult to come up with something that would represent what ethical practice means to me. Once I had a general outline to work from, the task became much easier."

In summary, we have found the use of an arts-based approach to ethics education in a health sciences curriculum to be an exciting and innovative approach to the education of future health-care professionals. The learning that occurs has the potential to contribute to the cultivation of deeply reflective and thoughtful practitioners, and to assist students to think "outside the box" and to explore creative aspects of themselves and their professional identities. In addition, many students indicated that the arts-based assignment is one of the most memorable and surprisingly meaningful projects they have engaged in throughout their higher education.

Disclosing a Personal Critical Incident

Inspiring Reflective Practice

STELLA NG

The idea for my approach to "keeping reflection fresh" was borne of a critical incident in my life as a practitioner. I was working as an educational audiologist, a unique role for a pediatric audiologist, and was tasked with liaising between clinical and school-based professionals to facilitate school-based health support for kids. One day, the phone rang. It was my boss, asking me to recount the events of the previous day. Another health professional had complained about my actions in relation to my interactions with them regarding a mutual patient. My employer conducted its own investigation, which resolved quickly with a dismissal of the complaint, and I moved on. Months later as I was working from home on my dissertation, the doorbell rang. I was handed a package and signed for its receipt. The package was from my professional college. Peculiar, I thought, that my college would send me something by registered mail. I opened the package, and so began eighteen months of uncertainty and incessant reflection as I underwent an investigation by my professional college.

I perform this very personal narrative to begin a workshop on reflection and reflective practice that I facilitate. I have given this one-hour workshop to audiences of audiology, speech-language pathology, and occupational therapy students and also abbreviated versions to colleagues in athletic therapy, dietetics, medicine, and nursing. I delivered the workshop for the first time six months after the complaint was fully dismissed. In my professional field of audiology, reflection and reflective practice are emergent; deep theorizing on reflection is minimal in comparison to other fields and relative to the application of tools and forms that have been adopted to perform and record reflective thinking. By walking students through my critical incident, sharing a personal disclosure that is seemingly gripping for students who hope to avoid a similar incident befalling them, I am able to introduce theories of reflection and reflective practice in an engaging way. The narrative that I weave draws upon reflective writing that I was encouraged (by critical companions) to produce as I experienced the incident. It also becomes a narrative performance as I reembody the experience and utilize imagery and metaphor to share themes of learning that I highlight during the workshop.

I devote the first half hour of this workshop to recounting my tale, highlighting themes I've extracted from my reflective writings on the matter, infusing my story with brief theoretical definitions and practical examples of reflection-in-action, reflection-on-action, and critical reflection. What went right in this incident? What went wrong? Where did misunderstandings emerge? What did I learn? In the second half hour, I delve more deeply into theories of reflection largely informed by the writing of Anne Kinsella, a scholar I consider to be my first mentor in the scholarly area of reflection and reflective practice.[1] I see this essay as a way to document the potential of transforming what could be viewed as a low point in one's professional life and career into a pedagogical tool and an opportunity to facilitate learning in others. We can all learn from misunderstandings, lawsuits, conflicts with patients and colleagues, and decisions taken in the past. We all carry around unmetabolized stories that can still teach us even years later, if we revisit and process their meaning. Themes I explore during the first part of the workshop include irony, stress, emotional self-care, critical reflection, and meaning making.

Irony: While I underwent investigation into my professional ethics and integrity, I was teaching future health professionals in a course titled Evidence-Based Practice and in another called Professional Issues and Practice Management. Moreover, I was working on my doctoral dissertation on the role of reflection in students' development as professional practitioners. Amidst this irony, I was also conscious of how fortunate I was to have this language of reflection and professional ethics to draw upon to help me transform this critical incident into a meaningful learning experience.

Stress: I was certainly in denial about the stress I experienced in the midst of this lengthy investigation. However, looking back, I recall that I constantly feared the arrival of yet another letter, notifying me of legal action as had been threatened. I was not concerned that I would be found guilty, because I had sufficient evidence to contradict the allegations; however, I knew that a lawsuit would be costly in terms of time, finances, and emotional toll. I developed idiopathic health issues during this time. This is not to say that this complaint process in and of itself was the cause of my stress and health concerns; however, it was certainly not helpful. I share with students that reflection was my ally as

I worked through the irony, sense of injustice, and frustration that I was being accused of unprofessional and unethical practice when I had, in my view, been attempting to uphold principles of ethics and quality care for a family. Further, because the complaint was from an unregulated health professional, there was nothing further I could do for the family in terms of reconciling their outstanding issues with the complainants. Would this happen again to another family?

Emotional self-care: While being overly hard on oneself is a potential outcome of incessant reflection, one that I did experience at times, I was able to use reflection-on-action to recall my engagement of reflection-in-action. This reflection-on-action upon reflection-in-action proved useful for my emotional self-care. In the midst of the incident that elicited the complaint, I vividly recalled the calm and quiet tone of voice and unassuming body language I deliberately adopted in an attempt to avoid escalating the situation. I also recall biting my tongue so as to not outwardly demonstrate disapproval of or disagreement with practices the other professionals had used (despite some of their actions being at odds with my clinical judgment, the family's wishes, and evidence-based practice guidelines). In using reflection-on-action to reflect upon reflection-in-action, I was able to engage in emotional self-care and to recruit support from others. But more interestingly, I can recall the power of having a language and theory, in the moments that this incident unfolded, with which to reflect in action!

Critical reflection and meaning making: Rather than patting myself on the back and assuring myself that my actions had been perfectly innocent and ideal, I engaged in critical reflection[2] to question how power dynamics did play into the interactions, in both how I interpreted the situation and how the other professionals interpreted my intentions. I questioned my assumptions going into the appointment and tried to wear the lens of the complainants to envision how I could have acted differently. Later in my reflective process, a scholar I had met in my academic life and who was well versed in ethics, narrative, reflection, and cultural competence prompted me to examine how I could be interpreted as "other" in such a situation. Until prompted by this scholar, I had not reflected on my position, relative to the complainant, as a member of a regulated health profession with a long history of "turf wars" with their unregulated profession, a young woman, and a visible minority.

In the more theoretically informed second half of the workshop, I explore with students Schön's reflection-in-action and reflection-on-action, and anticipatory reflection.[3] I also share pragmatic professional lessons such as the importance of the detailed documentation I had kept of all interactions with the other health professionals involved in this incident. In the end, this documentation likely was the most important evidence in the investigation, as it demonstrated inaccuracies and inconsistencies in the allegations.

While my own practice experience, a critical incident in particular, serves as the basis for the narrative that I weave, this approach to "keeping reflection fresh" can likely be of use to any practitioner-educator. I use my own story and transparency about it to encourage students and colleagues to think about their own difficult stories and encounters. With a thorough understanding of narrative ethics, narrative medicine, reflective practice, experiential learning, or other related theories, approaches, and concepts, a critical incident can be transformed not only into a powerful learning experience for oneself but also an engaging educational opportunity for others. Rather than serving as a mere confessional or act of contrition or vindication, imbuing one's experience with theory enables honest and critically conscious reflection.[4] In an age when students may resist or fear uncertainty, sharing imperfect experiences with others (rather than portraying a false image of infallibility) is imperative. Feedback on the session has been largely positive. Future work may explore the importance of the timing of such a session relative to students' experiences and place in curricula, and of follow-up sessions to delve more deeply into reflective processes with students by inviting them to share their own difficult accounts.

NOTES

1. Elizabeth Anne Kinsella et al., "Reflective Practice for Allied Health: Theory and Applications," in *Adult Education and Health,* ed. Leona English (Toronto: Univ. of Toronto Press, 2012), 210–28.
2. Stephen Brookfield, "Critically Reflective Practice," *Journal of Continuing Education in the Health Professions* 18 (1998): 197–205.
3. Donald A. Schön, *The Reflective Practitioner: How Professionals Think in Action* (New York: Basic Books, 1983); Kinsella et al., "Reflective Practice for Allied Health."
4. Brookfield, "Critically Reflective Practice."

Building Multigenerational Ethics Peer Mentors to Help Students Recognize and Manage Ethics Challenges

CATHERINE MYSER

As a founding member of a small faculty tasked with starting a brand-new medical school, I faced ethics education challenges both familiar and unique. Familiar challenges included figuring out how to (1) engage students in developmentally appropriate ethics learning and (2) effectively integrate the ethics curriculum with concurrent basic science and preclinical/clinical learning. Another familiar challenge was recognizing and successfully managing any informal/hidden curricula that might undermine the formal ethics curriculum. Unique challenges included addressing the fact that the basic science and preclinical/clinical curricula were being created contemporaneously—month by month—as the inaugural students completed their first semester and year. It was difficult, if not impossible, to integrate ethics meaningfully when the rest of the curriculum was not yet in place. In addition, the inaugural class had no multigenerational peers to support and guide them, as would any first-year class at an established medical school.

Due to the challenges highlighted above, our first-year ethics curriculum was inadequately integrated, seemed unduly "apart" and "abstract," and thus was not sufficiently compelling to students. I conducted a focus group at the end of our inaugural students' first year to learn from the students what ethical issues they had faced through the past year and where and how we might offer better support. Although not readily recognized by the students themselves, most ethics-related gaps fell into a category I was very familiar with.

During the 1990s, two medical students (Feudtner and Christakis) published a series of classic articles on the stage-specific ethical issues uniquely distressing medical students in their early clinical experiences.[1] These "ethics in a short white coat" (ESWC) issues included, for example, (1) novices performing procedures;

effects of ignorance; risks of coercing patients; (2) pressures to be a team player; (3) if, how, and when to challenge medical routine and hierarchy; (4) tensions of being closer to the patient as a person; and (5) witnessing unethical behavior. Feudtner and Christakis concluded that foundational ethics teaching should include focus on ESWC issues. ESWC issues were indeed felt as more familiar, troubling, and less supported by our inaugural students than the standard ethical dilemmas taught (for example, withdrawal of life-sustaining treatment) and are still too far from early clinical experiences to be as meaningful. This led me to begin building reflective learning communities—led by multigenerational Ethics Peer Mentors—as a possible solution.

Building reflective learning communities for ethics reflection, role modeling, and peer mentoring aimed to create an institutional community enabling and supporting vigilance and better management of various types and levels of ethics issues. It also aimed to foster empathy and support—by students and for students, and assisted by clinical teachers—to recognize and manage shared moral distress and ethical uncertainty. In addition, it aimed to help students recognize and address informal and hidden institutional curricula (for example, power and abuse) risking undermining (1) their formal ethics curriculum and (2) patient care. Building reflective learning communities across multigenerational (M1, M2, and M3) students furthermore aimed to maintain sustainability of such activities.

THE STORY OF ETHICS PEER MENTORING PILOTS, HIGHLIGHTING "ETHICS IN A SHORT WHITE COAT" ISSUES

In the summer of 2012, selected students and I created the Ethics Peer Mentoring pilot, whereby nine of our sixty-four first-year medical students in the inaugural class met the summer before their second year (June and July 2012) to identify key Ethics in a Short White Coat cases confronted in their first-year clinical and research experiences. Prior to brainstorming and writing cases, the M2s read Christakis and Feudtner's "Ethics in a Short White Coat: The Ethical Dilemmas that Medical Students Confront," now the required reading for M1s prior to this Clinical Learning Group activity. One student served as Lead Ethics Peer Mentor and not only helped select and recruit additional Ethics Peer Mentors but also helped organize meeting times and rooms. The cases students shared at our initial brainstorming session were later summarized, merged, and written up by me for use in the fall 2012 pilot Clinical Ethics teaching module as a new component of our formal ethics curriculum. As the M1s would by that time have had only a single ethics lecture on Core Ethics

Rules, including Veracity, Confidentiality, and Fidelity, and as an Informed Consent/Research Ethics case had also been included, I identified each case by ethics "type" for the fall 2012 pilot (later judged unnecessary and dropped).

Eight of these now second-year medical students co-facilitated/peer mentored these cases to the new class of sixty-four first-year students, alongside four clinical faculty, in one required, small Clinical Learning Group (these meet for one hour weekly throughout the year to reflect on M1 outpatient preceptors and Department of Health clinical experiences). I conducted faculty development and debriefing sessions, for the Ethics Peer Mentors and Clinical Learning Group faculty before and after the pilot module, to prepare co-facilitators and then reflect on benefits and outcomes.

Based on positive feedback from the first- and second-year medical students and clinical faculty in the fall of 2012, the next cohort of M2s and I evolved this Ethics Peer Mentor pilot module for fall 2013. Eight current first-year and I met several times in April and May 2013 to identify their own Ethics in a Short White Coat cases, which they co-taught as second-year students to the incoming first-year students in fall 2013. At that time, the Lead Ethics Peer Mentor took even more responsibility. She singlehandedly chose the Ethics Peer Mentors from among her classmates, scheduled a series of three one-hour meetings and rooms, and organized catered lunches—supplied by me. That year, the M2 students, who had been the learners during the fall 2012 ESWC Peer Mentoring pilot, were more prepared and proactive. They readily brainstormed, wrote their own cases, and added their own teaching questions and guidelines, completing all this in three planning sessions I supervised. We plan to coauthor further educational scholarship.

The Ethics Peer Mentors brought a unique student-driven creativity and positive energy—previously lacking for ethics—that heightened the engagement and learning of the whole class. This effectively transformed some of the negative attitudes that can undermine attempts to teach ethics to science and medical students. The student lead for each cohort of peer mentors assists in selecting students with the right blend of leadership ability, learning and teaching creativity, and positive energy to serve most effectively as peer mentors. These humanistic interests, positive energies, and reflective capacities otherwise risked lying fallow, and not being harnessed on behalf of ethics and related initiatives at our medical school. The peer mentors thus effectively transformed their own learning and professionalism, as well as that of their classmates. Several of our peer mentors are so enthusiastic that they have additionally served and/or volunteered in co-creating and co-facilitating further cultural competency and global health and global health ethics sessions I teach as part of our Foundations of Medicine course. They also continue informally to mentor peers in their own class as well as incoming classes. Thus, in addition to helping make ethics more meaningful, compelling, and better integrated at our new medical school, we created self-sustaining reflective learning communities of multigenerational Ethics Peer Mentors to offer crucial support and role modeling going forward. We believe that our Ethics Peer Mentoring program is readily reproducible and can offer similar benefits at established medical schools and other clinical faculties.

NOTES

In closing, I extend heartfelt thanks to our 2012 and 2013 Ethics Peer Mentors: Chris Nguyen, JD (Leader); John Ciotti; David Dillon; Eric Downes; Rachel Fowler; Juliet Meirs; Raffi Sturm; Rica Zantua (and JD Wilcox, who initially helped write cases); Lauren Spoo (Leader); Alex Casella; Jaclyn Klimczak; David Levine; Tony Nikolaev; Tiffany Olier; Cara Reitz; Whitney Woodhull (and M3 John Ciotti, who wrote one case). Without your extraordinary generosity and passion, we could not have so positively transformed our ethics curriculum.

1. Dimitri A. Christakis and Chris Feudtner, "Ethics in a Short White Coat: The Ethical Dilemmas that Medical Students Confront," *Academic Medicine* 68 (1993): 249–54; Chris Feudtner and Dimitri A. Christakis, "Making the Rounds: The Ethical Development of Medical Students in the Context of Clinical Rotations," *Hastings Center Report* 24 (1994): 6–12; Chris Feudtner, Dimitri A. Christakis, and Nicholas A. Christakis, "Do Clinical Clerks Suffer Ethical Erosion? Students' Perceptions of their Ethical Environment and Personal Development," *Academic Medicine* 69 (1994): 670–79.

Challenges in Reflecting on Story in a Four-Year Narrative Ethics Core Medical Curriculum

JEFF NISKER

The first challenge I experienced in developing a story-based, health ethics program as part of a four-year medical curriculum was to convince those responsible for the curriculum—usually trained in objectivity and comforted by principles and p-values—that a story-based learning program and evaluation method not only had merit but was worthy of the dedication of a large number of hours of jealously guarded curriculum time. What I had in mind over the first two years was a ten-module course, with each three-hour module beginning with an hour of theater or readings of poems or short stories to expose the ethical issue being explored (for example, professionalism, end-of-life decision making, resource allocation).

Believing that all students should reflect on the same stories at the same time, readings are not distributed in advance. Rather they are projected above the heads of their classmates who volunteer to read a few stanzas or paragraphs (except for theater, when the student volunteers would have previously rehearsed the play). Following the "narrative surfacing vehicle," the class would pose questions they would like to discuss, and I would write them on the board. The students would then break into groups to unpack the question of their choice for an hour. In the last hour of each module, the raconteur of each group would present that group's findings to the class for open discussion. Three hours was essential to do justice to the stories, the students, and the health ethics issues that were explored.

Because of the fierce competition for core curricular time, I had to start this Medical Ethics and Humanities program on Monday nights. I felt that medical students would be more attracted to reflecting on stories than those who control their bankers' hours and that most medical students would rather reflect on story than memorize minutiae on Monday nights.[1] Within three years, the core curriculum challenge was overcome through the efforts of the students who believed their Monday night reflections were essential for all their classmates and should be in the core curriculum. They lobbied our dean and associate dean undergraduate to this end.

Eventually, more than fifty hours of a core curriculum program in first and second year was devoted to our completely integrated Medical Ethics and Humanities course, with one module in third year revisiting informed choice through a video of a play performed by medical student actors and an Ethics Through Film selective in fourth year that was chosen by most medical students.

As the students learned health ethics by reflecting on stories, I believed it was important to evaluate their learning by having the students write stories themselves. At the end of second year, each student submitted an ethics exploration that they had worked on over the year. Students worked with me as individuals and groups during my office hours over second year. Students wrote short stories, poems, plays, and songs. Other students used paint or photography as the medium for their ethics reflection. All students were invited to present their work in an open forum with all students and faculty welcome, but some preferred to present only to me because of the personal nature of their reflections. Their reflections were beautiful, insightful, and poignant, and all received As or A pluses, as I did not force them to complete their reflections until they felt they were ready.

A challenge to evaluation through story came as a result of the publication of second-year narrative bioethics projects in important peer-reviewed journals like the *Canadian Medical Association Journal*. Increasing numbers of students, wanting to be published in order to improve their selection position in the Canadian Resident Matching Service, took on research projects more likely to be published rather than submitting narrative research studies and personal reflections that would be very difficult to publish.

In fourth year, the Medical Ethics through Film students were asked to write a reflection on an ethical dilemma they experienced during clinical clerkship. These narratives frequently explored injustices and had the potential to expose specific clinical services and individuals working on those services. Some students expressed their fear of repercussions for "telling secrets after being admitted to the club." I also believed that deep and honest reflection would require that I receive their stories confidentially. An anonymized, aggregate analysis of the narratives revealed that almost 20 percent of the students wrote very personal reflections on a patient without having adequate information for the informed consent they were required to obtain. Almost 20 percent of students reflected on the inadequate care they believed a patient received and their inability to better advocate for their patient.[2]

A challenge to the concept of learning and evaluating through reflecting on stories arose from an increase in class size from 86 to 154 and from the imperative to videoconference all lectures to an additional 50 students at our medical school's new satellite campus. Deep reflection on stories requires close engagement, with each student having considerable time for reflection and comment. Of course, I refused to videoconference our reflections as it would further deflate the passion of our engagement and shortchange the learning of the off-site students. In addition, the doubling of the class size necessitated adding more groups, making it difficult to provide enough time for each group's raconteur to report their findings back to the class and for the ensuing discussion. I trained a faculty member at the satellite campus to facilitate a curriculum using the same modules. We met frequently to discuss how it was proceeding and exchange ideas; however, I knew I was having difficulty ensuring the engagement of the 154 students in the main campus class.

Regarding evaluation, it was challenging to work with so many students on their second-year projects. Further, a new mandate for a uniform system of evaluations within and across both campuses of the medical school became an insurmountable challenge; as multiple-choice and short-answer evaluations demean reflection on story, I could not go there.

Securing funding for additional faculty members willing to dedicate significant time to learning about and facilitating health ethics learning through reflection on story was essential and difficult. Although I knew several former medical students who would have been wonderful in this regard and wanted to become faculty members, I was not able to convince the chairs of their prospective departments that such persons were worthy of funded protected time. Further, securing more funding from our dean, who generously protected two days a week of my time for Medical Ethics and Humanities, was difficult, considering a desire to develop new programs within the medical school. Trying to secure collaboration from other university faculties was attempted but did not work out.

Final Reflection: Just as there is no metric to accurately assess what medical students learn through reflecting on and writing stories, it is difficult for me to express, let alone quantify, the enormity of the gift that I have received from the students who reflected with me on stories and who shared their personal stories. I believe that the bidirectional generosity, which Arthur Frank insists is important in the physician-patient relationship, is important in the health educator–student relationship.[3] The generosity of my students' reflections in their comments in class and in the stories they wrote have made me a better clinician and a better human being.

NOTES

1. Jeff A. Nisker, "The Yellow Brick Road of Medical Education," *Canadian Medical Association Journal* 156 (1997): 689–91.
2. Emily Kelly and Jeff Nisker, "Increasing Bioethics Education in Preclinical Medical Curricula: What Ethical Dilemmas do Clinical Clerks Experience?" *Academic Medicine* 84 (2009): 498–504.
3. Jeff A. Nisker, "A Covenant Model for the Medical Educator-Student Relationship: Lessons from the Covenant Model of the Physician-Patient Relationship," *Medical Education* 40 (2006): 502–3.

The Humanistic Aspects of
Medical Education Seminar at
New York University School of Medicine

LUCY BRUELL, MICHELE SARRACO, FRED WERTZER,
AND JEROME LOWENSTEIN

Every Wednesday afternoon, a group of New York University (NYU) medical students break from their clinical duties on their medicine rotation to convene in a windowless conference room in the Division of Infectious Diseases & Immunology on the sixteenth floor of Bellevue Hospital. For the next hour, over snacks provided by their group facilitator, they put away their cell phones, pagers, and iPads and spend an hour talking about topics they bring to the table. That same afternoon, four other student groups are meeting with their facilitators. Unlike other requirements for the medicine clerkship, these seminars have no set agendas, no assignments, and no evaluations. Most importantly, all discussions are completely confidential.

Students sometimes refer to the seminar as "Feelings" or "The Touchy Feely Hour," rather than using its true name, Humanistic Aspects of Medical Education, or HAME. It began at NYU more than thirty years ago, initiated by Dr. Jerome Lowenstein.

As a member of the Bellevue house staff in the 1960s, when staff members worked around the clock every two or three days, Dr. Lowenstein joined his colleagues in a nightly ritual—consuming the day's leftovers in the hospital cafeteria. This midnight break provided an opportunity to discuss and to reflect on the day. "The midnight meal consisted of the day's leftovers," Lowenstein writes in his book, *The Midnight Meal and Other Essays*. "The real fare was the day's 'medical leftovers,' the thoughts and feelings that needed to be expressed."[1]

The HAME seminar provides a unique setting for students to grapple with what is sometimes considered unthinkable when administering to patients. In groups of eight to ten, students delve into their own vulnerability, disgust, and ethical dilemmas, as well as their own dedication, passion, and commitment to the field, as they care for people affected by illness or challenged by end-of-life issues. As a group, the students consider and reflect on ways in which a person's physical well-being is affected by emotional, social, economic, and psychological factors. HAME provides a forum for students to discuss the many complex patient-care challenges and dilemmas that may come up during the rotation, and it enhances the students' ability to deal with all facets of the work. Sometimes they share thoughts that give them pleasure or achievement.

This process doesn't happen automatically. Students come into the room after a day of rounding, presentations, and writing notes. They may sit silently, taking time to decompress. This silence is an incubator for topics to emerge. A casual comment about the weather prompted one student to ask why the weather mattered when as medical students they never have a chance to enjoy the outside. This in turn sparked a discussion of the expectations they have of themselves in striving to be "model" medical students. Topics that are discussed depend entirely on decisions made by the group.

Not to be confused with group therapy, the purpose of the seminar is educational. The seminar is intended to support students as they transition from the preclinical to the clinical years, a pivotal phase in their professional development. Students are encouraged to reflect on their feelings and reactions in developing understanding and insight that will help them in making clinical decisions and caring for patients. The confidential nature of the discussion helps to generate trust among group members so that they are free to discuss their own experiences and feelings with their peers. This experience of collegial support provides a model that they can emulate and engage throughout their professional lives.

Of the five facilitators currently in the program, four are social workers and one is a journalist. Over the years, a few of the facilitators have been NYU physicians. Although each of us has a unique approach, we share the experience of entering the room every week without a preconceived idea of what the students will discuss, what feelings they will express, and what responses might be shared. In any given week, a student might witness the death of a patient with whom they had a special relationship, work up a patient who was belligerent, or see a patient on the prison ward who was failing and had no one visiting him. The question of balancing the need to study and absorb as much medical knowledge as they can, while at the same time working full days as doctors-in-training is very much on their minds.

Issues of professionalism, of working as part of a team where there may be different perspectives on how to treat a patient, or of adapting to the culture of a hospital—seeing how things work or not—are all topics that emerge in the twelve weeks the students spend together. The observations of the students have led them to consider their own roles and values in relation to the institutional values and culture of the hospital. For example, a student questioned the use of derogatory phrases to describe patients by members of the house staff. "Most of the people in this room are saying they wouldn't personally say something like that. So, are we going to turn into those people? Maybe, I don't know." Another student had comforted a man who had been diagnosed with HIV after an extramarital affair and was afraid to tell his wife. This student, who instinctively spoke with her patient in a nonjudgmental way, helping him to accept his diagnosis and its implications beyond the hospital stay, later commented that had she met this person not as a doctor but as an acquaintance, she would have been furious with him. Her ability to acknowledge her dual role came as response to a comment about the supposed decline in empathy in the third year of medical school. Her story, together with the reactions of the other students, underscores how empathy is a basic element of their profession.

Some students distinguish between patients whose medical conditions are aggravated by the use of drugs or alcohol and patients whose illnesses are caused by so-called "chance" factors. Patients with addictions are frequently viewed as morally culpable in their own illnesses, and students tend to be less sympathetic to them. One group had discussed the importance of allowing patients to tell their stories as a means of gaining increased understanding of the context in which their health issues had developed. One student, who acknowledged that she was biased against patients with addictions, shared that she had listened to the story of a patient when she evaluated him at the VA Hospital. He shared that he had been wounded during the Vietnam War and was treated with painkilling medications while still in the combat zone. This occurrence was the beginning of his drug dependency. This revelation caused the student to be more circumspect and helped her realize that patients cannot be categorized into a group but need to be treated as individuals with personal histories. She encouraged the other students to learn more about the circumstances that may have contributed to a person's illness. Directly following this discussion, another student revealed her own father's struggle with alcoholism. She spoke with warmth about her father and his illness, his many unsuccessful attempts to overcome his alcoholism, and his frustration and despair. Eventually, he did find a program that was successful. This student also pleaded with the group to confront their prejudices and to attend to every patient as an individual. "You have to make your own judgment and avoid expecting that it is useless to try to help a patient."

The outcome of a successful humanistic group experience results in members' willingness to reflect on their own feelings and thoughts and to recognize how empathy and compassion are as essential as good diagnostic skills in healing a patient. Today, where conversation has given way to texting, the HAME seminar offers a safe place for honest discussion and the exploration of profound subjects that students will face as they develop into caring and competent doctors. At a time when people relate primarily via electronic connections, it seems to us that the seminars play an important role in developing a sense of community among learners and practitioners, a community that can contribute in important ways to the kind of physicians our students may become.

NOTE

1. Jerome Lowenstein, *The Midnight Meal and Other Essays about Doctors, Patients, and Medicine* (Ann Arbor: Univ. of Michigan Press, 2005).

Ethics as Work

MARK LACHMANN

In our geriatric psychiatry group we are tasked to teach a ninety-minute semi-nar on ethics to residents rotating through our service. This talk takes place nested in a series of lectures on topics such as cognitive assessment, types of dementia, and mood disorders in late life. In the psychiatry training program, this seminar is the only formal tuition in ethics for the six-month geriatric psychiatry rotation. By the time the residents meet with us in the seminar, they will have done four years of medical school and four years of psychiatry residency, not to mention premedical school academic training. The residents are well immersed in "the hidden curriculum," and a ninety-minute "ethics drive-by" is perfectly set up to play into the worst cynicism of the stifled adult learner. So what to do?

Our goal has shifted from having the residents come away from the seminar with a specific knowledge of a set of standard principles to an approach focused on empathy and the residents identifying in themselves the experiences of "moral distress." We work hard in the seminar at actually creating space for a group of about twenty adults to discuss how and when each of us experiences a feeling of moral uncertainty and what this may mean.

About a week prior to the seminar, I send an e-mail to the residents who will be attending with the invented Diagnostic and Statistical Manual diagno-sis of "Empathy Attrition Disorder," asking them simply to read it and come prepared to tell us what they think of it (see Table 2). At the beginning of the seminar itself, I introduce myself to each of the residents as he or she enters the room by shaking their hand. I then briefly introduce myself and frame the seminar as an exercise in exploring the role of empathy in psychiatric care for each of us in the room, linking this to ethics by simply asserting my opinion that the central ethical challenge of our profession is to preserve our sense of empathy over our careers and in our various institutional work environments. I talk personally about our professional formation as psychiatrists and relate several stories from my own life and from those of colleagues. The idea of moral distress (uncertainty as to the right course of action in a resource-constrained environment) is introduced, and I ask the residents to tell me when they have experienced this feeling.[1] This usually generates conversations about uncertainty, conflict, medical error, difficult relationships with supervisors, and concerns about boundaries. The feeling of moral distress is then explicitly linked to the experience of empathy, and we challenge the residents to come up with concrete responses in thought and action to address their own feelings of moral distress.

Table 2. Empathy Attrition Disorder: Description and Diagnostic Criteria

Description	Diagnostic Criteria
Empathy is an aspect of character which one seeks to foster over the course of a budding psychiatrist's training. However, empathy is well known to decline over the course of medical and residency training. Empathy Attrition Disorder (EAD) is a state of a gradual erosion of empathy over a several-year period, leading to a progressive disconnect from human suffering. Known risk factors associated with empathy attrition include: a) environmental influences (e.g., the "hidden curriculum," the corrosive effect of unrelentingly unrealistic official rhetoric for expectations of residents in the face of a chronic exposure to actual practice behavior of supervisors);* b) biologic predisposition (impaired serotonin transporter gene function, or other compromised autonomic stress mechanism). *Note: Early on in the disorder, some insight may be preserved, but this may soon be eroded by a lack of professional mentorship.	Criterion A. Pervasive sense of lack of connection from patients, colleagues, family, and friends, which has developed gradually over a period of years. Criterion B. Inability, despite direct encouragement or confrontation, to see the "self" in the "other." When questioned, the response is concrete and dismissive (e.g., "What are you talking about?"). Criterion C. At least 2 of the following must be present: 1. intense interest in cars; 2. intense interest in real estate; 3. intense interest in other expensive material possessions (e.g., shoes); 4. intense interest in Facebook and/or other social media, *but* reluctance to actually meet people. Exclusion Criteria: EAD is excluded if any other Axis 1 disorder is present, or if the individual owns a pet.

Moral distress is positively reinforced as a feeling that can inform our professional lives. This leads into a brief discussion of the origins of formal thinking through ethics and various traditions.[2] At the close of the session, articles are given out addressing in detail some "hot topics" in geriatric psychiatry ethics: sexuality, capacity, end-of-life care, and truth telling. The entire seminar is geared toward having the residents themselves relate moral distress and empathy to their own formation as members of a profession so that within the seminar we are working with their own questions and material.

Prior to training in psychiatry, I worked as a family physician for ten years in a remote setting in northern Canada. Central to this experience was working with a variety of physicians—other family doctors, anesthetists, surgeons, psychiatrists, and other specialists—in close quarters for extended periods of time as we all faced challenging clinical and personal events. The experience of isolation, uncertainty, and lack of resources emphasized to me the vulnerability of physicians as we manage our own selves in difficult situations. A part of residency training that can be strengthened is the development of a professional identity that is able to engage with uncertainty and personal vulnerability in a healthy way. This means explicitly promoting behaviors that decrease professional isolation (acknowledging uncertainty, asking for help, talking with colleagues) rather than increasing it (ignoring conflict, turning to substances). We have found it helpful in our own practice to talk with other physicians in order to validate feelings of moral distress as a way of beginning a deeper dialogue toward building a professional identity. By inviting the residents as colleagues, not in a learner-teacher dynamic, to explore moral distress, we hope to kick-start the engagement process for them. Frank discussion of moral distress is presented as a way to actively engage around empathy. The use of an "Empathy Attrition Disorder" serves to stimulate discussion in a tongue-in-cheek format with a serious underpinning and can also be used to critique diagnostic construction generally if the seminar goes in that direction.

An approach focused on having residents explore moral distress has transformed our ethics seminar. The seminar is now interactive and personal with a genuine feel of inquiry as to how the residents themselves will grapple with uncertainty, moral distress, and the preservation of empathy. Despite not reviewing a potted history of ethics or giving a principle-based case review, the residents by the end of the seminar are genuinely interested in how thinking through a variety of ethical traditions may be of some assistance to them.

NOTES

1. Bernadette M. Pauly, Colleen Varcoe, and Jan Storch, "Framing the Issues: Moral Distress in Health Care," *HealthCare Ethics Committee Forum* 24 (2012): 1–11.
2. Albert R. Jonsen, *The Birth of Bioethics* (New York: Oxford Univ. Press, 1998).

A Sweet Tradition

The Oath of Hippocrates on Lake Ontario

JACALYN DUFFIN

This sweet tradition came to Queen's University in late August 1996. Medical students in the class of 1999 were organizing orientation events for their new peers—the class of 2000. Confronted by that millennial shift—and well before Y2K raised the possibility of a future disaster, these students chose to celebrate by turning to the past. They imagined a torchlight historical walking tour of our campus capped by the "real" Hippocratic Oath.

The students identified five historic spots on our campus: the front steps of our hospital, founded in 1832 and the oldest continuously operating public hospital in English Canada; the curved stone back of an 1895 operating theater for teaching in-the-round; the doors of the Museum of Health Care, originally built as a nurses' residence in 1904; and the tiny park known as the Medical Quadrangle, surrounded by the old limestone buildings where medicine was taught from 1854 to 1979.

At each spot, a second-year medical student waited, garbed in black, armed with a tall bamboo torch, and primed with a historical tale—either about that place—or about the medical history of our community: cholera epidemics, mass graves, body snatching, admission of women students, exclusion of black students, and scientific achievements. Their stories were engaging, told dramatically, and short—each was three to five minutes in length. The tour became a sort of walking meditation for students. Reflecting on their new status, while learning a little about the history of their profession and their own medical school, allowed for a unique melding of past, present, and future.

The seventy-five new students of Meds 2000 held flickering candles inside paper cups. They assembled into five groups, each led by a second-year student with a big torch. They set out over the campus, moving from site to site, hearing the stories until all the groups coalesced at the end in the bowl of an outdoor amphitheater.

The second-year students had asked me to select a suitable rendition of the Hippocratic Oath and to lead its recitation. They explained that little solemnity had illuminated their own orientation one year earlier: it had been enjoyable and welcoming, but they were disappointed by the lack of ceremony around their momentous entry into medicine.

Many versions of the oath exist, modified to satisfy modern sensibilities, rejecting the outmoded, retaining the durable. In preparation, I read dozens of modifications. I also examined the Sponsio that Queen's students affirm on their graduation day, but it was about upholding the reputation of the profession and of the university. Modern gender-neutral renditions of Hippocrates seemed watered down and devoid of intrigue or connectivity. Finally, I decided to go with the original, except it would be in English, not Greek.

After the groups came together, I said a few words to explain the 2,500-year-old antiquity and mystery of the Hippocratic Oath. I warned that they might be surprised at some of its content and that they need not say anything that bothered them. I asked that they reflect about what parts we would now retain or reject. Then I invited them to discover the oath by repeating it after me.

The wind was stirring mildly in the rapid cool of that late summer night. Uncomfortable with the students' suggestion of a wizard costume, I wore my academic robe. Two tall students flanked me with their bamboo torches. I was nervous. What if no one replied? I took a deep breath and called, "Meds 2000, repeat after me: 'I swear by Apollo . . . '"

And to my amazement seventy-five voices responded in hearty unison, "I swear by Apollo!" Chills ran up and down my spine. When we reached the part about teaching the art to "the sons of he who taught me," there were titters; "without fee" brought laughter. But they kept on reciting. Voices dropped out at the promise never to use a knife, and only a dull murmur refused to give a pessary for abortion. But they waxed loudly again in refusing to do harm and in keeping holy secrets. Then there was silence. They stood still with their candles. I realized no one knew we had reached the end. So for lack of anything better, I said, "Welcome to medicine." Suddenly, all the students, both new and old, started cheering.

Such fun! Meds 2000 had been given the solemnity, a reflective ritual that Meds '99 had missed. Whether or not they would retain any of the history, they were existentially aware that they were entering an ancient profession on a historic campus. They even understood that ethical standards change.

A year went by, and in late August 1997, it was Meds 2000's turn to orient the members of Meds 2001. I was surprised to be invited back to participate in the same rite. The students must have liked it. And so it has continued every year without fail—as of this writing, for eighteen years.

The students do all the work of imagining and design, and I just wait to see if they will ask. Some modifications have emerged. The classes expanded to one hundred students; the groups are larger or smaller and more numerous. Sometimes new stations and stories are added; sometimes they are subtracted. Once in a while, the system for candles is frustrated by wind or by the odd paper cup catching fire. Twice, second-year students conducted deeper research on the history of the medical school and wrote entirely new stories for the walking tour that were handed down to successors. In 2002, a student selected a more modern version of the oath, which I read at her request; every year since, I ask the students if they have any preference. In 2011, a park bench appeared in the Medical Quadrangle—bearing a little plaque: "For Ruth (Meds 1957) and Peter (Meds 1956) who fell in love here in 1951." It too has been added to the tour.

The outdoor amphitheater vanished with the construction of a new research building. So for more than a decade, the oath has been recited on the southern edge of the campus, at the foot of the Murney Tower, an early nineteenth-century stone fortification on the shore of Lake Ontario. Often, the moon contributes to the setting, as silver light washes across the water.

Sometimes the tour, with or without the oath, is repeated during the year by special request, occasionally in winter and once on Halloween. On one occasion during my sabbatical, the ceremony was overlooked on orientation day. A second-year student grew anxious; his new colleagues, he said, "have not been Oathed," as if they lacked true initiation or some kind of magical protection against future sin. I had not heard the word used as a verb. Motivated by a sense of urgency, he ran the ceremony during a warm, sunny September lunch hour. We chose the Medical Quadrangle. He stood on the central rock above the crowd of newcomers, telling them that the oath was important because "a hundred generations of physicians cannot be wrong." I did not agree with this statement, but let it go.

Despite the changes, one thing always stays the same: the orientation is entirely owned and run by students; my participation is by invitation only.

Thus on August 26, 2013, one hundred students in the Class of 2017 completed their walking tour and gathered on the dark hillside with the Murney Tower looming behind. Rain had been threatening and the lake was shrouded in mist. The flickering of tea lights spread slowly across the crowd. Six bamboo torches were planted in the ground, I took my place in the middle, and, to my amazement, seventy-two students from the second-year class filed out of the dark to join in too, forming a great half circle behind me facing the newcomers. And once again, I took a nervous breath, called out, and heard from front and back the loud reply, "I swear by Apollo!"

Perhaps it will happen again next year.

Redrawing the Line on Professionalism

Reflecting on Professionalism across the Health-Care Continuum

PENELOPE SMYTH AND CAROL S. HODGSON

In the health professions, members of the health-care team may recount inter-actions and situations that appear unfair, unjust, unclear, and unprofessional. One may argue that a lapse in professional behavior often results from a lack of reflection on one's own actions. How then do educators develop a curriculum to enhance reflection in learners at all levels to improve communication on professionalism among members of the health-care team? Situated learning theory emphasizes the importance of interactions by individuals within a shared environment of work and learning, which suggests that a professionalism curriculum needs to be realistic and relevant, with the potential of exposing the hidden curriculum within the institution. The "Redrawing the Line on Professionalism: Views on Professionalism along the Health Care Continuum" project (funded by the Arnold P. Gold Foundation and the University of Alberta Teaching & Learning Enhancement Fund and approved by the University of Alberta Health Research Ethics Board) was developed to address our needs for an interprofessional curriculum that used self-reflection and group discussion.

Our first step was to develop a set of professionalism case vignettes that could be used to elicit reflection and sharing of personal views in a group set-ting. One goal was to determine if homogenous groups of learners could, after discussion, come to a consensus on whether or not the behavior described in the vignettes constituted professional behavior. Case vignettes were based on these components of the code of professional conduct for the Faculties of Medicine & Dentistry and Nursing at the University of Alberta: (1) honesty, (2) confidentiality, (3) respect for others, (4) responsible behavior, and (5) excellence and altruism (included in the Code of Ethics for registered nurses).

The process of gathering case vignettes from community members (that is, patients), medical and nursing students, residents, and nursing and medical faculty members was challenging. Medical students and residents were eager to reflect and provide personal professionalism experiences. The difficulty was in creating "gray" case vignettes in which the professionalism behaviors would be ambiguous enough for all levels of learners. Initially, physicians were difficult to engage—most expressed a lack of time to be able to participate. A different approach was needed. To accomplish this task, we arranged meetings with individual faculty members. Instead of asking faculty members to write about their personal experiences, we prompted them to recall their own stories with respect to the professionalism categories. We then asked questions, such as "Can you remember any time in your career where you had questions about your professional behavior or wondered about the behavior of others?" As physicians, they began the familiar pattern of reminiscing about personal experiences throughout their medical careers. Recollection of one case prompted recall of another. The cases were written down as they were described. Through this process, we gained a rich array of more than sixty professionalism case vignettes that were rewritten with all personal identifiable information modified/concealed to protect confidentiality. We engaged nurses in small groups and described the project. Following small-group reflection and discussion, they submitted cases through e-mail.

We then held a series of one-time in-person facilitated focus groups that lasted one and a half to two hours. Community members, first- and third-year medical students, nursing students, residents, and nursing and medical faculty members were recruited, with groups kept homogeneous with respect to profession and level of training. During these sessions, participants were asked to read and reflect on each professionalism case and then vote using an audience response system (ARS) to indicate whether or not the described behavior was "professional," "marginally professional," or "unprofessional." The ARS allowed participants to view the cases on a screen and anonymously record their numerical responses using a clicker.[1] The participants' responses were not displayed graphically until after all cases were read and votes recorded. After voting on all cases was completed, case-by-case results were graphically displayed and a group discussion followed on why participants thought the case described professional behavior or not.

What is innovative about this approach is the use of the anonymous ARS, which allows participants to commit to a decision and submit that opinion anonymously rather than potentially being swayed by others in the focus group. Each person can participate openly in the discussion or not, depending on their comfort level, after briefly reflecting and then committing to a response. No one was required to respond during the ARS portion, and yet we obtained a 99 to 100 percent response rate. This process allows for both individual and group participation, which is especially important when discussing sensitive issues, such as breaches in professionalism.

During the sessions, discussions sometimes resembled a debate with different students making diametrically opposed arguments for one side or the other. Some cases clearly caused more reflection than others. During one case, a faculty member commented that she herself had done the same thing for a patient but that she felt uncomfortable about it. She felt the action was marginally professional but that it was "necessary for the good of the patient." Another faculty member, who admitted to the same behavior, said that it was professional because it was righting an injustice perpetrated by an unjust health-care system. For the first-year students, discussion in their small groups was followed by a large-class discussion on the topic. The educational session ended with a discussion on the need to reflect not only on the behavior but on the context and motivations behind the behavior. We used Dr. Jonathan Bolton's "Can't, Won't, and Oops" model of unprofessional behavior[2] to discuss expectations of members of the health-care team and how there can be misunderstanding without proper reflection and communication.

In summary, using ambiguous case descriptions of behaviors in both small- and large-group settings can facilitate the use of self-reflection in learners across the health-care continuum. Prior to the discussions around our cases, all groups reported that they had a good understanding of professionalism. However, we believe that it is not through lectures but only through reflection on specific behaviors and ambiguity within the health-care learning context that we can begin to delve into the inner meanings and expectations that define the complexities of professionalism.

NOTES

1. Robin H. Kay and Ann LeSage, "Examining the Benefits and Challenges of Using Audience Response Systems: A Review of the Literature," *Computers & Education* 53, no. 3 (2009): 819–27.

2. University of New Mexico, Health Sciences Center (HSC) Office of Professionalism, "What Is Professionalism?" accessed June 5, 2015, http://hsc.unm.edu/admin/professionalism/behavior /index.html.

Two Processes for Reflecting on Clinical Moral Perception

CHRISTY A. RENTMEESTER

The processes I describe here are intended to help students reflect on their clinical moral perception, the capacity to discern how to respond with care to patients' and colleagues' vulnerabilities. I use a series of questions to help students cultivate awareness about their perception habits and to facilitate their metalevel reflections on how they are "trained" clinically and morally during their professionalization. The first set of questions was developed over several years of teaching third-year medical students in a classroom-based small-group discussion in a hospital setting. The second set was developed for teaching fourth-year medical students in a month-long seminar, an elective that includes two in-person small-group sessions at an art museum, led by an art historian and myself. Both sets of questions could easily be applied in a variety of settings with other groups of health professions trainees.

My long-term interest in how social and cultural features of organizations can influence, for better or for worse, clinicians' moral discernment of patients' and colleagues' vulnerabilities led me to explore my third-year medical students' habits of clinical moral perception in a formal, structured way. I developed reflection questions on students' clinical and moral responses to "difficult" patients, specifically those who are perceived as poor stewards of their own health.

Over seven years of bimonthly, hour-long small group discussions with third-year students in the hospital setting, the theme of frustration with patients who are poor stewards of their own health persistently recurred. My scholarly work on the phenomena of callousness and divestiture in clinicians[1] led me to categorize some important features of this theme, related to medical students' professionalization processes. First, at least some of the students' frustration is due to their perceptions and assumptions about what patients and colleagues "deserve" from them.

Another important feature of some students' professionalization is internalization of the belief that patients' health outcomes are valued more than their relationships with patients. The formation of students' patterns of clinical moral perception can be influenced by their faculty mentors' habits of responsiveness to this group of so-called difficult patients. Norms about what patients and colleagues deserve can be powerfully reinforced or powerfully problematized through either the formal curriculum or the "hidden" curriculum.

Rather than explicitly stating these subthemes to the students during our sessions, I tried to cultivate a learning environment in which they could reveal and explore these themes on their own terms. With this goal in mind, I developed and refined over several years a set of questions. I did not ask these questions in the same way for each group. Some questions came up prominently in some discussions and were, therefore, appropriate for more intense focus in those groups. Other groups explored these questions as I raised them in response to how I tracked the interests of students in a particular group over the course of the hour we shared.

In short, I found that exploring these questions with students required as much reflexivity from me as I was trying to generate in and facilitate among the students. Questions I asked them included: (1) Which kinds of qualities (behaviors, traits, communications, appearance features) of patients or colleagues influence what you think they deserve from you? (2) Which kinds of qualities narrow your conception of what another person deserves from you? (3) Which kinds of qualities tend to broaden your conception of what another person deserves from you? (4) What are your emotional and affective responses to these qualities that influence how you reason clinically and morally and how you respond to patients and colleagues?

Additionally, I asked students to consider the role of their mentors in influencing their responsiveness to this group of "difficult" patients. For example, I asked: (5) What are the behaviors of mentors you've had whom you think responded well or poorly to a patient who seemed to be a poor steward of his or her health? Students were asked to list these and talk about some of the behaviors they hope to practice and some they hope to avoid when interacting with "difficult" patients who have poor self-care habits. Finally, I also asked students these questions: (6) What do your patterns of perception and habits of mind suggest to you about your professionalization as a clinician? and (7) How do you respond to what you discern to be poor clinical moral perception, as might be expressed in colleagues' cynicism, biases, and value judgments of patients or other colleagues?"

Although not always the case, these questions sometimes generated intense emotional responses from students. Over time, I found it helpful to offer an explicit verbal iteration to students of the importance of cultivating awareness of their emotional responses to their learning, particularly with respect to their professional development. I also found it helpful to emphasize to students that we need not take a normative stance on an issue—such as whether and when an emphasis on health outcomes is nurturing or detrimental to the integrity of one's relationship with a patient in particular cases—in order to benefit from the exercise of trying to cultivate self-awareness about one's emotional responses to that issue. For example, I suggested that, for the sake of our discussions, we could be morally neutral about whether and when it is appropriate to value the promotion of positive health outcomes for patients above making patients feel that you are willing to have a relationship with them even if they will never achieve positive health outcomes. This enabled us to focus on the content of their reflections about their patterns of clinical moral perception and habits of mind without feeling pressed to offer arguments defending their views about the themes that came up during the course of those reflections.

I also found it helpful to follow the lead of several colleagues and use visual art to prompt reflection.[2] Observation, representation, and interpretation of both visual and narrative information are critical components of the clinical diagnostic skill set. Such skills also situate clinicians to be morally responsive—to respond with care to the specific needs and vulnerabilities of their patients. The fourth-year students who enroll in my elective, for example, can cultivate these skills by exploring art, narrative texts, and related interdisciplinary health-care ethics and humanities topics. With guidance from art museum staff and me, students (1) compile a journal of reflections in which they document their growth and development through the course. Students reflect in their journals, for example, upon patients, colleagues, or situations to which they experienced an aesthetic response. With guidance from me, students also (2) review selected scholarly articles on clinical moral perception, (3) identify and describe clinical cases from their own experience in which they observed poor and good patterns of perception in themselves or others, (4) write an article that draws upon the scholarly literature and their own experience, and (5) pose questions and state problems about clinical moral perception that might be clarified through further study and assessment.

Questions we have used to guide discussions during our museum visit sessions and self-study journal reflections include: (1) When looking at a piece of art what do you see first? What do you see second and third? (2) To which visual properties of the piece—colors, shapes, textures, movements, lines, curves, objects, subjects—is your perception drawn and why? (3) "What's going on in this piece that you can learn from its visual properties? What would you like to know more about in this piece? Since we focus on visual as well as narrative elements of discernment, I also ask the students these questions: (4) What about the story of this piece can you see by looking at it, and what about the story of this piece did you learn from information external to the piece? (5) How does the narrative information external to the piece influence your perception of the piece itself? and (6) What does your interaction with this piece suggest to you about your patterns of perception?

Students are asked to respond to this series of questions for several art objects at the museum and consider when, how, and whether their patterns of perception change or persist. Finally, I ask them to consider what their patterns of perception suggest to them about their habits of mind—their thought processes about processing visual and narrative information.

NOTES

1. Christy A. Rentmeester and Constance George, "Legalism, Countertransference, and Clinical Moral Perception," *American Journal of Bioethics* 9 (2009): 20–28.
2. Jo Marie Reilly, Jeffrey Ring, and Linda Duke, "Visual Thinking Strategies: A New Role for Art in Medical Education," *Family Medicine* 37 (2005): 250–52; Craig M. Klugman, Jennifer Peel, and Diana Beckmann-Mendez, "Art Rounds: Teaching Interprofessional Students Visual Thinking Strategies at One School," *Academic Medicine* 86 (2011): 1266–71.

PART 6

Spirituality and Mindfulness

Promoting Holistic Health through Reflective Learning about Spiritual Assessment

MARGARET B. CLARK AND JOANNE K. OLSON

Spiritual screening, history taking, and assessment require of professional practitioners an ability to reflect on interpersonal space. Some would call this space "transitional" and others "sacred in nature," essential to a therapeutic environment. Sadly, patient stories attest to incidents where spiritual harm has occurred in the face of nonreflective professional practice. Integrating self-awareness and reflective competence alongside approaches to spirituality, spiritual assessment, and spiritual care can foster the consciousness, empathic listening, and compassionate presence needed for optimizing whole-person healing and health promotion.

In designing a course titled Spiritual Assessment in the Promotion of Health, we asked ourselves: How can graduate students from various professional, clinical, and disciplinary backgrounds prepare to enter into fruitful discussions and deep learning about spirituality and spiritual assessment during an intensive two-week summer learning process? Three self-reflective precourse assignments have proven one of the best ways to invite students into spaces of deep listening to self, others, and Other/Divine/Deity. These exercises include (1) completing an online "Spiritual Self-Assessment" tool and reflecting on this experience; (2) writing a short descriptive paper about one's current understandings of the human person, health, and spirituality; and (3) preparing three bibliographic annotations from the literature. Five seven-hour class days follow. These focus on relationship-centered care and are organized around exploring three core concepts—person, health, spirituality—and six spiritual history and assessment models—from the early work of Ruth Stoll and George Fitchett to the more recent work of Gowri Anandarajah, Ellen Hight, and Christina Puchalski. During class time, students practice skills for spiritual assessment by working in groups, selecting a clinical narrative, and using an approach to spiritual history taking, or assessment, that fits the scenario. Group presentations incorporate discussion and feedback by the total class. Following their experience of the intensive seminar days, students complete a postcourse integrative paper in which they carry forward a spiritual assessment within their professional context and reflect on this experience by means of scholarly resources. This assignment requires students to integrate personal creativity, scholarly referencing, and critical reflective thinking so that course learning can be synthesized in a personal way.

This course has developed in the context of twenty years of interdisciplinary teamwork during which we drew on our professional differences (chaplaincy, nursing) in collaborative ways. We have researched literature in the field of humanities relevant to each of our academic backgrounds and interests, written a textbook on faith community nursing, coauthored a chapter on spirituality in a Canadian nursing textbook, and seen articles published in journals from both professions (on the spiritual dimension in Canadian undergraduate nursing education, collaborative interdisciplinary faith community ministry, and the education of faith community/parish nurses). Courses on faith community nursing and spiritual assessment have included lecture, clinical, and Clinical Pastoral Education (CPE) methodologies. Finally, our commitment to interprofessional competence in reflective practice has been underscored through shared keynote and workshop presentations (on compassionate care, advocacy in times of transition, and spiritual assessment as a collaborative task).

A specific teaching innovation arising from our collaboration centers on use of the McGill model of nursing as a place for interprofessional engagement. We read collected writings on the McGill nursing model.[1] We both appreciated the strengths-based, practice-derived, and relationship-centered principles upon which the model stood and saw the implications for spirituality and health. While the McGill model does not specifically address spiritual assessment or spiritual care, it highlights values of social learning, family filtering, promotion of inquiry, and the advantages of viewing patients/clients as active participants in decision-making processes that are easily translated to the realm of spirituality. In essence, the McGill model's health themes are also spirituality themes. Both faith and health are "learned" within family contexts. Likewise, just as health is filtered through family values so is faith filtered through a family's beliefs, codes of behavior, and spiritual teachings.

Translating theory into action through reflective competence in the fields of health and spiritual care enables practitioners to draw alongside patients/clients as they promote inquiry. Exploratory, working, and discovery phases of the professional/patient relationship can construct conditions for learning[2] and open *transitional space* in tandem with assessment, planning, implementation, and evaluation processes.[3] The skilled use of open-ended questions on the part of a nurse, doctor, chaplain, social worker, or other allied health professional can contribute to cultivating interpersonal and sacred space between practitioners and patients/clients such that collaborative reflection on health and spirituality occurs. Reflective practitioners are open to and respond to the curiosity, concerns, and emotional variances of the patient. In this safe, sacred environment of collaborative inquiry, patients can feel empowered to take an active role in their health decisions, adding to their resourcefulness as agents of change and health promotion.

Becoming a reflective practitioner takes both desire and discipline. Students in our course on spiritual assessment in the promotion of health choose to be there. When asked what drew them to the course, they speak of their desire to bring greater depth, sensitivity, wholeness, competence, and integrative awareness to their professional practice. We believe, and student feedback attests to this, that the pre- and postcourse assignments, together with classroom discussions and presentations, foster the students' reflective capacities and promote increased ability to listen deeply, engage the sacred nature of interpersonal space, and bring to their clinical environments an ability to both include and engage patients' and clients' spiritual questions and concerns.

NOTES

1. Laurie N. Gottlieb and Hélène Ezer, eds., *A Perspective on Health, Family, Learning and Collaborative Nursing: A Collection of Writings on the McGill Model of Nursing* (Montreal: McGill University, School of Nursing, 1997).
2. Marguerite Warner, "Learning to Be Healthy: The Workshop Approach," in *A Perspective on Health, Family, Learning and Collaborative Nursing: A Collection of Writings on the McGill Model of Nursing*, ed. Laurie N. Gottlieb and Hélène Ezer (Montreal: McGill University, School of Nursing, 1997), 146–54.
3. Margaret B. Clark and Joanne K. Olson, *Nursing within a Faith Community: Promoting Health in Times of Transition* (Thousand Oaks, CA: Sage Publishing, 2000).

Reflections on Interprofessional Education within a Spiritual Diversity Program

BETH SAWATSKY AND PATRICIA FRAIN

Mindful reflection is an essential component of the Spiritual Diversity Program offered at the Winnipeg Health Sciences Centre through Spiritual Health Services. The program consists of four courses, each available for full university credit. These courses include Hope and Healing (foundational elements), Supervised Practicum, Contemplative Presence, and Care in Trauma. Courses consist of three hours of class time and four hours of practicum experience a week at the bedside for a full term (twelve weeks). Each class encompasses three streams—theory, practice, and personal awareness.

In order to foster trust and collaboration, each course accepts eight to ten students, who come together to form a learning community based on personal experience, wisdom, and shared learning. Classes reflect a great deal of diversity, and have included undergraduate, masters, and PhD students. Classes also regularly include health professionals, such as nurses, social workers, occupational therapists, and complementary therapists, as well as professionals from other fields such as law, filmmaking, and education. The success of these courses can be attributed, in large part, to the interprofessional approach, which provides reflective teaching and learning experiences to all students, regardless of their professional affiliations.

In order to be accepted to the program, students must submit an application and attend an interview. One of the requirements for acceptance is for students to demonstrate an open and inclusive approach to spiritual and religious paths and traditions. The significant focus on mindful reflection is paramount to the success of the students as they journey through their learning experience. To achieve the reflective nature of the course, a number of approaches are utilized, including patient interaction reflections, journaling, specific class content, simulation laboratory, and final integration projects.

Patient Interaction Reflections: Students write a personal reflection outlining a significant interaction they have had with a patient (or a patient's family member) and then share this with the class. Students are encouraged to share an interaction that has not gone as well as they would have liked, with the understanding that reflecting on these moments provides them with an excellent opportunity for personal and professional growth. After describing the interaction, the students consider questions such as "Where did I feel stuck or wish I could have responded differently?" "What did I do well?" "What could I have done differently?" "What have I learned from meeting with this patient?" and "How has meeting this patient influenced me?" This mode of reflection reminds students that, ultimately, the patient is the primary teacher when we are mindfully present.

Journaling: These exercises invite students to spend time in intentional reflection. In the session on trauma, for example, the students write about their feelings and reactions immediately after they have been exposed to a traumatic situation. Further journaling and reflection help the students integrate their emotional awareness with the experience of being present with a patient in trauma. This is a powerful mode of reflection, as journal entries are shared weekly with course facilitators and allow for immediate response and conversation.

Specific Class Content: Intentional reflection themes provide students the opportunity to discuss and practice self-awareness in the face of ambiguity or fear. For example, the class topic "Confidence and Hesitancy" is a favorite with students. Here they reflect on hospital situations that caused them to hesitate and, in turn, consider practices that would help them gain more confidence in future practicum situations. Working together to brainstorm and reflect on their responses is a powerful learning opportunity for students as they realize that it is safe to share their hesitancies and that they are not alone in this inner experience. Each class incorporates time for both individual and group reflection—sometimes through presenting a question for reflection through art or poetry, or through viewing and discussing films.

Simulation Laboratory: Individuals from our local community volunteer to participate in simulated patient-care situations. These volunteers are provided with a scenario and act the role of patients in a hospital bed. Students take turns approaching the "patient" and practice providing care through a variety of scenarios. Scenarios can be tailor-made according to the learning goals of each student, and each student is given support and feedback by the patient, other students, and course facilitators. Students find this to be a valuable experience that helps them reflect on their skills, as well as their approach in providing spiritual health care. Many health-care professionals who are students in the program—for example, nurses—find it very challenging to allow themselves to be "with" patients and fully present without having to perform specific tasks for the patient. The "being with" versus "doing for" definitely requires practice.

Final Integration Projects: Students are expected to incorporate mindful reflection of their growth and self-awareness into an academic paper. This paper describes their practice of bedside care for patients and relates it to the content of each particular course and their individual journeys of learning and awareness. Students are also required to incorporate a research element into their papers, including source material and appropriate referencing of articles and readings according to the academic expectations of the accrediting university. If students choose, they may also incorporate a creative element into the project, such as painting, poetry, or sculpture.

While the Spiritual Diversity Program lends itself well to the practice of reflection, students come from a wide variety of backgrounds and at times are surprised by this focus and by the expectations for open and honest reflections. This emphasis on reflection is made known to students during the application and interview process, and success in the program depends in large part on the ability of students to both reflect on and integrate theory, practice, and self-awareness in their learning. Reflection is an essential expectation of the program.

Individuals in each course are encouraged to get to know one another in order to build a sense of safety and trust. Facilitators model respectful boundaries, risk, and vulnerability by sharing stories of their own that demonstrate to students that we are all human and we are all learners. This helps students take risks of their own when sharing their reflections. Ample time for storytelling and encouraging students to recognize the wisdom in the group invites them as individuals to deepen their reflection and sharing.

Once students feel safe in this reflective environment and are open to sharing and learning in this way, the innovation of the program and the spontaneous learning environment it fosters become evident to them. Students share their successful interactions, as well as those that may have left them feeling inadequate. They offer their wisdom and challenges to one another in the form of thought-provoking questions. In the ten years the program has been offered, each class has noticeably become a community of learners willing to reflect and grow together.

As the courses progress, students explore themes such as the difference between religious and spiritual care, vicarious trauma, ethics, self-care, diversity, mindful approaches to patient care, and death and dying. Specific themes related to each individual course, such as the archetypes we unconsciously rely upon to guide us, are also explored. A variety of guest speakers participate in the program, including speakers from various religious and spiritual paths, hospital professionals reflecting on their experiences, and others from a wide range of backgrounds. Students engage in mindful expression with artists, listen to stories from those who have lost a loved one, and hear from patients describing their personal journey with mental and physical illness.

The Spiritual Diversity Program offers students, professionals, and interested participants the opportunity to learn and reflect together. As a result of this program, health-care professionals have indicated that their careers have been enhanced. Some students have gone on to become professional Spiritual Health Specialists, while others have noted that the program has enriched their individual course of study. In addition, many opportunities for relationships and further conversation have developed within the wider community, after leaders from many different religious and spiritual communities have participated as speakers within the Spiritual Diversity Program.

Spiritual Health Services at the Winnipeg Health Sciences Centre are excited to continue to offer this program, which changes and grows as new ideas and opportunities arise. Since 2005, reflection has become the essential center of the program. Without dedicated attention to reflection, within both class and practicum, the program would not be as successful.

Chair Sculpture of Suffering Exercise

KENNETH FUNG AND MATEUSZ ZUROWSKI

Suffering is part of life. It may be caused by intractable, chronic medical conditions or unwanted emotions or thoughts. However, the relentless pursuit to avoid pain or control subjective experiences may actually exacerbate and augment suffering. Acceptance is an alternative that can be cultivated in the face of suffering. While acceptance of what cannot be changed can be intellectually grasped, it is harder to appreciate and apply. Acceptance and Commitment Therapy (ACT) is a third-wave psychotherapy that is specifically based on promoting acceptance and makes use of experiential and mindfulness exercises to cultivate it.

The Chair Sculpture of Suffering is an experiential ACT exercise that has been developed to help individuals (1) identify and reflect on the use of avoidance and control strategies to deal with aversive, unwanted experiences or physical sensations; (2) reflect on the observation that despite best efforts, the aversive stimuli persist and are only compounded by the use of avoidance and control strategies; and (3) foster acceptance as an alternative strategy to face suffering. The exercise can be used in group psychotherapy or in training workshops to experientially demonstrate the concept of acceptance. A group size of ten to twenty people is ideal.

Chair Sculpture of Suffering Instructions:

1. Set up the Space: Participants' chairs are arranged to form a circle or semicircle. The facilitator initiates the exercise by placing his or her chair in the center of the circle or semicircle where it will immediately draw the attention of the group. (The facilitator does not sit in this chair but rather joins the group in the circle.) Have participants get in touch with an aversive stimulus

they are trying to avoid, and project this onto the center chair. When used in group therapy, the aversive stimulus may be physical, emotional, or cognitive internal experiences, such as pain, anxiety, sadness, anger, negative thoughts, etc., that participants are trying to suppress, avoid, or control. When used in training workshops, the health-care professional's struggle and frustration with challenging patients can be the target stimulus. The more the unwanted experience is present and immediate in the room, the more this exercise will resonate with participants.

2. Form the Chair Sculpture of Suffering: Ask the group what strategies they personally use to cope with the aversive stimulus represented by the center chair. As individuals take turns responding, ask them to get up and use their chairs to physicalize the strategy and place their chairs in a representative relationship to the center chair. The participants then return to their own spots in the circle, where they now stand. For example, a participant may share that she tries to "forget about the problem" and then stack her chair upside down on top of the center chair. During this process, facilitators may clarify and thank the participants for sharing, but they do not comment, judge, evaluate, or discuss the coping strategies. As participants contribute their coping strategies, the pile of chairs stacked and placed haphazardly in the middle of the room will grow, and many participants will be left standing. Depending on the size of the group, the time allotted, and the engagement of the group, the facilitator may elect to involve most or all group members.

3. Reflect on the Sculpture: Begin with open-ended questions and ask the group to reflect on what they see, feel, or experience. Reflect with the group on the amount of effort and the diversity of strategies used. Notice that the unwanted stimulus represented by the center chair continues to exist, albeit buried under and surrounded by an unwieldy pile of other chairs. The pile of chairs may appear quite precarious and in danger of toppling over. Instead of sitting, participants will now be standing in the periphery. The space of the room is now occupied and diminished. The chair sculpture draws attention away from other aspects of the room. The suffering is now expanded to include the efforts and strategies (other chairs) that are used to cover or conceal it (original chair). Focus on the additive function of the coping strategies as opposed to judging them. Give the sculpture a name—for example, the "Sculpture of Pain," the "Sculpture of Anxiety," or the "Sculpture of Frustration with Patients."

4. Dismantle the Sculpture and Release the Chairs: Thank the participants for sharing their personal struggles and coping strategies. Invite them to take back their own chairs to reform the circle and to have a seat again. This will reveal the lone chair in the center. Pause for a moment and direct the participants to

compare the presence of the single chair to the chair sculpture that was just dismantled. Reflect on the difference in allowing the lone center chair to be present—the stance of acceptance.

Acceptance of aversive internal stimuli is a challenging concept to teach for the instructor or therapist and may be difficult to appreciate for the learner or patient. Some may equate acceptance as a form of submission or admission of defeat and therefore dismiss it as weak and undesirable. However, from the ACT perspective, acceptance is the willingness to experience (rather than to avoid) the internal emotions, physical sensations, and thoughts, including judgments, memories, evaluations, etc., that may be present.

This exercise experientially helps participants to physicalize their suffering as well as to observe symbolically the natural consequences of avoidant coping strategies. The inevitable additive function of these strategies becomes apparent, regardless of whether they are "poor" coping strategies—such as drinking alcohol, taking painkillers, or avoiding the problem—or "positive" coping strategies—such as problem solving, getting help from others, physical exercise, etc. Some who have been exposed to the concept of mindfulness and acceptance may similarly be using mindfulness strategies as yet other tools to suppress, avoid, or control. The key point is that we are not here to judge the relative merits of the coping strategies; many of them may indeed be helpful or beneficial. However, when these strategies are used with the explicit goal of eliminating suffering, they may ultimately augment it.

We have found this exercise to be emotionally powerful and engaging, especially when it is facilitated in an empathic, nonjudgmental, and accepting manner. It highlights that everyone in the group encounters the same challenges and struggles and increases group cohesion. It also emphasizes that the failure of these strategies to overcome aversive stimuli is not from the lack of trying. These are powerful messages, especially for patients with chronic illness who are frequently told (through self-blame or implicit blame from others) that they are not trying hard enough to manage their illness. The exercise validates their struggle and reminds health-care workers that we also use similar defenses to avoid suffering in our work and in our own lives.

The point that entanglement with a problem can fully occupy participants' energy and indeed their entire lives usually resonates deeply in patients with chronic illness. This is dramatically represented by the imposing and sometimes precarious chair sculpture and the fact that participants are left without seats and pushed to the periphery. Participants often spontaneously discuss their losses and how much they have given up in terms of time, energy, activities, and opportunities in the service of avoiding or suppressing their emotional or physical pain. The sculpture contrasts greatly with the single chair when the sculpture is eventually dismantled. In a symbolic way, the participants are removing their coping strategies together and allowing the emergence of acceptance to occur.

This exercise has received very positive feedback from diverse participants, including patients living with chronic illness (chronic pain, anxiety, and depression); participants facing other kinds of life challenges (parents of children with autism, or stigmatized populations, including people with HIV/AIDS in ethnoracial communities); and health-care providers. For some, the exercise has been transformational. Many commented on the lasting visual impact of the sculpture, and some participants have used portable phones to photograph the sculpture as a personal aid and reminder of what they have experienced in the group.

The Chair Sculpture of Suffering exercise uses a physical metaphor in a group setting to facilitate reflection on the common human tendency to fight adversities and persist in this endeavor even in circumstances where it is futile or counterproductive. Through this exercise, the alternative stance of acceptance, conceptualized as the willingness to experience, is cultivated through collective exploration.

SUGGESTED RESOURCES

1. Hayes, Steven C., et al. "Acceptance and Commitment Therapy: Model, Processes and Outcomes." *Behaviour Research and Therapy* 44, no. 1 (2006): 1–25.
2. Hayes, Steven C., Kirk D. Strosahl, and Kelly G. Wilson. *Acceptance and Commitment Therapy: The Process and Practice of Mindful Change.* New York: Guilford Press, 2011.

"My Aesthetic Moment"

Interprofessional Narratives

JENNIFER L. LAPUM AND JASNA K. SCHWIND

It is vital that interprofessional relationships are fostered to ensure effective collaboration. These interprofessional relationships can be cultivated through creative reflective capacity. As part of an interprofessional group, we collaborated to create an undergraduate course aimed at storytelling and "deep listening" within an interprofessional context. The focus of this essay is to elaborate on the use of one particular assignment, "My Aesthetic Moment," which we designed to promote students' capacity for reflective practice through storytelling.

The inspiration for this assignment emerged as a result of an article by Jacyntha England, in which she recounts her story of searching for a pedagogy that is open to the aesthetic.[1] England crafts a series of interrelated stories, in which she surrenders to both imagination and the "pedagogy of the aesthetic"—that is, a "moment of feeling truly alive." England recounts hearing Maxine Greene's words running through her head about feeling, imagining, and searching for meaning. Drawing upon the aesthetic, one is invited to find beauty and passion by writing without boundaries and resisting any sort of judgment. Imagination can foster an envisioning that repositions self and shifts one's frame of reference to that of another person.[2] This shifting of one's frame of reference is important in order to understand another person's perspective and foster interprofessional collaboration. JL shared an experience about a workshop by Laurel Richardson, which she attended several years earlier.* It involved writing a story and then rewriting it using a different perspective, character, method, or place in time. She found this activity to be a method of inquiry that for her promoted deep reflection of self.

---

*The initials refer to an author of this essay.

The purpose of the assignment was for students to engage in reflective practice, linking it with interprofessional narratives. Students were required to reflect upon and tell two interconnected stories. Prior to being introduced to the assignment, students read and discussed England's article, which recounted her first-person experiential account of finding the aesthetic in day-to-day life. JS engaged students in Narrative Reflective Process,[3] which is informed by F. Michael Connelly and D. Jean Clandinin's narrative inquiry research methodology.[4] Students were encouraged to reflect on their experiences and then craft a story, choosing and drawing a metaphor to represent that experience. Actively engaging students in these reflective activities allowed them to more deeply open up to their stories, in ways they might not have considered previously. In class, instructors provided students with various storytelling media, including images, video clips, poetry, prose, and physical movement. All of these activities served to open up students' imagination and to lower resistance to ways of knowing based on the arts.

Assignment Guidelines: First, students were asked to draw upon their own aesthetic moment and compose a story about an experience, using the prompt "What makes me feel truly alive?" As we developed the assignment guidelines, JL reflected upon a moment: "In the oppressive heat of summer, out of country, the rain pours down. Torrential. Drenched. I can barely see. Worries, anxieties, memories—wash away. I stand laughing, with the three people that know me best." As students were crafting their story, they were asked to consider: How does your identified moment make you feel truly alive? How did you capture this? Why? What in your life led you to this moment? Who are the characters in your story? What are the key situations and events? How are pain, passion, and happiness a part of your story? Who is not in this story? Why?

The second component of the assignment asked students to rewrite the story of their aesthetic moment using a different method to tell the story, a different way to capture that moment, or a different perspective from which to recount the event. For example, this might involve writing the story from someone else's viewpoint or writing it in second- or third-person voice. JL reflected again, shifting her perspective to an "Other," another character: "I wish we could stay in this moment. Look at her. Unbound. Nothing weighing her down. Pure joy, soaked. Feeling so alive, so far away, and so close to it. I know it's fleeting."

The final component asked students to explore how awareness of this moment might shape their future practice. Asking students to rewrite their story (as in component two) lays the groundwork for them to become open to different perspectives, an integral component of cocreating interprofessional narratives. Students can use this capacity to shift perspective in practice with colleagues and persons in their care. Students were invited to consider how awareness of this moment might allow them to see certain attributes in people or layers of their practice. For example, what might it reveal and what might it hide? Like the students, we know that storytelling is a vulnerable act. Thus, JL only provides a glimpse of what she is willing to reveal:

> Laying open my soul through stories is a partial act, some of my reflections remain mine, but that does not mean that I am not aware, that I have not reflected. Telling the partial story and shifting to retell from a different character provides space to imagine the other person's story. Like England, I also remember Maxine Greene's words that imagination provides an opening into the world beyond our own experiences. I want to throw myself, fully, into imagination.

Students voiced intrigue about the assignment and hesitancy about what to write. As teachers, we shared their feelings, but we were also hopeful. We encouraged students to craft their stories in the way they could best articulate. Storytelling was also being used as a pedagogical tool in the classroom so that students were experiencing what it was like both to tell stories and to deeply listen to stories. Thus, the classroom became an entry point into the reflective and interactive nature of storytelling within academia and practice.

We received students' papers with anticipation about whether this assignment would achieve what we hoped it would. As we began to read, we were drawn into their stories with curiosity. There were stories about family hardships, (un)belonging, connections, immigration, mental health, and disability. JS recalls her feelings when reading students' papers:

> I felt invited to walk along with each of the storytellers. Their poignant moments articulated through written, as well as through artistic expressions, moved me into my own reflection. I was able to look into my own moments of when I felt truly alive. One story prompted me to recall the joy of sitting quietly with my father on top of Grouse Mountain, having hiked for several hours; while another helped me reflect on when I immigrated to Canada as a young girl, standing on the precipice of my future.

Additionally, JL recalled: "I was drawn into their stories with such intensity. I felt fear, sadness, surprise, shock. I came as close to their moment of feeling truly alive, without being there. And, I was also thrown back into my moment to reflect, to re-story, to change my way of seeing."

Students noted revelations about the power of reflection through storytelling and how it cultivated an awareness that repositioned how they saw the world and interacted with others. They voiced aspirations and hopes that reflective storytelling would continue in their practice and remind them to suspend assumptions because we all experience and examine interprofessional relationships from multiple standpoints. Students became more engaged into their own reflective process, as well as with one another, regardless of what discipline they were from. They first encountered us and each other as human beings with unique perceptions of what matters and what is beautiful and then explored our and their professional affiliations.

We cannot be sure about how this assignment will impact the future practice of these students, many of whom have graduated. A couple of students noted that even two years after the course, they still reflect on the assignment and the moment when they felt "truly alive." We ourselves imagine that students will have to consciously remind themselves of the moment when they felt truly alive, since it is easy to become caught up in the routine acts of life and work. It is our hope, nonetheless, that the creative narrative reflection they engaged in will continue into their practice and that they will remind themselves to reflect and imagine the world of their colleagues as a way to foster interprofessional relationships.

NOTES

We are pleased to acknowledge all members of the teaching team, as well as funding we received from the Ryerson University Interprofessional Grant.

1. Jacyntha England, "Capturing the Aesthetic Moment, Even in a Winter of Discontent: A Performative Narrative," *Educational Insights* 12 (2008), http://einsights.ogpr.educ.ubc.ca/v12n02/articles/england/index.html.
2. Jennifer L. Lapum et al., "Employing the Arts in Research as an Analytical Tool and Dissemination Method: Interpreting Experience through the Aesthetic," *Qualitative Inquiry* 18 (2012): 100–115.
3. Jasna K. Schwind, "Accessing Humanness: From Experience to Research, from Classroom to Praxis," in *From Experience to Relationships: Reconstructing Ourselves in Education and Healthcare*, ed. Jasna K. Schwind and Gail M. Lindsay (Charlotte, NC: Information Age Publishing Inc., 2008), 77–94.
4. F. Michael Connelly and D. Jean Clandinin, "Stories of Experience and Narrative Inquiry," *Educational Researcher* 19, no. 5 (1990): 2–14.

Two Voices: One Intention

GORDON GIDDINGS AND JANET FINLAY

THIRTEEN YEARS (GG)*

"You've got 12 years max, and the clock starts now," she said. "Make of it what you will." It was strange to hear those words coming from a mentor, colleague, and friend, especially on my last day of palliative medicine residency. As a palliative physician herself, she was somewhere around her ninth or tenth year. She talked about the "average lifespan" of a palliative physician based on what she had observed from her own colleagues and experience. Practitioners working in the field of death and dying are well known to carry a heavy burden, which can sometimes become emotionally and physically exhausting. This is known as "compassion fatigue" in recent literature. And in true palliative fashion, my mentor was giving me a prognosis—one I had not asked for and didn't much care for.

Like many young graduates, I was confident that it would not happen to me. I was certain that my resilience was beyond that of this physician in her late fifties, who perhaps had not had the benefit of living in as many diverse, metropolitan areas as I had. I was always quick to point out that I was raised in Brooklyn, which I felt gave me more "street credibility" than most of my contemporaries. Certainly I was at least as capable of a reasonably long and satisfying career as she was, if not more so. As a matter of principle, it would be at least thirteen years for me—or perhaps twenty or even twenty-five years. Like many of my own patients, I was determined to beat the odds.

After a few years in the field, however, I began to see some cracks in the surface of my carefully crafted professional exterior. It was not necessarily the routine exposure to death, dying, or suffering that was the problem. It was professional isolation, feeling overworked and underappreciated, and ultimately, finding

*The initials refer to an author of this essay.

my place in the structure of an organization with limited resources that did not see the field of palliative medicine as I saw it. So when it came my turn to mentor young physicians and head an academic palliative program myself, I felt somewhat guilty piloting medical learners into a field that many said would give them a relatively short "sell by" date. If I were going to encourage them in the practice of palliative medicine, I would also have to give them tools that would help them to process their experiences when caring for dying patients. These tools would also be necessary to sustain them in their personal lives.

This concern led me to enroll in a workshop in therapeutic writing to see what I could learn about using narrative as a means of reflective practice and self-care. The workshop inspired me to write a memoir focusing on a period of sanctuary at a Buddhist monastery, as well as reflection on my patients who shared their stories with me.

The memoir led to a pilot project in Narrative Competency and Reflective Practice for the palliative medicine residents in our program, all of whom had similar hopes of beating the twelve-year curse.

CRAFTING THE NARRATIVE COMPETENCY/REFLECTIVE PRACTICE SEMINAR (JF)

I first became aware of Dr. Giddings from an article in our city magazine about this local palliative care physician who had written a book about reflective end-of-life care. Having attended a retreat program in Santa Fe, New Mexico, the author was inspired to tell his story about his medical practice. Saying Santa Fe to me makes bells ring because it's a place where I've also spent time writing reflectively and seeking spiritual renewal. As a college professor of writing who had just published my own book, I was looking forward to attending Dr. Giddings's book launch. Even before meeting, we already had three things in common. We were both writers, inspired in Santa Fe, and now living and working in the same Canadian city.

As I introduced myself to Dr. Giddings after his reading, he suggested we have coffee and I gladly took him up on the offer. My motive? A physician who writes narrative is unusual and I was intrigued. Two weeks later in a neighborhood café that, as it turned out, we both frequented, I asked Dr. Giddings, "Is there anything you're doing where you could see an English teacher/writer contributing?" He reflected seriously for several seconds before replying, "Yes, I think there is." This led to my involvement with the pioneer program for Narrative Competency and Reflective Writing Practice where the learners were palliative medicine residents at our local hospital.

I began with Susan Bauer-Wu's work,[1] written for terminally ill patients. *Leaves Falling Gently* was filled with activities for reflective thought, or meditation, and reflective writing. In this book, improving a patient's reflective practice was grounded on three overlapping aspects: mindfulness, compassion, and connectedness. It occurred to me that walking in the patient's shoes through thought and writing would be a way to help medical learners develop their own reflective practice skills. Bauer-Wu's book was set up in twelve chapters, which I adapted to twelve monthly three-hour sessions.

During our time together, we worked through a three-part process of meditation, writing, and discussion. The meditation took various forms. We started with deep breathing as a way to transition from the often-overwhelming schedule of the palliative care resident. Breath as well as prompted thoughts were our focus. I led with phrases such as, "I am grateful for my life," "I share my talents with others," and "I face my fears by simply acknowledging them." We also meditated on food, chewing slowly, and being aware of the taste of dates, the texture of almonds, and the smell of mango chutney, for example. Meditation also took the form of a body scan, releasing tension in tight shoulders, a stiff neck, or a throbbing lower back through deep breathing.

After meditating for about fifteen minutes, participants were provided with a writing prompt. The five senses were often a focus. "Write about what you hear," for example, evolved into a suggestion to take this awareness of sound to work every day. Or the writing prompt might be "Focus on others' expectations of you" or "What do you need more of?" About twenty minutes was allotted to writing.

Then participants were invited to share their written narratives aloud. Initially, we simply read our own work and then continued with another meditation-writing-sharing round. But as the writing sessions progressed, we became comfortable enough to comment on each other's work. The discussions evolved as the writing evolved. This meditation-writing-discussion cycle was repeated two or three times in a session.

Initially, the reflections were general observations and linear outlines of the occurrences in a day's routine. But gradually over the year, changes occurred. As the sessions progressed, I could see a deepening mindfulness as the meditations on breath, body, thoughts, sounds, sights, movement, eating, and, significantly, silence led to writings focused on awareness of bodily sensations, thoughts of the past, worries about the future, and focus on the present moment. The writings moved from thoughts of personal life to patients' lives and patients' conditions. The medical learner asked questions about patients' lives before they became ill.

This seemed to increase the quality of communication, as seen in the writings, between resident and patient and between resident and family members.

Scanning one's own thoughts and emotions, setting priorities, asking for and giving help are all crucial aspects of being human. When medical learners are comfortable with these aspects of life, they are able to recognize these needs in others. At the end of the year, one resident commented on beginning to "feel more comfortable leading difficult conversations with patients and family regarding end-of-life issues and feel[ing] . . . more capable of bringing families together during this time."

Dr. Giddings's concern about the emotional burden and physical exhaustion experienced by so many palliative medicine practitioners and learners is understandable. But as I watch medical learners become more mindful, reflective physicians, I am happy to be part of a process that helps them to go the distance.

NOTE

1. Susan Bauer-Wu, *Leaves Falling Gently: Living Fully with Serious and Life-limiting Illness through Mindfulness, Compassion, and Connectedness* (Oakland, CA: New Harbinger Publications, 2011).

Reflective Space

The Medical Library as a Mindfulness Sanctuary

RUTH WONG, VENUS WONG, JULIE CHEN, AND L. C. CHAN

Like their fellow medical students around the world, at the University of Hong Kong (HKU) medical students' minds are also occupied with acronyms for differential diagnoses, timetables, lunch plans, their Facebook pages, and the incessant inner chatter that clutters minds. Mindfulness is an increasingly evidence-based approach to decluttering the mind, bringing about present-moment awareness, and enabling attention in difficult situations. It can be practiced in any setting but is best facilitated in a physical space that mirrors the peace and calm being sought. Thus, the natural coupling of a deliberately designated reflective space in the library for such practice is presented as a fresh approach to reflection.

Mindfulness for Medical Students: Medical training and clinical practice are associated with anxiety, stress, and burnout. Mindfulness-based programs targeting medical students were shown to be effective in reducing psychological distress.[1] Several studies suggested that psychological distress linked to a "loss of meaning or lack of control in practice (or student) life" can be countered with the development of "mindfulness—the quality of being fully present and attentive in the moment during everyday activities."[2] The experiential training of mindfulness practice cultivates a person's persistent ability to witness whatever physical sensations, thoughts, or emotions come up from moment to moment, without being carried away by them. Apart from dealing with stress and burnout, mindfulness practice has evolved and is now being considered as a way to nurture the positive qualities that are essential for human service work. These include qualities such as attention, awareness, a capacity to cope with witnessing human suffering, and compassion.

The Mindful Practice Curriculum at HKU: Beginning in the 2012–13 academic year, all students enrolled in the six-year undergraduate medical program completed the Medical Humanities curriculum as a compulsory element of their first-year studies. This included mindfulness training under the theme "culture, spirituality, and healing," specifically aimed to foster well-being and resilience traits, which are helpful in reducing anxiety, stress, and burnout. The entire first-year class (210 students) attended a one-hour introductory lecture, followed by a three-hour workshop, in which forty-two students per group learned and practiced techniques to help develop the mindfulness skills of attention and awareness.

Evaluation of the workshop revealed that a great majority of the students found their mindfulness workshop experience enjoyable, with requests for continuation of the practice outside the classroom. We felt this was an opportunity to identify another physical space outside the formal classroom, to strengthen the practice of mindfulness, and to facilitate its development into a habit. As medical students spend a lot of time in the library, we talked with the medical librarian about identifying a quiet and protected space in the medical library for mindfulness practice.

The "Third Place" of a Library: A library's image, function, and service change with time. Thirty years ago, scholars in the library world talked about libraries without walls. Ten years later, library professionals were excited about and invested tremendous time on the new developments of the information superhighway. In the late 1990s, digital collections and virtual services were dominant enterprises. Libraries globally moved from print to digital and to networked-based collections and services. With such a move, library users could use resources and services without even visiting the library building during their course of study. In the early 2000s, the design of library services became more client-centered, with an aim to better fit services into students' lives. For instance, to reduce college students' stress levels, some libraries in the United States will even have dogs that students can "check out" as a form of pet therapy.

With the gradual recapturing of physical library space and a client-centered outlook, the "third place" becomes a prominent concept in the planning of library space and offering services. The "third place" is defined as a space where users choose to go to meet and create a sense of community of their own. Such a space in the library for human connection is different from a coffee shop because it is not only welcoming and enjoyable but is also perceived as a serious destination known for a respect for silence.[3] The idea of the "third place" echoes students' needs, which have been identified from various studies overseas. From these studies, students expressed that they spent most of their time in class or preparing for class. Apart from classrooms and home, they wanted a place to relax and to do something meaningful.

A biannual survey on users' needs and library performance has been conducted since 1996, and optimal use of space has consistently been one of the top ten concerns raised, because space is, of course, a prime issue in Hong Kong. We felt that creative allocation of space within the library would fulfill the needs of students for a place to reflect, relax, and do something meaningful. The idea for a Mindfulness Practice Space in the library was discussed with the dean of medicine, who gave his full support. Stakeholders got together to design plans leading to the identification of a study room within the library to be set up as a temporary home for structured mindfulness drop-in sessions, welcoming all users of the medical library. A future physical space is also in planning to be transformed into a Mindfulness Sanctuary. Its design is intended to evoke a sense of peace and well-being and it will be well equipped with books, audio-recordings, and videos on enhancing well-being. It will also provide meditation cushions and a Zen-like tranquil space, which most of the students would find difficult to arrange at home or in their student dormitory. A private group space for mindful practice will be incorporated, as shown here.

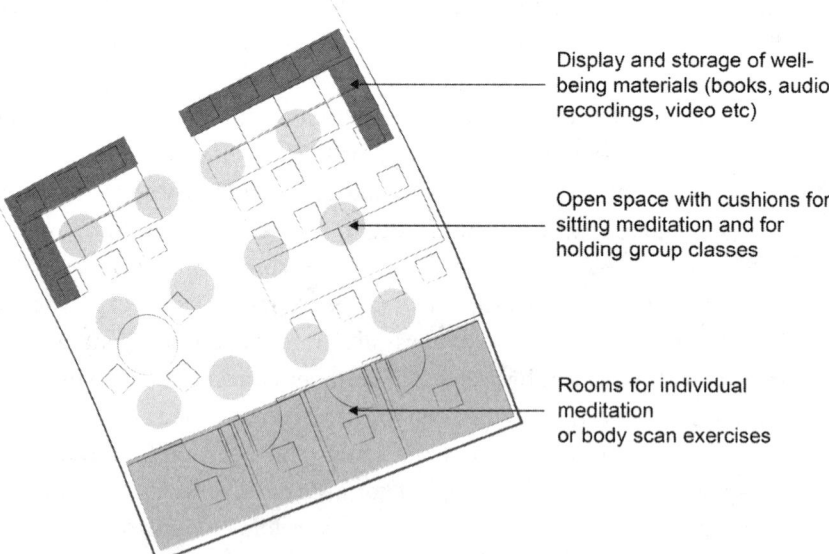

Display and storage of well-being materials (books, audio recordings, video etc)

Open space with cushions for sitting meditation and for holding group classes

Rooms for individual meditation or body scan exercises

Proposed plan for the "Mindfulness Sanctuary" superimposed on a small reading area in the medical library at the University of Hong Kong.

NOTES

1. Shauna L. Shapiro, Gary E. Schwartz, and Ginny Bonner, "Effects of Mindfulness-based Stress Reduction on Medical and Premedical Students," *Journal of Behavioral Medicine* 21 (1998): 581–99.
2. Michael S. Krasner et al., "Association of an Educational Program in Mindful Communication with Burnout, Empathy, and Attitudes among Primary Care Physicians," *Journal of the American Medical Association* 302 (2009): 1285.
3. Susan E. Montgomery and Jonathan Miller, "The Third Place: The Library as Collaborative and Community Space in a Time of Fiscal Restraint," *College & Undergraduate Libraries* 18 (2011): 228–38.

Growth beyond Borders

Exploring the Role of Reflection in Global Health

AMY R. BLAIR AND VIRGINIA MCCARTHY

Loyola University Chicago Stritch School of Medicine holds reflection central to the personal and professional development of future physicians. Reflection is woven throughout the vertical curriculum, encouraging students to begin reflection practices during the preclinical years and continue into the challenging clinical years. The hope is that students trained at Stritch will incorporate the practice of reflection into their personal development and professional practice as a lifelong tool, much in line with the charism of the Jesuit tradition of Ignatius of Loyola, living a life of contemplation in action.

In a similar vein, service outreach at Loyola stems from the charge to live a life in the service of others. For over twenty years, Stritch has been an active member in international service, forming partnerships abroad and introducing students to their global citizenship through immersion in the field. Graduates continue to work with underserved populations in reducing health disparities locally and internationally. A more concerted effort to provide students with the necessary tools to engage in the global arena responsibly and ethically came through the establishment of the Global Health Honors (GHH) program in November 2011. Reflection is incorporated throughout the honors program and has served as an innovative tool to evaluate the outcomes of the program. All reflections quoted here are included with student permission.

Reflection in global health occurs on several levels and serves as the gateway between appearance and meaning. As the experiences occur within the interpretive framework of an individual, global health experiences filter through a lens formed by personal values, as well as previously held assumptions and beliefs. Participants' understanding of the way the world is or ought to be may be either confirmed or challenged by an experience in a new culture, geography, or population. Prior beliefs may be reinforced, shattered, or altered. Reflections such as the following reveal a complexity that is not captured in superficial observation: "Walking into the [Central American] prison I expected challenges. I expected to run into some significant clinical issues, and to face some difficult patient encounters. What I did not expect was that the biggest challenge would be me and my own struggle with internal bias and discomfort. How do you treat patients with dignity and respect when you yourself feel uncomfortable, out-of-place, and guarded?"

When reflection is required, the expectation alerts learners to pay close attention to their experiences and allow themselves to enter into contemplation that reaches beyond simple observation. This expectation is most effective when it is conveyed through structured and consistent feedback and mentorship. Mentorship is most successful when guided by the concept of critical reflection as defined by Louise Aronson: "the process of analyzing, reconsidering and questioning experiences and of making an assessment of what is being reflected upon for the purposes of learning."[1] Aronson encourages clear guidelines and expectations for reflection, followed by targeted feedback on the structure of reflection instead of focusing primarily on the subjective content included in a reflection. This emphasis allows for the development of a comprehensive practice of reflection as a lifelong skill.

The following example shows how a senior student has independently refined the structure of her own reflection:

> I believe my feeling of guilt is why I have avoided writing this reflection for so long. I did not want to disappoint anyone by talking about the more difficult experiences I had in [West Africa]. I literally wrote two other versions of my reflection over the last two months, yet I felt disingenuous by only writing about my positive experiences. Part of me was not ready to admit that my trip . . . wasn't a 100% positive experience. I realize now after having written this reflection and having finally allowed myself to process some of the more difficult experiences in an honest way that I should have just talked to someone about how I was feeling sooner. I absolutely feel that by writing this reflection, I have been able to process my complex feelings and can let go of the guilt that I have been harboring.

In global health, structured reflection and appropriate mentorship bring into conversation the personal, medical/professional, contextual, and systemic factors that converge in the new, or newly reaffirmed, worldview that evolves from field experience. This example illustrates this convergence of personal and professional values that were challenged in the global setting:

In total, this experience not only shaped the type of physician I want to become, but it also has helped shape the kind of person I want to be throughout residency . . . [I want to always] go the extra mile to learn more and do more for those people in my life. This rotation also reemphasized to me how important it is to think about a patient's individual context in society when prescribing a treatment for that person. This is especially important when treating those without as many resources.

What is the role of reflection in the Global Health Honors program? GHH students begin reflecting from the moment they consider a global health experience. Students are asked to share their motivations for participating in the program, the factors that initiated their interest in global health, an anticipated area of emphasis for their scholarly project, and how they hope global health will be incorporated into their personal and professional trajectory.

These early reflections help clarify motivations prior to participation, including recognizing that motivations may not be purely altruistic. Introductory level, institutionally sponsored trips are accompanied by a trip chaplain or coordinator who encourages the incorporation of reflection into conversation. After participating in an introductory experience, participants submit written reflections on their experiences and are asked to address how the trip compared to their expectations. They share thoughts about the ethics of short-term global health experiences and ways that this experience has affirmed or restructured their envisioned trajectory in global health. In-person debriefings with faculty and staff cover superficial feedback on logistics but often evolve into deeper reflection. These sessions often reflect students' evolving concepts of their position of privilege, both in country of origin and in economic position. Effective debriefing sessions include "best practices" of global health, which focus students away from habitual medical tourism and toward participation in sustainable solutions to reduce health disparities.

In later years, GHH students take those lessons and transition to a student-driven model of engagement in global health. Reflections are required from each experience and are reviewed by the faculty mentor, who provides direct feedback on their reflections in addition to any conversation surrounding the experiences. This approach aims to incorporate the reflection process more deeply in personal and professional growth structures.

While I knew I would be entering the field of pediatrics prior to my trip, the experience has me thinking more about what I want to do with my career. Since returning I've tossed around the idea of going into pediatric critical care which is a prospect I was terrified of prior to going to [West Africa]. However, surviving a month of working with really sick kids showed me that maybe I'm tougher than I thought. Whatever subspecialty I go into, I want it to be something that will be useful to the department of Child Health when I return to [West Africa] one day. Yes, despite the rolling blackouts, 90 degree weather and bucket showers, I want to go back. I want to learn all I can during the next few years in residency so that I can share what I know and undoubtedly learn from the [West Africans] as well.

While the GHH program utilizes reflection to achieve goals and evaluate outcomes of the curriculum, there is ample room for improvement of reflection practices. Desired improvements include (1) standardizing the model of critical reflection throughout the entire medical curriculum; (2) devising a quality-improvement protocol to maximize programmatic enhancements extracted from the wisdom of reflections; and, perhaps most importantly, (3) acquiring protected time for faculty development and training to optimize mentor training. The benefits of mentor training spread far and wide for students dedicated to a life of global service.

This experience definitely changed my life. [Sub-Saharan Africa] opened up my eyes to the harsh realities of the world that I had previously only read about but never experienced. I realized there are so many problems in the world that one who wants to change it for the better could find themselves insanely frustrated. However, I realized that if I find my focus, my small piece I can add to the endless abyss of problems and hopefully make the world just the tiniest, tiniest bit better in maybe the tiniest amount of people, then I will die both happy and fulfilled.

NOTE

1. Louise Aronson et al., "A Comparison of Two Methods of Teaching Reflective Ability in Year 3 Medical Students," *Medical Education* 46 (2012): 809.

Service Learning and Reflective Practice

LYNN-BETH SATTERLY

I have long held the belief, reinforced now by many years of teaching clinical medicine and practice, that one way to help ensure that health-care professionals behave in humane and compassionate ways is to provide training experiences in which they are treated in this way by their faculty and in which they witness faculty and staff interacting in this manner toward each other and patients. Ideally, such experiences would also provide ample opportunity for reflection, with faculty behaving in this manner and guiding their students to do the same. In addition, they would reinforce the value of intuition and acumen, along with factual knowledge and technical expertise, so that real healing could be facilitated as treatment is delivered. Anyone who has been through medical training in the United States knows that such experiences are few and far between. When they do happen, they are generally fortunate accidents and not intentionally designed educational experiences. I have also always valued the tenet of professionalism that charges the professional, where universal health care is unavailable, to compassionately serve a certain number of needy or vulnerable individuals during the course of a career, with no expectation of ever getting compensation.

In 2007, Amaus Medical Services at the Cathedral of the Immaculate Conception was founded to provide primary care for the economically vulnerable and medically marginalized in Syracuse, New York. Amaus was to have a dual mission of service to the poor and education of health-care professionals in service and relationship-centered professionalism. Reflection and self-care were to loom large in the praxis of the educational goals.

Since those early days in 2007, Amaus staff have cared for up to 1,000 patients annually and have provided educational experiences grounded in the above-mentioned philosophy for medical students, physician assistant students, nurse-practitioner students, nursing students, seminarians, and social work students. This educational philosophy and the workplace values of the clinic are grounded in the tenets of *Gaudium et Spes,* the Vatican II document that delineates well the tenets of a Catholic Social Theory in terms of justice, mercy, and human dignity and how people of faith are called to engage and to serve the world.[1] Finally, techniques are informed by curricula that I designed for another course, and also by the Healer's Art course developed by Dr. Rachel Remen.[2]

Relationship-centered professionalism can be defined as professional practice in which benevolent and effective interpersonal interactions are reflected upon and become intentional and normative for an individual or group. Training in this concept is experiential at Amaus, with staff and providers modeling this practice and with preceptors and staff interacting with students in the same manner. For instance, feedback to students at Amaus is always delivered with kindness, focusing specifically on what the student did well and also on opportunities for growth. Students are given the opportunity to debrief about what they feel during the course of their time at Amaus and are asked to journal nightly about their feelings and reactions to what they experience at the clinic. They are encouraged to look insightfully at the doctor-patient interaction in particular encounters and reflect upon their reactions to it and what they would do similarly or differently. They are encouraged to pay attention to how a particular encounter felt and how the "energy" in the room changed during the course of the encounter, and to utilize this information to hone their own bedside manner. Students are encouraged and guided to harness their own emotions and reactions, to insulate themselves from burnout and to interact more effectively with the patient. Students are encouraged to be sensitive to the power differential between patient and provider and also the cultural divide that might exist. Students are encouraged to consider the profound trust that patients and society place in health-care providers and the responsibility and integrity it demands.[3]

Many students over the years have sought out an experience at Amaus to help them regroup after a particularly difficult semester or to spend some time considering if they do, in fact, wish to continue in their chosen profession. Amaus students consistently report that the experience at Amaus reminds them of why they pursued a career in health care and encourages them to continue on to make a positive difference in their own way, knowing that the sometimes dysfunctional, even emotionally abusive, dominant culture in health-care education is not necessary in order to achieve excellence and mastery. Students from all health-care disciplines at Amaus find themselves on what the Amaus team calls a "level playing field," on which all disciplines are valued for their unique contributions and no one is held in more esteem than another. For instance, professionals of all disciplines work together in a deeply collegial fashion and at the highest level of their professional function to deliver care effectively and efficiently to a given patient in need. Students are trained by the volunteer team and deliver care with direct supervision beside them. Students notice and often comment positively on this truly collegial and team approach to care, as students from the various disciplines are trained in its milieu.

Periodically at Amaus, an evening is set aside for a discussion dinner, for which staff and students select a topic related to professional practice and come to dinner with a dish to share and a poem, story, or piece of art, for example, related to the topic, which serves as a point of reflection and discussion. Such topics have included prejudice, power and professionalism, self-care, and vulnerability. In addition, periodic movie nights feature films and subsequent discussions and debriefing as a means of professional reflection and self-discovery for students and staff. It is intentional to include students and staff together at these events to expose both groups to each other's lived experience and insights; feedback generally indicates that the groups enrich each other and that sharing in this manner fosters better collegial relationships.

In the end, Amaus is first and foremost a practice that seeks to provide excellent primary care, free of charge and with absolute respect for the patient's dignity, to the most vulnerable in the Syracuse region. Staff are highly qualified and passionate about the work, and they volunteer their services. This is the personification of service professionalism. It is fertile ground in which students can feel safe and are encouraged to practice reflection, self-care, and compassion toward self and others.

Time and time again, in caring for the patients of Amaus, students are exposed to our common humanity, which transcends economic and cultural differences. Patients, health-care professionals, and students work together as equals in sharing stories and making meaning. Many students have expressed that their enthusiasm for their chosen profession or their desire to serve with generosity has been ignited or augmented by the Amaus experience. In its educational role, Amaus is not merely a figurative Band-Aid for the current health-care crisis in the United States. We hope that it is a healing balm and catalyst for positive change as we expose the next generation of health professionals to a powerful philosophy of care.

NOTES

1. The Holy See, "Pastoral Constitution on the Church in the Modern World—*Gaudium et Spes*—Promulgated by His Holiness, Pope Paul VI on December 7, 1965," accessed June 6, 2015, www.vatican.va/archive/hist_councils/ii_vatican_council/documents/vat-ii_const_19651207_gaudium-et-spes_en.html.

2. Lynn-Beth Satterly, "The CDC Model of Clinical Instruction," *Family Medicine* 37, no. 5 (2005): 313–14; also see Institute for the Study of Health and Illness, "The Healer's Art Course," accessed June 6, 2015, www.ishiprograms.org/programs/medical-educators-students.

3. Lynn-Beth Satterly et al., "Inner-City Healthcare and Higher Education: A Partnership in Catholic Social Teaching," *Journal of Catholic Social Thought* 7, no. 1 (2010): 115–30.

PART 7

Curriculum Design and Innovation

Reflection across the Curriculum

JOHANNA SHAPIRO

The program in Medical Humanities & Arts is a small but vital component of the educational curriculum at the University of California Irvine, School of Medicine. At its core, this program is a reflection curriculum. Its goal is to cultivate self-aware, self-reflexive physicians who are able to critically situate themselves and their patients within the culture of medicine as well as within larger societal contexts; challenge themselves and the health-care systems in which they function; pay empathic attention to disenfranchised, marginalized voices in health care; recognize how their stories and emotions, as well as those of their patients and colleagues, influence the patient-doctor encounter; and ultimately treat their patients with greater presence, emotional connection, and respect for personhood.[1]

In pursuit of these goals, my physician colleagues and I routinely draw on various forms of reflective practice. Our primary method is reflective writing on topics such as difficult patient-doctor interactions, cross-cultural encounters, ethical dilemmas, loss and grief, medical student/resident burnout, and finding meaning in medicine. Exercises may include point-of-view writing, letters to patients, poetry, and essays. Some students have kept a "parallel chart," recording all that they notice, imagine, wonder, and feel about a patient, everything that does not have a place in the official patient chart. This writing is guided by principles of reflexivity as articulated by Wald et al., including an emphasis on both transformative and confirmatory learning.[2]

We also have students create original projects using a variety of artistic media (poetry, art, drawing, video, skits, music, dance) as a means of reflection on their awe, ambivalence, or guilt about cadaver dissection; on pediatric and adult patients' various experiences of illness and hospitalization; on patient-doctor and family member–doctor relationships; on aging, disability, death, and dying; and on the socialization process involved in becoming a doctor.[3] Other forms of reflective practice include participation in medical readers' theater and attendance at theatrical performances, followed by expert panels and facilitated group discussion to ponder the implications and ramifications of their experience. Students also learn visual-thinking strategies through examining representational art, followed by reflection on the relevance of these practices to patient care. As part of a doctoring class, students break into groups, receive a medically themed poem, and reflect on how they would interact with the patient it portrays. Participating in an elective, students watch a video of *Wit* (2001), a film of the iconic play about a woman dying of ovarian cancer, and then argue about the nature of medical professionalism. The thirty students enrolled in the fourth-year "Art of Doctoring" capstone elective work in teams to make a creative statement reflecting on how the past four years of socialization into the profession of medicine have changed them in positive and negative ways.

All medical humanities courses and course components routinely incorporate "reflection on reflection" by sharing students' original reflections in small-group sessions, followed by comments and insights from fellow students and faculty, thus deepening and extending the reflective process. All written materials produced by students are read and responded to in writing by at least one faculty member. Whenever possible, as in the example below, we have one physician and one non-physician provide written and/or verbal feedback so that students can receive different perspectives on their thoughts.

An excerpt from a fourth-year medical student essay (used with permission): "Why was I exhausted? Helping people was supposed to bring me joy and satisfaction; shouldn't those things energize me? My attitude was the antithesis of an attitude of service. While I couldn't deny my feelings, I hated having them. I realized after working with Mrs. G. that not being used up is going to be more difficult than I anticipated."

Excerpt from a non-physician psychologist: "Such terrific thoughtful questions. They lie at the core of medicine. It might be worth actually noticing when service to the patient 'fills you up' and when it depletes you." Excerpt from internist/geriatrician: "Now that you have asked the questions, perhaps you can give yourself time to consider, 'What can I do to take care of myself that will lessen this feeling?'"

As is suggested in these brief snippets, faculty both attempt to support students, while helping them to go more deeply into investigating their own processes and those of their patients. Within the time constraints of busy medical students, we encourage ongoing dialogue (either in person or by e-mail) to continue the exploration of topics that are uncertain and ambiguous and that require more than one answer. Interested physician faculty have been trained in reflective methodologies through faculty development workshops, but we rely primarily on an iterative process of mutual role modeling and feedback to help faculty hone reflective skills. For example, written comments are shared not only with students but with colleagues so that we can learn from each other's styles and strengths.

Through this variety of reflective processes, we are concerned with exploring issues we consider essential to the training of physicians in the twenty-first century. Using a developmental model, we first focus on identity formation—how bright, idealistic college graduates are transformed into physicians. We next move to an examination of the ideals of professionalism, including the primacy of patient care, respect for patient autonomy, and the principle of social justice, as well as how the hidden curriculum can compromise and subvert these ideals. In the clinical years, our teaching attempts to interrogate assumptions about patient-doctor interactions based on race, ethnicity, class, gender, ability, and power, as these attributes are manifest in the doctor-patient relationship and within the wider health-care system. Other goals in the clinical years include tackling moral distress, ethical dilemmas, physician and student burnout, and compassion fatigue. In examining these themes, our intention is to help students become more familiar with confronting uncomfortable truths about personal, interpersonal, and systemic limitations.

Perhaps immodestly, through exposing students to reflective practices, we hope to influence the culture of learning at our institution, to make space for questioning, uncertainty, and, in poet John Keats's term, "negative capability." Medical students are used to expecting right and wrong answers. They are used to expecting *answers*. When questions are posed, they frequently react defensively, afraid that their instructor is interested in embarrassing them by highlighting the limits of their knowledge, rather than understanding that, in reflective practice, their teachers are asking questions because they themselves are uncertain about the answers.

Students coming to medicine from biological and other science majors can be uncomfortable with reflection and sometimes may question its value. These attitudes stem primarily from lack of familiarity with such activities and a pervasive discomfort with ambiguous, uncertain situations. By creating a supportive, nonjudgmental, trusting context that encourages curiosity and exploration, most students become excited when presented with an opening to think about their experiences and the experiences of their peers. The focus of this reflective work is not on evaluation (reflective learning activities are not graded), but we encourage critical thinking and reasoning in our learners. The whole point of reflection is not to be satisfied with initial impressions, assumptions, and conclusions but to dig deeper to discover nuance, complexity, and moral ambiguity.

These reflective activities comprise a very small part of the overall medical school curriculum at UC Irvine. But because they are diverse and spread across all four years and because they are designed to build on prior exposure, the MH program provides serious training for students in the skills of reflection. We believe this curriculum offers an alternative to lecture-based, multiple-choice, test-directed learning. As a result, we hope that our students graduate with certain habits of mind that give them greater self-awareness and insight; sustained ability to understand patient stories and how they intersect with their own stories; sensitivity to the role of both their own and others' emotions in medicine; and attentiveness to how clinical interactions are part of a larger sociocultural fabric that often makes unwarranted assumptions about vulnerable, marginalized others. We will have succeeded in educating reflective practitioners when our students embrace the cultivation of phronesis, the practical wisdom needed to interpret and guide their daily clinical interactions.

NOTES

1. Johanna Shapiro, Deborah Kasman, and Audrey Shafer, "Words and Wards: A Model of Reflective Writing and Its Uses in Medical Education," *Journal of Medical Humanities* 27 (2006): 231–44.
2. Hedy S. Wald et al., "Fostering and Evaluating Reflective Capacity in Medical Education: Developing the REFLECT Rubric for Assessing Reflective Writing," *Academic Medicine* 87 (2012): 41–50.
3. Arnold K. Kumagai, "Perspective: Acts of Interpretation: A Philosophical Approach to Using Creative Arts in Medical Education," *Academic Medicine* 87 (2012): 1138–44.

Stanford Medicine

Cultivating Creativity and Reflection through Intensive Arts, Humanities, and Social Science Opportunities

AUDREY SHAFER

I preach to the choir. Not literally: unlike some medical centers or schools, we do not have an established choral group. Figuratively, however, the metaphor works for the Medicine and the Muse Program (formerly: Arts, Humanities and Medicine) of the Stanford Center for Biomedical Ethics, as the bulk of our health humanities efforts at Stanford University School of Medicine are elective in nature. The health humanities do not have a massive presence in our medical school grid curriculum. We don't have a mandatory thread through all years of training for all students. But we do have an extensive elective program in which students can do anything from enrolling in a workshop to spending years on a reflective, intensive, scholarly project funded by the medical school, or receiving a co-terminal degree. It's up to individual students whether they prefer to remain mostly silent, hum along, or go for the whole "Hallelujah Chorus" experience.

Before describing the elective experiences, I will note that our school has had, and continues to have, reflective experiences that are mandatory for our students, including Doctoring with Care small-group discussion sessions throughout medical school. The two-year required preclinical course, "Practice of Medicine," embeds health humanities. Within that course, for years, every student read Anne Fadiman's chronicle of a Hmong family in California's central valley, "The Spirit Catches You and You Fall Down," followed by a live session with the physicians featured in the book. Filmmaker-in-residence Dr. Maren Grainger Monsen shows and discusses her films from the Bioethics and Film Program. We have taken the entire class to the Cantor Arts Center on campus for observation skills training and to San Francisco to hear a staged reading of Molière's *The Imaginary Invalid* by the renowned American Conservatory Theater. In Advances and Perspectives in Medicine, a two-year required course for all clinical students, which I codirect, students have heard from a law professor and a humanities professor about the context of medicine. But I would say that, compared to the time invested in anatomy and pharmaco-patho-physiology courses or clinical rotation training, time mandated to study the arts, humanities, and social sciences in relation to medicine has been relatively small in our curriculum.

This brings me back to the "choir" and how we developed a program that provides in-depth learning opportunities for students. Our program began as a couple of elective courses on literature and medicine and creative writing, and a few scattered events at the medical school, such as readings by poets and writers Adrienne Rich, Billy Collins, Dr. John Stone, and Dr. Perri Klass. These nascent efforts reflect not only the origins of health humanities as literature and medicine but also my interest in writing. At the end of the 1990s, an opportunity arose to become a part of the Medical Scholars Program, an established research grant program for Stanford medical students. The scope of the program, originally designed to foster the development of physician-scientists, was enlarged due to the vision of then senior associate Dean Phyllis Gardner. It was a case of "if you build it, they will come." In our first call for proposals in 2000, worthy applications for Arts and Humanities Medical Scholars grants materialized.

In 2001 I held the first celebration of student projects at my home, and by 2002 we had launched "Medicine and the Muse," which became an annual spring symposium to highlight student project presentations, promote student creative work and performance, and feature a keynote speaker. As a result of orientation announcements and word of mouth, a medical student committee forms to organize the event, with student directors and other opportunities for student leadership roles. Perisymposium events for the keynote speaker include a medical student lunch, a committee dinner, and an interview for the student journal, *H&P,* which our program also supports.

Flexibility, adaptability, proactive forecasting, and teamwork are all key features of my profession of anesthesiology, and I have found these to be helpful as well in medical education. As soon as we began to feel comfortable with the Arts and Humanities Medical Scholars Program, the medical school underwent curriculum reform. The Medical Scholars Program was subsumed under a new scholarly concentrations program. We approached the Stanford Center for Biomedical Ethics and joined forces to offer one of the original concentrations, Biomedical Ethics and Medical Humanities (BEMH), in the rollout of the scholarly concentration program in 2003. The number of concentrations has since exploded to fifteen, and, despite the science-based, research-intensive nature of our small school (only in the last year did the number of matriculating students exceed ninety), we continue to attract up to ten students per year to our concentration.

As in all the concentrations, BEMH students are required to pass core courses (ours are Medical Ethics and Medical Humanities and the Arts), take elective courses, and complete a project, which can be funded by a Medical Scholars grant. We are in an advantageous position in that our medical school is on the same campus as the rest of the university. Our students enroll in a huge range of courses; project mentorship includes faculty from a wide range of departments, such as history, art and art history, and anthropology. Exposure to faculty and nonmedical students through courses and collaborative work is a way to broaden perspective on health and illness, deepen understanding of the context of medicine, and question medical culture as students progress through their education.

The Medicine and the Muse Program offers a considerable number of other opportunities for not only students but also faculty, staff, alumni, and the community at large to reflect on the meaning of embodiment, suffering, communication, transcendence, resilience, and other issues through events and seminars, writing workshops designed to level the inherent hierarchy of an academic medical center, and writing groups. Pegasus Physician Writers consist of faculty, house staff, and medical students in dedicated, ongoing writing groups that meet monthly.

Medical students utilize the Medical Scholars grant program and the scholarly concentration project requirement to delve into topics such as the meanings of medical education and doctoring, illness and patient perspective, history of medicine, and global health. Students use a variety of genres and approaches, from academic investigation to creative arts. These projects have resulted in books, articles, exhibits, web resources, and curricula. Although this "choir" of students performing intensive health humanities work creates profound opportunities for self-reflection, the "music" they create is heard by many and, I believe, contributes to a culture of medicine that celebrates diversity, creativity, questioning of the status quo, and a greater understanding of the human condition.

Using the REFLECT Model for Reflective Practice and Action Research

BEV TAYLOR

I have been involved in teaching reflection in academic and clinical settings in Australian nursing and midwifery since 1988. When reflective practice was introduced to Australian nursing and midwifery in the late 1980s, it was the latest new strategy for bridging the practice-theory gap, so it was embraced with fervor when the disciplines were being established in tertiary educational settings at that time.[1] In the ensuing decades, reflective practice has become enshrined in nursing and midwifery curricula, and most students will have at some time been required to reflect on their practice. My main involvement now in teaching reflective practice principles and processes is as a guest lecturer to undergraduate students, and as a facilitator of participatory research projects.

In undergraduate teaching, I center my teaching around the REFLECT model, which evolved from the publication of three types of reflection[2] and subsequent research projects testing the model.[3] The model uses the mnemonic REFLECT to represent Readiness, Exercising thought, Following systematic processes, Leaving oneself open to answers, Enfolding insights, Changing awareness, and Tenacity in maintaining reflection. The REFLECT model gives students a process for how to reflect, so they can make sense of their experiences as they amass their skills, knowledge, and expertise.

In clinical research, I integrate the REFLECT model with the cyclical action research process, as they are both based on critical reflective thinking and they fit together very well. Experienced clinicians as research participants are delightful to work with because once they trust the group process, they share their practice stories generously from a wealth of clinical experience. The process within the REFLECT model guides them in how to reflect effectively, while they develop an action plan to improve their practice.

Readiness involves being silent, centering oneself in stillness, and setting the intention to reflect. Being silent creates a space of internal quietness in which energy can be gathered and the busy mind can be stilled momentarily. Setting the intention is done by confirming to oneself the most immediate task at hand, so one's focus is set on that activity, clearly and directly.

Being silent, centering, and setting the intention can happen as internal processes in minutes or in a microsecond. It all depends on the situation. Having some reflective knowledge and skills, taking and making time to reflect, making the effort, being determined, having the courage to reflect, and knowing how to use humor as a means of putting situations into perspective can also contribute toward a person's readiness for reflection and action.

Exercising thought activates thinking processes by focusing actively on experiences while using inspiring and guiding strategies, such as writing in a journal or speaking with a trusted friend. Being spontaneous as one thinks, speaks, or writes about experiences means that more ideas come forward, unedited, from a bountiful source. Expressing oneself freely takes away the restrictions of overly edited and "sanitized" sentences and concepts so that ideas are articulated creatively and candidly. Remaining open to ideas allows space for thought expansion and prevents early foreclosures on possible ideas, strategies, and solutions to problems. Thought will probably be exercised more effectively when one is not tired or stressed, so choosing a place as conducive as possible to reflective thought is important.

Following systematic processes means that a person chooses a suitable reflective practice model and follows it carefully. For example, I advocate systematic questioning processes in the form of technical, practical, and emancipatory forms of reflection. The types of reflection differ according to the questions they pose in relation to work issues. Technical reflection focuses on issues relating to work procedures and policies. Practical reflection focuses on communication difficulties, and emancipatory reflection focuses on power relationships.[4]

Leaving oneself open to answers involves not jumping to early conclusions; being prepared for twists and turns; finding tentative, multiple answers; and learning to live with uncertainty while working through reflection. The first answer is not always the best one, so by not jumping to early conclusions, more possibilities may emerge. Also, many twists and turns in thinking may be necessary and advisable. Rather than locating one answer, it is possible that tentative, multiple answers may be useful and ultimately more helpful, and that might mean learning to live with uncertainty for some time. Some work puzzles do not have quick-fix answers, and some complex issues need time to be unpacked. Learning to leave oneself open to answers creates space and time in which potential answers can come into form conceptually as possible multiple options for decisions and actions.

Enfolding insights involves mixing new insights into present understandings to create richer possibilities. At this stage, it may be helpful to use a variety of group or individual reflective processes, such as using creative art and performance work and enlisting critical friendships. When insights rest a while in the enfolding process, they have the potential to become more integrated and ideas may develop into deeper and more meaningful possibilities. The enfolding of insights brings together many ideas from various sources, all of which combine to create improved understanding and thoughtfully directed action.

Changing awareness comes about through making small, manageable changes in preference to making no changes at all. Unexamined cultures may be difficult to alter, and it may not be possible to "change the world" through reflection, especially in locations where reified power is exercised as control. However, sometimes small and local changes can make a difference, and that can be a good start. Self-reflective questions need to be asked to get to the foundation of emotions. What was the emotion I felt? Why did I feel this emotion in this particular situation? How do the particular aspects of this situation "cut across" my values of what I feel is ideal or appropriate? By naming an emotion, identifying its source, and analyzing the nature of the conflicted personal value that has caused the emotion, it may be possible to reach new insights and change one's awareness. If this is possible, changed awareness comes by reflecting effectively at the intersection of our emotions and the actions.

Tenacity in maintaining reflection is about holding on lifelong to reflective processes. Through tenacity, it is possible to reaffirm oneself constantly as a reflective being, through creating a daily reflective habit, constantly seeing things freshly, and always staying alert to practice. It helps to remain "unblinkered" by personal habits and preconceived attitudes so that one sees things freshly in every situation and stays alert to whatever transpires in any given moment. Maintaining a reflective mentality may also be assisted by finding support systems within the workplace, or within personal friendship circles, to find avenues for sharing reflective issues and insights with others. In work settings, it may also be possible to incorporate reflective processes into research projects—for example, in action research or other collaborative approaches.

In summary, the REFLECT model can be used to teach students the fundamentals of how to reflect to prepare them for practice, and it can also be applied to the experiences of practicing clinicians to help them to improve their practice. The model fits well with action research because both approaches share a common interest in assisting practitioners to describe, unpack, and change their practice.

NOTES

1. Dawn Freshwater, Beverley J. Taylor, and Gwen Sherwood, *International Textbook of Reflective Practice in Nursing* (Oxford: Wiley-Blackwell Publishing, 2009).
2. Beverly J. Taylor, *Reflective Practice for Healthcare Professionals,* 3rd ed. (Berkshire, UK: Open Univ. Press, 2010).
3. Joanne Rowley and Beverley J. Taylor, "Dying in a Rural Residential Aged Care Facility: An Action Research and Reflection Project to Improve End-of-Life Care to Residents with a Non-malignant Disease," *International Journal of Nursing Practice* 17 (2011): 591–98.
4. Taylor, *Reflective Practice.*

Curating a Reflection Course
in Postgraduate Medical Education

ALLAN PETERKIN

Four years ago, I was asked by our postgraduate education director to create a new course on reflection for second-year psychiatry residents. These trainees had just completed a year of medical internship and were "coming home" to full-time study and clinical work within our department. The new course would be part of their compulsory Wednesday afternoon lecture series, which included content on psychotherapy, bioethics, and psychopharmacology. I was to fill eight one-hour seminars.

I was excited by the prospect, as reflection in medical education is one of my areas of interest, but then I got to "reflecting on reflecting." I became curious as to how other, nonclinical disciplines defined refection and turned to scholars in our local health, arts, and humanities learning community for examples. I put out feelers to find out who would be willing to share with resident learners their critical lens on health care in general and reflection in particular.

My ("modest") draft of learning objectives was as follows: (1) to encourage "thinking outside the box" and a tolerance of ambiguity; (2) to honor right- *and* left-brain learning (critical thinking and subjective/emotional ways of knowing); (3) to have learners challenge personal assumptions, biases, values, and blind spots; (4) to consider how reflection enhances self-care as well as empathic care of patients; (5) to enhance narrative competence; and (6) to identify how arts-based learning can shine light on power dynamics and the "hidden curriculum."

I was relieved to hear from a number of fearless volunteers, primarily educators in other faculties across the university, willing to have a go. We e-mailed and met and e-mailed some more and decided that sessions would have to involve some form of onsite writing/reading or recitation/viewing/drawing exercises to contrast with the less participatory quality of the other lectures they were receiving on Wednesdays (for example, on topics like serotonin receptor subtypes).

The first-year curriculum included the following topics: (1) An Introduction to Reflection—What? When? Where? Why? How?; (2) Narrative-Based Care—How Reading and Writing Enhance Reflection; (3) A Sociologist Looks at Reflexivity; (4) Medical Hubris—How Medical History Keeps Us Honest; (5) A Psychoanalyst Looks at Film; (6) Visual Reflection—Working with Images and Nonverbal Cues; (7) Ethics and Storytelling; (8) Playback Theater—Actors Reflect on Your Reflections. (Titles have been enhanced for illustrative purposes.)

Subsequent iterations of the course have replaced Playback Theater (as the residents didn't like it) with Mindfulness as Reflection, taught by a social worker who is a local expert trainer in the area. (In hindsight, our first group of residents was not adequately prepared for the method and goals of playback theater, which has been used to great effect in other training settings.) Poetry and Reflection—Keats and Negative Capability, taught by Mount Sinai Hospital's poet in residence, got slotted in when our sociologist was unavailable.

The residents completed evaluations in which they were asked to share what worked, what didn't work, and what needed fine-tuning. Their anonymous feedback to each session was submitted to the course director, who then discussed it with me at the end of the course each year. Apart from the less than enthusiastic response to the one reflective Playback Theater session, resident feedback suggests that they highly value the course overall. They consider the sessions to be a safe space to examine, critique, and unpack meanings and concerns, as they explore the acculturation they experience as young doctors and ponder inequities in the teams and hierarchies of their chosen profession. They share stories of being silenced and, at other times, being misread by their attending staff, or of how they did (or didn't) advocate for patients. They enjoy talking about the role the arts play in their lives, and some rediscover (and revalue) long-lost pasts as artists or as students of the humanities.

As an educator, I've coined the phrase "curating as creating." I think we can foster reflection by stepping outside of our own comfort levels and providing learning experiences that extend our worldview and allow us to see what is truly beautiful in what we offer as healers. Reflection has to have an end, a purpose, or it becomes navel-gazing. We reflect to provide better care to our patients and their families. In so doing, we step back to find renewed meaning and balance in our work. Hopefully, we also remain honest about what we do and why.

How Family Medicine Residents Go Crazy over Passport Stickers, and Their Impressive Cultural Self-Reflection along the Way

JEFFREY M. RING AND JULIE G. NYQUIST

The White Memorial Family Medicine Residency Program takes its cultural medicine curriculum very seriously, dedicating over thirty hours to multifaceted training experiences over the course of a one-month residency orientation.[1] This training priority rests on a strong commitment to eliminating health inequities and to empowering our physicians to provide excellent patient-centered and culturally responsive care to all of the patients they will encounter during their careers. This paper aims to describe the key components of a one-month cultural medicine orientation and how a "Passport" serves to inspire and collect residents' reflections on their experiences and on themselves along the journey. The reflective processes used are in line with recommendations made in the international literature for best practices in reflection and journaling.[2]

New residents participate in a number of different cultural medicine orientation activities. These include preparing and presenting their own family genograms and deliberate immersion in the local community of Boyle Heights to learn about the environment where their patients live, shop, eat, work, and pray. They spend half a day rotating through, reflecting on, and then debriefing at seven fifteen-minute training stations. This experience includes the opportunity to draw conclusions from health disparity data, to explore implicit associations, to respond to poetry that explores cultural and linguistic barriers to care, and to discover how physical appearance can often incorrectly distract from one's own personal ethnic and racial identity.

The Passport is a twenty-one-page journal that contains an array of questions to encourage self-reflection at the beginning stage of their residency educational journey when their identity as a family physician is forming. Examples of these questions include (1) Describe at least one of your stereotypes that you discovered in this exercise and one way you will stretch yourself to enhance your awareness, attitudes, knowledge, or skills to manage your own stereotypes; (2) What were some things that surprised you in either the preparation or presentation of your genogram? (3) Tell a story about how you felt when one of your physical characteristics (gender, height, weight, features, skin color, etc.) led to stereotyping by someone else; (4) What beliefs do you hold that might conflict with those of patients in this community? Describe one that relates directly to decision making in patient care; (5) What unique strengths or characteristics do you bring to the team?

Some examples of resident self-reflections from their Passport entries included the following:

- "I don't think I fully recovered or grieved after the death of my close family member—my ex-fiancée's mother. I didn't get to fully cry to get all my emotions out."
- "[Presenting my genogram] was more emotional than I imagined."
- "Culture is a very big and important part in my life. I do not want to disrespect others by not being culturally responsive."
- "I learned that even well-intentioned physicians have bias that can be detrimental to delivering great health care."
- "I will try to stop myself from making assumptions and ask patients directly how they identify themselves. . . . [I will] ask them if there are any cultural or family traditions that I should be aware of. Asking them about sexual orientation as well."

Passports are collected several times over the course of the orientation month for faculty to read and provide supportive written feedback to the learners. In other words, the faculty member enters into a dialogue with the residents about their reflections. When the faculty members feel that a resident has not directly answered the question, or when the faculty member believes the resident should deepen their reflection in a certain area, he or she directly requests additions and revisions. It has been our experience that this direct, respectful feedback loop serves to greatly enhance the quality of writing and reflection on subsequent entries.

At the conclusion of the month of orientation, the Passports are collected and saved in resident files. Smaller self-reflection pieces are collected at the conclusion of the monthly cultural medicine teaching session and added to learners' portfolio collections. These monthly pages often ask residents to make a commitment to how they intend to change their attitudes and practice in providing excellent, culturally responsive care based on the content presented.

Every June, as the academic year draws to a close, a special session is dedicated for residents to reread their Passports and portfolios and to do additional writing about how they assess their progress and professional development. These assessments become additional elements of the portfolio.

The residents report surprise at revisiting who they were at the beginning of training and often celebrate the many advancements they have made. At the same time, they are able to identify new future goals to strive for. Here are a few examples of these annual reflections on their reflections:

- "I am more aware of my facial expressions when I know that I have a patient that complains too much."
- "[I strive to] spend the same time with patients that are challenging and those that are not."
- "I need to learn more about other cultures. Sometimes I just don't open myself enough to learn about other cultures."
- "Sometimes patients have certain beliefs that are very solid (especially religious beliefs) that should be respected and honored. For instance, I have two patients who had potential reversible problems, but refused interventions because they put their faith in God."
- "I plan to self-reflect when I am judgmental, take inventory, and provide the best care possible."

At the conclusion of each of the eleven cultural medicine sessions included in orientation, we ask the residents to select stickers to place at the back of the Passport to indicate that they have completed this portion of their journey. Our sticker collection is wide and varied, including animals, places, happy faces, and other images pillaged from our children's and grandchildren's collections. This moment is always greeted with laughter, smiles, and some feisty grabbing of stickers out of colleagues' hands! We witness the joy of moving forward, the pride of accomplishment, and the shared warmth that comes from dedicated team building—along with playful and creative learning. We witness the fruits of an invited self-reflection process that is met with faculty who read everything they write, mull it over, and write back to students in a respectful manner that invites additional reflection and growth.

In summary, the Cultural Medicine Passport and Portfolio serve as a coordinated strategy to invite, encourage, and instruct learners in the skills of written self-reflection. It was built using solid educational principles and continues to evolve as the lead faculty members evolve in their own skills. Our learners tell us that this is a very rich learning project that continues to provide benefits over the years. The faculty who facilitate these exchanges also report how moved they are by the depth and emotionality of the Passport entries and how rewarding it is to engage in this shared learning journey—not to mention the pleasure gained in watching the residents snap up their sticker collection!

NOTES

1. Jeffrey M. Ring et al., *Curriculum for Culturally Responsive Healthcare: The Step-by-Step Guide for Cultural Competence Training* (Oxford: Radcliffe Publishing, 2008).
2. Louise Aronson, "Twelve Tips for Teaching Reflection at All Levels of Medical Education," *Medical Teacher* 33 (2011): 200–205; John Sandars, "The Use of Reflection in Medical Education: AMEE Guide No. 44," *Medical Teacher* 31 (2009): 685–95.

The Scavenger Hunt

Writing about Medicine's Unmapped Territory

SUSAN J. SAMPLE

They've tested, they've matched, and they've (almost) passed the rigors of medical school; one final block of courses remains before graduation. That's been the most productive and exciting time for fourth-year students at the University of Utah School of Medicine to take a reflective writing elective. Offered by the Division of Medical Ethics and Humanities for the past ten years, Writing the Doctor-Patient Relationship has proven to be a unique way to bridge medical school and residency. The elective, which consists of ten three-hour sessions, offers students an opportunity to define and shape the kind of doctor they would like to become by reading poems, personal essays, and memoirs and by engaging in reflective writing. They explore different types of relationships with patients, particularly in terms of empathy, altruism, compassion, and caring. To imagine how they can develop these relationships, however, students must allow themselves to—in the words of Emily Dickinson—"dwell in possibility," which, in the context of medicine, may be understood as the unmapped regions of uncertainty and ambiguity, clouded with the emotions of patients and physicians alike. An approach we have found highly effective in this regard has been a fieldwork exercise and writing prompt we refer to as the Scavenger Hunt.

On the first day of Writing the Doctor-Patient Relationship, students are sent to five specific locations in the university hospital: the inpatient rehab unit on the second floor, the general surgery waiting room on the third floor, an ICU nurses' station of their choice, an outpatient clinic waiting room on the first floor, and a visitor elevator. Once they arrive, they follow instructions provided on a handout. In the rehab unit, they are directed to walk down the halls and record and describe a sign, poster, or note that they see taped to the outside of a door of a patient's room. At the ICU, they are instructed to stand at the nurses' station for several minutes and then write down what they smell. In the surgery waiting room, students are directed to walk around, note the different textures, and describe the texture of one item that they touch. In the outpatient clinic, students are instructed to sit down, observe the patients and others who are waiting, and describe in detail what one individual is wearing. In the elevator, they are asked to write down a phrase, sentence, or fragment of a conversation that they hear.

Three additional requirements make the experience not only challenging but, for some students, risky. They must go to each site alone; they must spend at least five minutes at each location; and, most importantly, they cannot wear their identification badge, name tag, or white coat. In other words, they venture anonymously, which transforms the familiar territory of the hospital into the unfamiliar—the unknown, where they can suddenly feel "out of place," as one student noted. Yet it is precisely in this space where medical students may gain access to a renewed sense of self-awareness, essential for their professional development as interns and residents. In her poem "Out Of Place," Lynn Dakoulas effectively articulates this heightened sense of self-awareness, which was inspired by her experience of the Scavenger Hunt exercise: "Uncomfortable, the greater part of four years / This is not my outfit, these are not my clothes / Why am I here? / Why are you here? / Who are you? / Hiding behind blue scrubs, covered in a white coat / Pretending, following in fake skin / Cold interactions with strangers, the greater part of my week."

Before physician-trainees can develop meaningful relationships with patients, many students find it valuable to reflect on aspects of their own identity and experiences that, by necessity, became off-limits during medical school. Although his parent died during his second year, one student felt like he never had the time and space to grieve until the writing class. For him, as for most others, reflection led to discovery and the possibility of reexamining his life, past and future.

One of our intentions in having students experience the Scavenger Hunt has been to help them reintegrate their bodies and minds through writing. The "absent-presence" of the body in medicine is well-documented.[1] Medical students spend far more time concentrating with their minds than considering empathic, relational aspects of caring for patients. Students across all disciplines also frequently consider writing to be essentially a mental activity, rather than an embodied process. However, writing well requires using all five senses—seeing, hearing, touching, smelling, and tasting.

Scavenger comes from the Flemish word *scauwen,* which is akin to the German *schauen,* "to look at." In this reflective exercise, students use their vision to see but also use their other physical senses to understand their experience; in doing so, they gain access to a fully embodied learning experience. When he visited the surgery waiting room, fourth-year student Nick Hurst made the following notes about a chair: "Squeaky, soft, cushioned / Wanted it to be comfortable / Looked like it would be / But the dry squeaky noise / Was more irritating than comforting / Was it the new stiff vinyl upholstery? / Was it the old springs? / No peace / No comfort / Instead, a grating noise / To mock the fear and apprehension in the room? / Maybe that is why no one sits in it." Hurst focused on how the chair looked, felt, and sounded. But more importantly, he used what poet W. S. Merwin refers to as our sixth sense: imagination. In wondering about the chair, the student touches upon the silent but palpable quality of the waiting room that the families of patients undergoing surgery know too well: "the fear and apprehension." Now he, too, empathizes and can begin to understand their position.

Student responses to the Scavenger Hunt prompt have been overwhelmingly positive, as in the following examples:

- "I didn't know writing was such fun!"
- "[Reflective writing is] a much desired change from our routine training, but still focused on being a physician."
- "I think it was fantastic in letting us explore compassion and caring about patients by reflecting on our relationships with them."
- "I think my goal personally for this course was to try and reflect on medicine, But often I found my mind was focused on other aspects of myself, which I find to be beneficial. . . . I have opened up to seeing the value and beauty of *different* styles of language."

The Scavenger Hunt provides a fun and safe exercise that encourages students to consider different aspects of medicine and their own developing sense of self as a physician. Reflective writing promotes thoughtful exploration and discovery of self and others: an awareness that will be helpful to graduating medical students as they prepare for the transition to the rigors of residency.

NOTE

1. Michael Bury, *Health and Illness* (Cambridge, UK: Polity Press, 2005); Chris Shilling, *The Body and Social Theory*, 3rd ed. (Los Angeles: Sage, 2012).

Meeting a Future Cadaver

Humanities as Touchstone for Reflection during Anatomy

RACHEL HAMMER AND J. MICHAEL BOSTWICK

At Mayo Clinic College of Medicine, first-year medical students take a longitudinal human development course titled Disruptions in Development. We seek to incorporate into the course a humanities curriculum with a unifying theme proceeding from the assumption that medical procedures—life-saving, life-enhancing, or not—affect normal development, often disruptively. The course material is primarily conveyed through live and videotaped patient interviews in which patients describe how their lives have been affected by illness and treatment. Into their stories we weave the humanities—film, literature, theater, visual arts, and creative writing—to address intangible skills such as professionalism, healthy detachment, attunement, and empathy. Our methodology is heavily influenced by paradigms established in the field of narrative medicine.

This essay describes a two-and-a-half-hour session called Meeting a Future Cadaver: Respecting Humanity out of Context in Medical Education, timed concurrently with Gross Anatomy. Gross Anatomy commonly generates anxiety, as students confront mortality in the lab. Students frequently experience cognitive dissonance in having to confront the humanity of their cadavers as they are literally cutting them apart. In some students, memories are aroused of deceased loved ones or other experiences with death, with minimal outlets in or out of the curriculum to explore their discomfort. Our Meeting a Future Cadaver session uses excerpts from literature as touchstones for student reflection.

The session begins with an overview of the history of anatomy that underscores how the practice of dissection has evolved over the centuries—from a public spectacle for the curious, to a punishment for criminals, to its current status as an act of altruism. Students then watch a videotape of an elderly woman relating her reasons for bequeathing her body to a medical school. The video reminds students that their cadavers were once fully alive, with stories of their own, including personal reasons for wishing to donate their bodies. Class discussion then invites students to imagine their cadavers as living people and to share their candid reactions with their classmates.

In addition to the lecture, video, and discussion, we select one of the following three reflective exercises using literature: (1) after reading from Paul Harding's novel *Tinkers,* about an elderly man with dementia in his final days,[1] students are asked to write a character description of a corpse; (2) after reading Sylvia Plath's poem "Two Views of a Cadaver Room"[2] and viewing Brueghel's painting *The Triumph of Death,* students are assigned to write about at least two incongruous images in the poem, the painting, or both; and finally, after reading an extract from the introduction to Mary Roach's *Stiff: The Curious Lives of Human Cadavers,* students are assigned to respond to the prompt "Let me tell you about my first cadaver" and invited to share their written reactions with the group.[3]

After each exercise, students discuss their responses to the prompt in small groups before the discussion expands to involve the entire class. No one is required to share their writing aloud, but students are required to submit their reflective writing to the instructors for feedback. Frequently, through these submissions, the instructors identify pressing topics for discussion or issues to clarify in the next class session.

One dominant theme that students express is that the instructors have managed to create an oasis from "the rest of medical school." We believe the humanities exercises contribute most to this effect. Many students state their gratitude at having an opportunity—rare in or absent from their other classes—to integrate their subjective experiences with the objective data that they are learning elsewhere in the curriculum. One student wrote, "I thought today's discussion was therapeutic. Buckets of information, most of it not applicable to our future practice, are dumped on us continually day after day. It's important to reflect on the process of development we are going through as anatomy students. The course feels like a rite of passage."

Many students mention that it is difficult to foster a disciplined practice of reflection on their own time and so appreciate the prompt to do so during mandatory class time. In the following excerpt, a student expressed that for her, medical school is a dizzying whirlwind. She appreciated the invitation the class affords her to take a moment to stop and contemplate what is rushing by:

> Yesterday was a great opportunity to reflect on our cadavers after a whirlwind first few weeks of anatomy. The course consumes so much time that I have often

found myself just working and memorizing without realizing what I am actually doing and the significance of my activity. It really is a privilege to work on a human body to establish our baseline medical knowledge, but until yesterday I hadn't taken the time to reflect on the decision of my cadaver to give his body to science after his life ended.

We have found that the human element emphasized in literary texts—explored in class discussion and reinforced by reflective writing—inspires ruminations on what it means to become a professional. Maybe that is the equilibrium I am slowly beginning to appreciate: professional in the moment but still connected enough to not forget the humanistic aspect, or the story, behind each patient.

Many student reflections take the form of personal goal statements or pacts with a future self. We hope that students will someday reread what they have written in Disruptions in Development to mark the passage of time and the evolution of their professional identities. Other reflections document the turbulence stirred up in students' internal climates in response to Gross Anatomy. Many students worry that they are losing an innocent part of themselves. Some write with the pressured voices of beleaguered individuals struggling to hold on to a sensitivity and humanity they fear they are losing, as in the following example:

> Since the day anatomy started, I have dreamt of and dwelled plenty on my cadaver. He visits my dreams. I think I am beginning to be desensitized to the fact that this cadaver was a living and breathing human being. I look at it as a piece of meat and when I dwell too much guessing about this person's life, I get queasy or weak at the knees. I have been confused by the professors of anatomy and whether they want me to empathize or desensitize.

We believe that the free form of the reflections is central to our method. We neither tell students how to respond nor how to reflect. We merely give them the space to react and the promise to receive whatever comes with equanimity, giving them our honest responses to what they have written. We find students hold themselves to high standards even when few expectations are given. We are repeatedly impressed by the fluidity with which many students navigate between reflections on their cadavers as physical corpses, as philosophical embodiments, and as tools for accessing their innermost feelings. Many assignments are elegant works of improvisatory creative writing:

> Let me tell you about my first cadaver. He was an older gentleman. I wish I was more emotionally attached to him but lately it has been really hard to become

emotionally attached. Class is stressful and I have seen a couple different dead people and have come to terms with the fact that they are dead. Back to my cadaver, he is older and seems to remind me of an old English fellow with a bowler hat. His stubble on his face shook me to the idea that he was a real person. Sometimes I dream of him grabbing me while I am dissecting and him saying stop. This dream isn't as scary as much as it is my mind trying to humanize this patient.

Many responses retain a healthy mood of uncertainty. In reflection, students are freed up to explore their immediate reactions—however irrational, without the "irritable reaching after fact and reason." We delight in establishing a setting in which students feel safe to say what they must, not what they think is "right." It seems only proper that a human development course should make every effort to help students examine their own developmental trajectories.

NOTES

1. Paul Harding, *Tinkers* (New York: Random House, 2011).
2. Sylvia Plath, *The Collected Poems* (New York: Harper Perennial, 1992).
3. Mary Roach, *Stiff: The Curious Lives of Human Cadavers* (New York: Norton, 2004).

A Narrative Companion for
the Medical Curriculum

DEBRA HAMER, JESSE KANCIR, JONATHAN FULLER,
AYELET KUPER, PIER BRYDEN, AND ALLAN PETERKIN

As we can all attest, the road to becoming a doctor is paved with privilege, challenges, and adversity. Students and physicians repeatedly confront their academic, physical, and emotional limits. Through the process, we often feel overwhelmed, desensitized, and lost. Perhaps what we are most at risk of losing as we acquire our professional identities are our distinct, individual identities. Yet we have the opportunity to weave both together through caring, reflective practices.

Within the medical education literature, narrative medicine and the medical humanities have been proposed as educational strategies to encourage learners to examine their relationships and to reflect on their attitudes when caring for patients. A narrative has the power to reach its audience through the transmission of language, ideas, imagery, experiences, and emotions, providing that audience with an understanding of other lived worlds—what we call "empathy." The use of narratives in medical education may encourage learners to think critically not only about their experiences but also about their own shifting identities. A critical disposition and reflective capacity can serve to support trainees and doctors as they grapple with uncertainty, assumptions, and conflicts—both personal and professional.

At the University of Toronto, a group of students and medical educators—ourselves included—came together to evaluate how the undergraduate medical curriculum could better develop capacities for empathy, caring, and critical reflection. The medical humanities and narratives seemed to offer a way, but how could this approach compete for curriculum time with established pillars of the curriculum? Was it possible to create a humanities accompaniment to the biomedical curriculum that would be genuinely integrated and adopted by learners? And how would the students take it up? It was out of this mélange of questions and challenges that the Companion Curriculum was born.

The Companion is a curriculum that links the science-focused undergraduate medical curriculum with relevant narratives selected from literature, visual art, and audiovisual texts. It provides an introduction to narratives created by writers, physicians, and patients with a talent for evoking reader responses. The selections aim to enrich the perspective that is brought to didactic biomedical lectures or to act as a commentary on the medical profession's approach. The collection also aims to expose students to a variety of uses of language so as to enhance clinical description of illness and remind students of the power of communication and connection. In this way, the Companion allows students to develop curiosity and reflective capacity, while also fostering a community for reflection among their peers. Like any good companion, the humanities pieces support the core medical curriculum, giving it new perspectives.

The Companion was first conceptualized and supervised by Dr. Allan Peterkin at the University of Toronto. The project then grew to involve Drs. Michael Roberts, Ayelet Kuper, Pier Bryden, and Elizabeth Berger (faculty members); Drs. Debra Hamer and Caitlin McKeever (residents); Jonathan Fuller and Jesse Kancir (medical students); and Joan McKnight (our administrative coordinator). The project has also involved countless medical students from all four years of study who have shaped the selection of narrative pieces as well as how the pieces are used and distributed to learners. Unlike reading lists generated by faculty in other medical schools, our Companion is a student-generated project, which is crucial to its uptake and integration as well as its sustainability.

The Companion is divided into preclerkship and clerkship curricula to match the two distinct stages of medical education at the University of Toronto. The preclerkship Companion complements the first two years of medical studies that explore health and disease through the basic medical sciences, such as anatomy, physiology, and pathology, as well as the medical management of disease. The Companion mirrors the weekly lecture architecture, providing narrative content that parallels the learner's biomedical studies. For each biomedical lecture, there are a few select pieces of literature, reflective essays, poetry, or other media that echo elements of the medicine being taught.[1] Learners can thus come to imagine encounters with patients and their families despite minimal clinical exposure in the first two years. Some faculty members involved with this project initially selected pieces for this curriculum; later, a group of twelve students assumed the effort of collecting suggestions, finalizing selections, and obtaining permissions for distribution. We released the first-year preclerkship materials in September 2011 and began distributing the second-year materials in September 2012.

In preclerkship, the Companion pieces have been printed and distributed as a preface to the weekly lecture note packages that are provided to students. The students are encouraged to use the humanities selections in whatever way they wish. Some read them during the breaks between lectures, while others find them to be a welcome place to encounter something beautifully written and to rest their minds as they prepare for exams. However they are used, the humanities pieces remain with the students as a reminder of a wider, human-istic perspective that otherwise may become lost among facts and mnemonics.

The clerkship Companion is structured differently from the preclerkship Companion to reflect the transition at this stage in training to more inde-pendent clinical experiences. The clerkship Companion captures this change by presenting more clinically directed narratives, accompanied by probing questions that can be used for self-reflection.

At the University of Toronto, clerkship is currently 77 weeks and is divided into Year 3 (51 weeks) and Year 4 (26 weeks). During that time, clinical clerks rotate through different specialty areas (internal medicine, pediatrics, surgery, psychiatry, etc.) for up to eight weeks at a time. The clerkship Companion offers two to three narrative pieces for each clinical rotation. The clerkship Compan-ion subcommittee included ten medical students who worked collaboratively with Dr. Hamer (resident) to select appropriate pieces. Each group member was assigned a specialty area and was responsible for finding pieces for that area of interest. Once pieces were found, they were brought to the group for vetting and discussion, with a focus on finding pieces that would be interesting for learners as well as clinically relevant. The group then developed the series of reflective questions to be included with each piece.

The clerkship Companion has thus far been distributed to learners by either e-mail or in print form at the beginning of each rotation. We have encouraged clerkship directors to use these materials as they see fit, allowing student access in a manner that reflects the demands of the rotation. While at this time most rotation coordinators simply send students the materials at the beginning of the rotation, we have also suggested sending a reading every one to two weeks, thereby creating a reminder for students that these materials are available and encouraged. More recently, there has been a growing focus on faculty and resident development, in order to generate more interest and competence in using these narrative pieces as part of clerkship teaching. For example, within the psychiatry clerkship rotation, there is growing interest in starting a resident-led teaching module based on the Companion materials in order to engage more students with the materials and to allow for deeper guided reflection.

The Companion is an organically grown humanities curriculum that takes as its primary source the perspectives of successive cohorts of medical students. At this time, new students are adding and changing the selected texts to reflect their interests and annual curricular changes, as well as looking at new ways to distribute the materials. In preclerkship, we have begun to integrate the Companion using online social media platforms on a new website called ArtBeat, which has blogging capabilities. This allows students to extend the discussion beyond the classroom and generates more spontaneous and authentic reflection.

Since its inception, the Companion has been propelled by the interest and passion of students, educators, and administrators at the University of Toronto. Support from all three levels is essential for the sustainability of the Companion Curriculum and for the success of any similar initiatives that we hope it will encourage. Interest in our project has been gaining momentum, including growing collaborations and student involvement. We are currently evaluating the Companion through student focus groups, which we expect will reveal its impact, as well as challenges, surprises, and important lessons regarding our strategy of narrative as companion to the curriculum.

NOTE

1. For a complete list of Companion texts, see www.health-humanities.com.

Recognizing Learning Opportunities in the Workplace

Encouraging Clinical Supervisors to Think Big in Their Teaching

NATALIE RADOMSKI AND PAM HARVEY

In clinical placement settings, learning and teaching opportunities are embedded in day-to-day health-care encounters and activities.[1] The insights and complexities that inform health professional work with patients and colleagues may be unseen or taken for granted. Clinical supervisors may not recognize the unique learning and teaching opportunities afforded by their health-care environments. Making clinical learning and teaching experiences more explicit helps learners make sense of what is happening and why, creating a richer context for understanding and involvement.[2]

Our reflective teaching strategy comes from our professional development work with Australian rural and regional clinical educators located in a range of health-care settings in our clinical placement area (including hospitals, primary care, and ambulatory health services). We wanted to encourage our supervisor participants to see and appreciate their health-service settings as learning environments—to identify and, importantly, analyze the potentially rich learning and teaching opportunities in those settings. As one of our rural supervisor colleagues commented, "Some of the most valuable teaching takes place unexpectedly and you need to be able to utilize and capitalize on those opportunities."

In devising our pedagogical approach, we took the view that the health-service setting (including the health-care tasks, patient situations, and workplace relationships occurring in that setting) can encourage or limit opportunities for participation and active learning. Our reflective strategy incorporates three workshop activities and has been conducted with groups of eight to twenty clinical supervisors. Prior to the workshop, we ask our participants to take a few minutes during one of their work shifts to observe and record brief individual responses to the following questions: How many learners are there in your health-care setting (that is, your particular ward, clinic, or community practice setting)? Who are they and what are they doing? How are patients involved in teaching? Can you describe any learning and teaching opportunities that are not being utilized?

Our educational aim for this preworkshop activity is to encourage clinical supervisors to notice the educational activities actually occurring in their work environments and to identify potential learning opportunities that could be developed. We build on this observation activity with a reflective workshop designed to analyze the workplace-based learning and teaching opportunities generated by our participant group. Participants are invited to share their learning opportunities, and we capture these on the whiteboard (for approximately 30 to 40 minutes). We then ask the clinical supervisors to work in pairs (for about 20 minutes) to explore what they think their learners might learn by participating in one of "underutilized" opportunities they have identified (such as involving students in discharge planning or asking them to follow a patient on their medical journey). We encourage participants to choose a workplace-based learning opportunity that is of particular interest to them. To support a deeper level of analysis for the paired activity, we devised a written template to help tease out specific practical skills, conceptual knowledge, and health professional interactions and contextual learning experiences that could be developed. Information recorded in the template provides a practical starting point for writing clinical learning objectives and clinical teaching plans.

We conclude our reflective workshop by encouraging our clinical supervisor participants to harness the rich learning opportunities available in their practice settings. We also highlight important workplace-based teaching concepts, such as educational signposting, focused observation, guided learning, and thinking aloud.

Our professional development approach is deceptively simple in its pedagogical intent and implementation. Its effectiveness in engaging busy clinical supervisors in thinking differently about the learning opportunities in their workplace settings has been encouraging so far. Our approach aims to acknowledge and build on the educational strategies already in place in our local health-service settings. Rich, context-specific learning and teaching opportunities are generated by the clinical supervisors themselves (rather than imposing additional educational requirements or curriculum tasks). Innovations that have come from this workshop include (1) using the ward communications book to suggest clinical tasks for learners so that other staff members can assist with teaching, (2) asking learners to do appropriate tasks manually rather than using technology to consolidate their procedural skills, and (3) keeping clinical objects, such as de-identified investigations and treatment plans, in an onsite teaching "toolkit." One challenge for the future is to work at both an individual and organizational level to facilitate community-based learning approaches that span health-service departments, encourage shared supervision, and extend learning into the local community.

NOTES

We acknowledge funding made available by Health Workforce Australia and the Department of Health, Victoria, Australia, which made publication of our guidebook possible.

1. Helen Rainbird, Alison Fuller, and Anne Munro, eds., *Workplace Learning in Context* (London: Routledge, 2004).
2. Natalie Radomski and Pam Harvey, *Workplace-based Teaching for Rural and Regional Clinical Supervisors: Guidebook* (Bendigo, VIC: Monash School of Rural Health, 2013).

Reflective Practice

A Longitudinal Course for Medical Students

JOSEPH ZARCONI AND DELESE WEAR

The Northeast Ohio Medical University has had a strong curricular commitment to humanism and professionalism since its inception. Just over eight years ago a new course, now called Reflective Practice (RP), was developed as a longitudinal course through the four-year curriculum. Elsewhere we have proposed that "reflection be approached . . . as part of a larger ongoing process in the education of physicians—that is, as an ethos in the medical environment."[1] This course is an attempt to create such an ethos.

The RP course is comprised of a series of small-group reflective discussion sessions that examine themes related to humanism, ethics, and professionalism. Assigned materials for these sessions are drawn from fiction, creative nonfiction, essay, poetry, film, case studies, medical literature, and contemporary journalism. Materials are chosen with the following goals:

- To promote critical reflective thinking, writing, and discussion aimed at preparing students to recognize and resolve issues/dilemmas relating to a life in medicine
- To engage in discussions that promote respectful and trusting relationships with colleagues and a sense of community
- To develop a broadened understanding of a wide range of human experiences
- To recognize and be fully conscious of the forces intrinsic to their own professional identity development and socialization in the culture of medicine,
- To develop a broader understanding of the commitments and obligations that attend the privilege of service in medicine.

Twelve to fourteen students are assigned to each group, with each group precepted by two faculty members, at least one of whom is a physician. Topics and materials in each session are linked to the curriculum as much as possible. Students are expected to arrive having reviewed the assigned materials and prepared to discuss their responses. The importance of confidentiality is emphasized at the outset. For most of the sessions in the first two years, students are required to submit a one- to two-page essay one week in advance of the sessions. Faculty are expected to read and respond to these essays in advance of the sessions as well.

In the M1 and M2 years, there are five or six ninety-minute sessions. Our medical students participate in three two-week open, online blogging sessions as they rotate through their core clerkships in their M3 year. During these sessions, students are required to enter at least two substantive responses to assigned material. These electronic conversations are also enjoined by their faculty preceptors. In the M4 year, there is a closing gathering of the RP groups and faculty in the weeks just prior to graduation. For sessions for which essays are required, students are instructed to focus on the themes, issues, or dilemmas that arise from the assigned materials. They are encouraged to describe their personal feelings, insights, and supported opinions as they relate to their sense of medical work and their own professional identity development. The course is pass/fail, and to pass, students must attend all sessions, arrive on time, engage meaningfully in responding to assigned materials, and submit appropriate essays by assigned deadlines.

An M1 class orientation to the course is presented in September. There are then six ninety-minute sessions throughout the year, with themes including narrative medicine, the patient-physician relationship, narrative ethics, the cadaver experience, emotions in medicine, and impairment of professionals. As an example of one of the M1 sessions, the cadaver experience session is conducted while students are engaged in anatomy and dissection, and they are assigned a number of cadaver poems as well as Perry Klass's essay "Invasions." For this session, students can opt to write their essays in the form of letters to their cadavers.

Prior to the start of the M2 year, students are assigned Rebecca Skloot's *The Immortal Life of Henrietta Lacks* as required reading. The first session in the M2 year focuses on research ethics, with this book as the assigned material, but issues of poverty, race, and socioeconomics in medical care and research surface rigorously in the discussions. The remaining sessions focus on themes including patient responses to cancer, health disparities, and physician biases toward obese patients. The final session allows the students to select their own topics and materials for reflection. In this most recent year, topics for this session have included technology in medicine, self-care, fears related to residency, end-of-life care, physician shortage challenges, and specialty choice, among others.

The themes of the M3 online sessions include derogatory clinical humor, the "e-patient" (focused on how electronic clinical tools impact the patient-physician relationship), and finally, professionalism. For the final session, students are asked to consider how their conceptions of professionalism have evolved through medical school, and what has influenced these conceptions. The final group meeting occurs during the Clinical Epilogue and Capstone Course late in the M4 year. While this is largely meant to allow the groups to come together with their faculty preceptor one last time before graduation, the session frequently focuses on issues related to preparedness for residency and conscious reflection on how students hope to develop as residents and new physicians.

Prospective course faculty are identified by course directors and existing RP faculty, largely based upon the extent to which they are perceived as reflective, humanistic, and professional teachers. Faculty have been selected from a broad range of departments and clinical or academic specialties in the College of Medicine. For those faculty not employed by the university, modest per session honoraria are paid by the Office of Academic Services. Each year, all new faculty members meet with the course directors for orientation. When a faculty member takes on a new group in the M1 year, it is hoped that he or she will commit to staying with that group through the four-year curriculum, and most are willing.

Immediately prior to each small-group session, all RP faculty are invited to a thirty-minute meeting with the course codirectors. Attendance is optional but most attend regularly. In these meetings, the codirectors review important themes to explore in the group discussions. But mostly these meetings allow the faculty to discuss issues that may surface in the student essays or concerns they may have about a particular discussion. Faculty members seem to enjoy the opportunity to share ideas in this way. For example, when a faculty member cited student concerns that they perceived too many of the assigned readings as "doctor bashing," course directors were able to guide faculty to relate to the students that such readings are not selected to "bash" doctors but rather to stimulate students to examine doctors and the culture of medicine critically. Such critical examination is important to students as they reflect upon how they wish to practice medicine. This discussion also led faculty to search for readings that depict laudable or inspiring physician caregiving for future sessions.

In addition, these meetings have led to a sense of community and comradeship that is helpful not only in sustaining faculty engagement but also in identifying "best practice" ideas for faculty development. Clearly, faculty learn from and energize one another.

Annually, the directors convene a half-day faculty retreat to review the curriculum and the student evaluations of the course and to discuss challenges faced by the faculty. Faculty are encouraged to surface new materials for consideration and to assist in the identification of additional faculty. While there are always students who do not find RP useful or worthwhile, in general students have responded quite positively to the course. Over the seven years of RP, about 94 percent of students believe the course is well taught, 85 percent believe RP helped them think about themselves in relation to professional issues, 94 percent report greater self-awareness regarding the patient-physician relationship, and 84 percent agree that the assigned materials stimulated their thinking. Every year, a number of students identify RP as their favorite part of the larger doctoring course—and some as their favorite course in the curriculum.

Faculty consistently enjoy their participation in this course, and most sign up for new M1 groups when their groups graduate. Clinical faculty members remark that they derive great meaning from this work, feel that their sense of calling toward medicine is rekindled, and indicate that they return to their work as better physicians. Faculty report that they become "more aware, sensitive, and reflective of their lives, within and external to, medicine as clinicians, teachers, and lifelong learners."[2] In addition, many report developing close mentoring relationships with a number of their students and enjoy following the progress of their professional identity development, even into residency and beyond.

NOTES

1. Delese Wear et al., "Reflection in/and Writing: Pedagogy and Practice in Medical Education," *Academic Medicine* 87 (2012): 604.
2. Ellen Whiting et al., "Teaching Softly in Hard Environments: Meanings of Small-Group Reflective Teaching to Clinical Faculty," *Journal for Learning through the Arts: A Research Journal on Arts Integration in Schools and Communities* 8 (2012), https://escholarship.org/uc/item/5381g6c9.

Reflection for Practice-Based Learning

MARGARET L. STUBER

Over the past century, medical schools have moved from an emphasis on teaching facts to an emphasis on teaching medical students and residents how to think, find evidence for a particular practice, and learn from their experience. This last is referred to as "practice-based learning"; it is trickier than it sounds. It requires that the learner not only note whether or not something worked but also analyze the factors that were salient to the success or failure and consider how to do things differently the next time. It requires students to move beyond the patient-caregiver interaction to think both more personally and more broadly.

For the past four years, an interprofessional education course at UCLA has used reflective writing to promote practice-based learning for third-year medical students and advanced practice nursing students. Groups of eight or nine students from the two schools meet together once or twice a month for nine months (three quarters), along with two seminar tutors. Each session has a theme. Each student is assigned a different reading. The students are also provided with a prompt for reflective writing on the theme. Students write a half page to a full page on the theme of the session, and then send their writing to the group and tutors at least forty-eight hours prior to the session. During each session, one of the students acts as a facilitator, linking together the readings and the written experiences and promoting a lively discussion.

The focus of the course is systems-based health care. All of the students are actively involved in clinical placements or clerkships during this year, so they are immersed in real systems of health care. They are also receiving clinical instruction and are regularly interacting with patients. The topics that are selected are chosen as controversial, or "hot," topics that they are likely to encounter in their clinical work. Readings include editorial sections of the *NEJM* or *JAMA*, essays by physician writers such as Atul Gawande or Jerome Groopman, and policy statements of professional organizations, such as the American Academy of Pediatrics. The prompts for reflections encourage students to write about an experience they had, as either a consumer or provider of health care. They are asked to describe a situation and their response to it, analyze the factors that contributed to the situation and response, and then describe how they would handle things differently in the future as a result of this experience.

The students start the year with a session in which they read and write about teams and teamwork as they enter into work with their interprofessional learning group. In the second session, they begin reading and writing about situations in which they experienced a challenge to their personal moral beliefs. Topics in the past have included working with a woman seeking repeated abortions as her method of birth control, caring for a seriously ill older patient who asked not to be told his diagnosis or prognosis, and being asked to prescribe pain medication to a patient who is obviously in pain but also appeared to be abusing narcotics.

This sort of discussion is only successful if the students feel safe within the group. The students therefore spend some time in the first session setting expectations for confidentiality and mutual respect. Students are encouraged to say what they think but also to listen actively to others and be open to other points of view. Students set their own limits on how much of what happens in the group can be talked about outside the group, but they generally decide to keep everything within the group.

Other topics raised during the year include conflict of interest, end-of-life issues, medical error and apology, sexuality and the workplace, implicit assumptions and biases, health-care economics, boundaries, and burnout. Readings are updated each year, and written prompts are designed to elicit personal experiences on the wards or in the clinics.

Tutors are meant to be facilitators, not lecturers, in this course. Students watch carefully to see if there actually is a "correct" viewpoint, so tutors have to be careful about anything that may come across as judgmental. To this end, the course directors meet with all of the tutors immediately before they meet with the students each session. As a group, the tutors discuss the approach they will use to guide the overall group discussion, adjusting according to the experiences in the student's reflective writing.

There is some argument each year among the tutors about how much focus there should be on writing skills versus reflective skills. It is difficult for many tutors not to correct grammar, syntax, and spelling. However, the primary goal of the written aspect of the course is to increase skills in practice-based learning. To that end, tutors are encouraged to give feedback on the student's level of analysis of the situation—the extent to which they can see the impact of larger systems—and their thoughtfulness about future plans. It is tempting for many of the tutors to focus on the personal reaction of the student from a psychological standpoint, but this is not the only goal. Developing insight into one's blind spots is important but often difficult and can require encouragement before it is expressed in the written reflections. It is common for the students to initially maintain a relatively impersonal writing style and to describe more emotional aspects of their experience in class only when they feel it is safe to do so. Although most students find the course to be very helpful in providing social support, the course has to be respectful of students who need emotional privacy as well.

Course directors meet with a representative from each of the groups two or three times each year. Students also submit midpoint and end-of-year written evaluations of the course. Despite the faculty's concerns and dire warnings that students do not like to write, students have been very positive about writing and sharing their narrative reflections. The most serious critiques of the course occur when students feel that their tutors or other students are critical or judgmental, or if they feel the tutors talk too much. Students want to know that their writing is read and they want feedback, but they do not want to be told which opinions are "right." This can be an issue if a student takes a position that faculty feel is rigid or unprofessional. The course directors will sit in to observe groups in which there are these types of issues. In rare situations, a student will need to be moved to another group if conflict with one or more of the tutors negatively affects the learning for the group.

This course has included advanced practice nursing students and nursing faculty since 2009. In 2013, third-year dental students and dental faculty were added to the course. The interprofessional competencies outlined by the Inter-professional Education Consortium in 2011 (team/teamwork, values/ethics, roles/responsibilities, and collaboration/communication) are now incorporated into the topics for the readings and reflective writing. Ongoing meetings with the leadership, faculty, and students of the three schools have supported the utility of this approach to students' professional as well as interprofessional education. We are now exploring the possibility of including students and faculty from the UCLA School of Public Health.

Prompting Reflection in Small-Group Learning

"Things I Thought about in the Car"

DEBBI ANDREWS

Anyone who has ever taken a writing course will be familiar with the idea of "writing prompts." These are short suggestions of things to write about, such as a description of a situation or a lead-in sentence. Writing gets better by practicing—the purpose of prompts is to encourage the habit of daily writing to improve one's craft. A writing prompt can provide a suggestion when you can't think of something to write about or a challenge or constraint when you want to increase your versatility or try a new form. A daily practice increases fluency and skill. It becomes easier to write.

"Things I thought about in the car" is a collection of arts- and humanities-related prompts I have collected over the past five years while serving as a small-group tutor for second-year medical students during their neurology block. I initially thought of this material as "humanities enrichment," but I now recognize the items as being "reflecting prompts," short suggestions of things to think about to encourage the students to connect didactic material in their cases with their knowledge of the patient's experience of illness and with what they may already know from areas outside of medicine.

I love these problem-based learning sessions in neurology. I am not a neurologist. I don't see strokes or dementia in my day-to-day work, but I do take care of children with developmental conditions based in the nervous system. Each year for ten weeks I welcome the opportunity to revisit stroke and dementia and other neurologic disorders and try to learn a little bit more of the neuroanatomy and neurophysiology that I didn't master in medical school. I attempt to link together what I know about developmental language disorders in kids with the stroke-based language deficits seen in adults. I look for parallels in the stepwise manner in which the nervous systems builds complexity in child development and how that complexity is unsystematically lost in adult neurodegenerative diseases. How the beautiful minicolumns and neuronal layers turn into tangles. How myelin disappears, taking with it speed and efficiency.

Neurology is interesting for me, but it is not always easy for the students to connect with the material. Some students revel in mastery of the folding and crossing of pathways, but many struggle. What's worse is that neurology is full of untreatable diseases that steal one's essential personhood and don't give it back. In neurology, the problem is not attached to a part of the physical body, a part that can treated or repaired or even replaced. The problem is within the brain, the seat of all our thoughts and feelings, and with its connections with our corporal self. The problem may be with our mind. You can't transplant a mind. Students find this depressing.

I wanted ways to help students engage in learning about these disorders and reflect on the implications of neurological disease for the patient. Simply talking about this in the abstract or even in the guise of the paper case personae was not achieving this engagement, but serendipity stepped in. One of the cases we were using back then presented with foot drop. As I was driving from campus back to the rehab hospital where I work, I thought about the television show *House,* whose main character has a limp. So in my weekly e-mail to the group, on a whim, I added a single postscript question: "Does Dr. House have a foot drop?" I didn't think that anyone would even notice the question, but when I arrived for the next session, one of the students immediately said no, that it wasn't a foot drop, and proceeded to explain why and what the character was supposed to have instead.

The next week the case included differentiating delirium from dementia. This was at the time one of the Harry Potter movies had just been released, and as I drove across town, there was mention of the "Dementors," the evil beings who guard Azkaban prison. Harry has an acute change in his mental state whenever he encounters these creatures but reverts to baseline after they go away. Should they then be described as *dementors,* or was there a better term? I put the question to the students in the weekly e-mail, along with some bits and pieces about the etymology of *delirium* and *dementia* and how that might help them remember which is which. The numerous hours driving to and from campus provided much time for me to consider the discussion that was going to occur (or that had just taken place). My e-mail content evolved naturally, expanding to include four to six items related to each week's case, drawn from all aspects of the human experience of that condition—from memoirs and illness narratives, fiction and poetry, visual arts and video presentations.

Medical students are busy, and this was not part of the formal curriculum. It was important that this material was not perceived as an assignment but as an opportunity. In the e-mail, students were invited to pursue prompts for fun or interest, but told they had no obligation to read any of it and could delete the e-mail if they were too busy or just not interested. Many chose to save messages until after an assignment, but often there would be an informal discussion going on when I arrived at the day's session. We did not allow this to infringe on scheduled work time, so that their important learning objectives for the day were covered.

What makes for good content? Biographies of famous people describing their experience of specific neurologic conditions are a good source (for example, *No Laughing Matter* by Joseph Heller, in which he describes his bout with Guillain-Barre syndrome). Whole volumes are often not practical, but abridged versions, such as Jill Bolte Taylor's *My Stroke of Insight* distilled down into an eighteen-minute TED talk, are manageable. Shorter pieces are best—Oliver Sacks's essays are a rich source of neurological cases.

Full-length feature films are also too long for a course like this, but often students have already seen movies that are pertinent (for example, *I Am Sam* [2001] about an adult living in the community with an intellectual disability, or *The Notebook* [2004] and *Away from Her* [2006]) for themes related to dementia. There are also many short videos on YouTube, such as the British fantasy writer Sir Terry Pratchett's address about his diagnosis with early onset dementia. The TED website offers numerous good choices, including Temple Grandin talking about what it is like to have autism.

Sometimes wandering the Internet will result in good finds. The search engine Google makes it is surprisingly easy to find whole websites of famous people "who died of X" or "who have Y," but make sure that the content is verified by cross-checking with other sources. Patient support sites often contain narratives and may include video content, original artwork, and poetry. I look for interesting facts and unusual juxtapositions and present them as trivia questions (for example, Name the Canadian mystery writer who had a stroke that presented as loss of his ability to read). I investigate the history of eponymous conditions and the people for whom they were named (for example, Who is the third person who originally described Guillain-Barre besides Guillain and Barre?)

I listen to the news. I use the students' interests and follow their leads. After a student's casual joke about alien abductions, I discovered an entire journal volume on the neuroscience of this experience as well as the "neglect phenomenon" called "alien hand."

Do students really reflect? Students regularly mention things included "in the car" that week, sometimes in case discussion per se and at other times in the pre- and postsession chat that occurs as the group is assembling or departing. It strikes me that what I am doing in the car can serve as prompts to reflection and that, by thinking explicitly and publishing this in an e-mail, I am modeling reflection.

SUGGESTED RESOURCES

1. Heller, Joseph, and Speed Vogel. *No Laughing Matter.* New York: Putnam, 1986.
2. Bolte Taylor, Jill. *My Stroke of Insight: A Brain Scientist's Personal Journey.* New York: Penguin, 2008.
3. Sacks, Oliver. *The Man Who Mistook His Wife for a Hat and Other Clinical Tales.* New York: Summit Books, 1985.

Crises of Empathy

Practicing Having the Body of an "Other"

SARA K. SCHNEIDER

Take the body: It is not merely a system of mechanical pulleys, levers, squeeze bottles, and intricately connected tubing. Nor is it simply a miraculous electrical communications system. The lived body is much more, much that is real in experience and in relationship. It is an artifact constructed through its culture— a system trained in particular ways to stand, sit, and walk; to respond to touch and attention, authority, and power; to experience pain; to embody particular views of modesty; and to decide its future. And, just as the mechanical and electrical bodies may react differently to the same medications or treatment regimens, the cultural body responds in unique ways to its encounters with Western health-care providers and Western medicine.

My workshop, "The Bodies of 'Others': Compassionate Cross-Cultural Care," was presented at three national conferences to help health-care professionals "cultivate their sensitivity to the increasingly diverse needs and expectations of patients and families in the multicultural physical dramas of examination, consultation, and treatment rooms." These workshops, including two day-long and one half-day sessions, were offered as preconference professional development days in 2010 and 2011. The numbers were small at the workshops, perhaps because of the "hard skill" offerings against which they competed: in all, I had five holistic nurses, eight occupational health nurses, and four school counselors. We rearranged the hotel conference room settings to create intimate dinner table–style seating.

One might imagine that health-care professionals taking a workshop in culturally sensitive health care would want to come away with a toolkit that would help them take concrete steps and know what to say when dealing with a patient or client from another country, ethnic group, or immigrant status.

However, such an objectifying approach would only exacerbate the already instrumental approach taken in much of Western medicine.

I wanted "The Bodies of 'Others'" to help each practitioner to view herself also as an "Other," as reflected in the eyes of her patients and clients. The workshops foregrounded the cultural identities of practitioners, helping them to see themselves as culturally encoded beings who bring their own perceptions, histories, biases, filters, and norms to their encounters with others. The idea came in part from my work at National Louis University in the Teaching, Learning, and Assessment (formerly Interdisciplinary Studies) Program, where I have worked with practicing teachers going on for their MEd degrees in a two-year professional development program. In the Teaching, Learning, and Assessment (TLA) Program, as teachers conduct extended action research in their work settings, we examine the personhood of the teacher and its palpable influence on students' behavior, engagement, motivation, and achievement.

When they enter the program, teachers typically see themselves, like many health-care professionals, as invisible: they are objective deliverers (and, if fortunate, inventors) of curriculum. Certainly, with their herculean efforts, they don't much influence or impede its delivery. Yet over the course of our extended work together, they come to see themselves as personal and cultural actors in their classrooms, with powers to influence students that are unique to their own gifts, biases, histories, and talents. As these professionals become visible to themselves as beings with unique personalities and cultures, they are empowered to make more conscious choices in relationships with those for whom they assume some responsibility for well-being of body, mind, and spirit.

Unlike the TLA Program, "The Bodies of 'Others'" was to last just one day, not twenty months, yet I wanted it to have lasting impact. I began by teaching participants about *tonglen,* a Tibetan Buddhist meditation practice in which each breath becomes a practice of compassion. One breathes in the suffering of others and breathes out a sense of compassion. One might argue health-care practitioners are all too attuned to the suffering of their patients and clients: why emphasize that by purposefully inhaling it? The body of the tonglen practitioner becomes a crucible within which suffering is transformed into healing through the body of the practitioner. She symbolically shares her wellness, humanity, and love with the patient. In succeeding cycles of tonglen, one may move from offering compassion to loved ones, whose suffering is saddening for the practitioner, to offering compassion to strangers or enemies, whose suffering either seems to matter less or to be deserved. Through tonglen, the practitioner can become a little more aware of where her empathy hits a wall, thus limiting her effectiveness as a caregiver.

Then, after I briefly explained the anthropological concept of the Other, participants shared experiences for fifteen minutes in safe pairs of having been "otherized," perhaps in a health-care setting. Perhaps perception of one's gender, one's skin color, or a language difference created an occasion for objectifying treatment. Perhaps it was not clear what had been the basis for a distancing, but it was felt nonetheless. Universally, participants encountered no difficulty recalling such an experience.

I then invited participants to return to the group table to spend twenty minutes writing a poem about their own cultures, as revealed in their upbringings and homes of origin. It's a rare adult who accepts gladly the task of writing a poem in public, yet a poem template that is often used in educational settings—variously called "I Am . . ." or "I Am From . . . ," originally written by George Ella Lyon—relieves much of the threat of that task. Writers are asked to merely supply things like a saying from their parents, or the names of household objects or store brands from their childhood. By the end, each person has created an evocative and highly sensory portrait of the flavor of her upbringing.

While no one was required to read their poems aloud, everyone did. Safety was ensured by emphasizing respect, listening, confidentiality, and nonintrusive questions and remarks. Not infrequently, tears of remembrance were part of the writing process or of the sharing afterward, as participants connected with each other across the table. Finding commonalities in food was a typical feature of the discussion: "You had Cheez-Its after school, too?" The "I Am From . . ." template emphasizes habitualness, pattern, and things that tended to happen, thus highlighting family choices and proclivities that, over and over again, distinguished them from and joined them with others. Through this exercise, even those who assume that only recent immigrants or non-native speakers of English have a "real culture" discover that they, too, are cultured beings, graced with specific worldviews and experiences that affect how they relate to so-deemed "Others."

Further activities, including journaling, role-playing, brainstorming, and discussion, were featured throughout the day. During even more top-down instruction—for example, about the elements that distinguish culture—I reinforced the participants' earlier learnings from self-reflection. Perhaps most eye-opening of these later activities for participants was when the group worked together to construct a mind map of the cultural features of their workplaces—also significant, along with their families, in shaping their workplace selves. The model allowed participants to see, many for the first time, their workplaces' emphases on such things as efficiency, a distinctive hierarchy, and thorough documentation as features of specific work and professional cultures rather than as universal values that should be embraced by patients, clients, and providers.

It should be noted that the health-care providers in these workshops tended not to be the power players in their institutions. These nurses and school counselors might be expected to recognize the artificiality of, and pinpoint the features of, a culture that serves others' power interests more fully than their own.

Participant evaluations showed the importance of acknowledging and understanding one's own cultural self in order to fully meet the cultural "Other." One nurse wrote that she left the workshop with a "newfound appreciation for my 'own' culture and how I affect others." Another connected her personal and professional cultures: "Because we are generally the type of people that have a need to 'help' or 'solve' problems for others, I have discovered that health-care professionals need to recognize their own 'culture' and how it affects [their] job performance."

Being able to see one's view of the "Other" as a projection goes a long way in owning one's own power and one's cultural humility as a health-care professional. We are all working in a diverse universe where perhaps the only truly useful question to have for working with a patient whose culture is unfamiliar is psychologist Sukey Waller's all-purpose "Is it okay if I . . . ?"[1] If we are okay as practitioners finally to be able to see ourselves as cultural objects, we may at last be able to see others as cultural subjects and to bridge across and breathe into our own crises of empathy.

NOTE

1. Anne Fadiman, *The Spirit Catches You and You Fall Down: A Hmong Child, Her American Doctors, and the Collision of Two Cultures* (New York: Farrar, Straus and Giroux, 1998), 95.

Promoting Patient-Centered Care

The Intersection between Interprofessional and Complementary/Alternative Medicine Education

ANASTASIA KUTT AND SUNITA VOHRA

Patient-centered care requires that health-care providers be aware of all the therapies a patient is using and communicate effectively with each other as well as the patient. Interprofessional education is mandatory for many health professions, teaching collaborative team skills to promote high-functioning health-care teams. Due to high rates of patient use of complementary and alternative medicine (CAM), some of which could interact with conventional treatment,[1] patient-centered care demands that conventional health-care providers also be comfortable communicating about CAM treatments and evaluating their safety and efficacy.

At the University of Alberta, "Interprofessional Health Team Development" (IntD 410) is a mandatory ten-week, thirty-hour course for all undergraduate health sciences students (for example, dental hygiene, dentistry, dietetics, medical laboratory science, medicine, nursing, occupational therapy, pharmacy, physical therapy). Core learning competencies include collaboration, communication, role clarification, and reflection. The CAM stream of the course includes learner evaluation of CAM safety and effectiveness, and a patient-centered, evidence-based approach to patient CAM use. Most of the time is spent in interdisciplinary small groups, focused on case-based learning, augmented with large-group lectures and opportunities for experiential learning.

One goal of the CAM stream was to shift the students' perception of health care from a profession-centric model to a patient-centric model. The profession-centric model may describe the viewpoint of students who have so far only been exposed to the views and perspective of their own professions. They may collaborate with other conventional health-care practitioners; CAM providers are often thought of as separate, if at all. In IntD, students are encouraged to shift to a patient-centered model in which they recognize that patients make their own health choices, some of which are self-initiated (for example, self-care with over-the-counter therapies such as herbal medicines), while others may be based on health-care provider advice (whether conventional or CAM). The students realize their professions are only one part of the team supporting the patient and his or her health-care choices. Effective communication with both the patient and other health-care providers is recognized as key to promoting coordinated care.

During this course, reflective essays were given as assignments to encourage students to recognize knowledge gaps and to shift their approach to being more patient-centered. Three individual and two team reflective essay assignments were given to the students (described below).

Individual Reflection 1 (initial reflection): On the first day of class, students were asked to create a table, listing the perceived strengths and weaknesses of (1) their own profession; (2) three other "conventional" professions (that is, their colleagues in IntD); and (3) three CAM disciplines. This assignment was eye-opening for many students, who understood that they could not effectively work together and draw from each other's strengths if they did not know what those were. They recognized knowledge gaps, such as perceptions based on television or popular opinion; some students felt unable to complete the table. This reinforced the need to learn about each other's strengths and weaknesses, and better understand each other's scopes of practice.

In a follow-up class, students gave a ten-minute presentation to their teammates about their own profession, addressing some common assumptions. Students realized patient-centered care was a common goal they all shared. Students reported that this exercise allowed them to put the value of this course in context from the beginning and to move forward as a team more quickly.

Individual Reflection 2 (natural health product vendor visit): Using case-based learning, students explored relevant issues for patients using natural health products (NHPs), such as NHP-drug interactions. Students were required to visit an NHP vendor—for example, a pharmacy, supermarket, or health food store—so they could see the world through their patients' eyes. They were asked to explore information available to patients in the store and online and note how this varied in terms of product recommendations, quality, and cost. We asked them to discuss and compare their experiences. We also provided students with a list of reputable sources for information on NHPs so they could evaluate the suggested options themselves. Each student wrote a reflective essay and reported surprise at their interactions with NHP vendors (such as the vendors' receptiveness to questions and varying education levels), at the low cost of some NHPs, and at the varying quality of information available. The recommended resources challenged student assumptions that there is little evidence regarding NHP safety or efficacy. Most importantly, students learned to see NHPs and their related issues from the patient's point of view.

Individual Reflection 3 (CAM provider practice visit): Using case-based learning, students considered patients wishing to use CAM practices, such as massage and acupuncture. Students were provided with a brief summary of educational requirements, industry regulations, and credentialing requirements for eight CAM therapies. Students then attended a CAM fair held at our university, a one-day educational event featuring local CAM providers from a variety of disciplines—specifically acupuncture, art therapy, biofeedback, chiropractic, massage therapy, mindfulness-based stress reduction, music therapy, naturopathy, Reiki, and yoga. Students interviewed CAM providers at the CAM fair to learn about their training, scope of practice, and clinical experience. Students were also invited to participate in experiential activities—workshops (for example, yoga, qi gong) and mini-treatments for acupuncture, massage therapy, and Reiki. In addition, students visited CAM provider offices to better understand what patients experience through direct observation; students then discussed and compared their experiences with their teammates. Student reflections suggested practice visits better reflected the patient experience; however, attendance at the CAM fair was a more efficient learning environment. Overall, both CAM providers and students alike expressed appreciation for the opportunity to communicate with and learn directly from one another.

Team Reflections: Team reflections focusing on interprofessional teamwork and CAM were assigned at the middle and end of term. Team reflections suggested that the course helped students recognize how each team member contributes unique information to help the patient and how valuable interprofessional collaboration is. We recognize that there may be a positive response bias, that students may have felt obliged to respond in a positive fashion when discussing their colleagues. Students wrote about their awareness that there is heterogeneity in the amount and quality of evidence about CAM therapies (more for some, less for others) and felt more confident in their ability to find and evaluate this evidence to inform patient care.

Overall, we found that reflective exercises enabled students to identify and challenge assumptions. CAM can be taught concurrently with interprofessional education and can promote a patient-centered evidence-based approach. It was a rewarding experience for us as educators to witness this shift in perception, and it will be interesting to see how the effects ripple into the community when these students enter the workforce.

NOTE

1. Joan Gilmour et al., "Natural Health Product–Drug Interactions: Evolving Responsibilities to Take Complementary and Alternative Medicine into Account," *Pediatrics* 128, Suppl. 4 (2011): S155–60.

A Traditional Departmental Grand Rounds Format Shifts a Health System Culture toward Reflective Practice

ALICE FORNARI AND BARBARA HIRSCH

A relatively new medical school, the Hofstra North Shore–Long Island Jewish School of Medicine (SOM) has included reflection as one of its ten guiding core values:

> We are committed to embedding in all of our learning experiences the time and skills necessary to consciously examine, interpret and understand the thoughts and feelings that emanate from intense patient encounters. Through this process of mentored self-reflection and assessment, we ensure the development of a true learning and professional community capable of nurturing the transformation from student to physician.[1]

In anticipation of welcoming our inaugural class of medical students in 2011, a Narrative Medicine Working Group formed in 2010 that included professionals from the SOM and North Shore–Long Island Jewish (NSLIJ) Health System partnership.

This working group was assembled after an invitation was sent to practitioners across diverse health professional disciplines to attend a narrative medicine training workshop at Columbia University. With members representing many of the twenty-one hospitals in our health-care system, our working group currently functions as a "community of reflective practice" (CORP), which is focused on discovering how to bring teaching and learning moments supporting reflection into mainstream academic health-care environments. We have multiple aims and purposes: (1) networking among like-minded individuals; (2) representing our discipline, setting, and learners at the table; (3) sharing ideas and feedback on developing and implementing new learning opportunities that include reflective practice; (4) educating each other and keeping current in the literature of humanities and reflection; (5) supporting research interests and projects; and (6) documenting and sharing all we accomplish with our larger health professions education community. An early challenge we faced was how we might effectively advocate for this value and help to incorporate it as an "alive" aspect of our undergraduate and graduate educational environment.

Introducing the conceptual framework of reflective practice into multiple clinical departments using an experiential pedagogy that is compatible with clinical education has been an early goal. With a faculty development role and associated responsibilities for both the SOM and NSLIJ Health System, the chair of our working group introduced a grand rounds series titled Reflective Practice as a Lifelong Learning Tool, which has been directed to a wide audience of clinicians and educators across the medical school and health-care system since 2013.

We approached the chairs of all clinical departments and offered to present a framework and experiential exercises as part of a traditional grand rounds presentation to introduce reflective practice. Members of the CORP working group offered to lead the presentation, which would include approximately fifty minutes of content delivered to a large and diverse group of faculty, trainees, students, and supporting clinical staff. Our grand rounds presentation begins with a fifteen-minute introduction we use to define reflection and summarize relevant literature and evidence supporting reflective practice as a tool to enhance learning from one's own experiences. We have found these introductions to be important, as most attendees knew very little about reflective practice, as either a concept or skill. The interactive aspect of our presentation begins with a relevant reading that is then followed by a writing exercise and the sharing of the individual reflective writing. These participatory, interactive aspects of the session are designed to experientially introduce the audience to the value and benefits of reflective practice.

With respect to specific rounds presentations, we select a discipline-specific short story. After reading the story aloud, we introduce a verbal prompt to create an opportunity for a reflective dialogue. A writing prompt created specifically for the attendees' clinical specialty is then introduced, followed by a five- to six-minute writing exercise. Two to three volunteers are invited to share their writing to elicit discussion among the audience. The session concludes with closing slides that briefly summarize how the participants could apply this pedagogy as an educational strategy in future departmental teaching sessions.

For example, for one of our grand round presentations, we selected the poem "In Line at the Hospital Coffee Stand" by Tabor Flickinger.[2] This poetic narrative contrasts a serious experience of hearing about the death of a chronically ill patient juxtaposed with the mundane act of getting a cup of coffee at the hospital coffee shop. The presenters felt that all trainees and attending physicians could relate to this poem. The prompt that followed was to "write about a time you wish you had said more to a patient." This has consistently proved to be an effective prompt, with some older participants drawing on memories from fifty years earlier and others recalling more recent events. It easily crossed generations of physicians.

In reflecting on our progress to date, we feel that we have been successful in introducing reflection as an educational pedagogy in departmental grand rounds. We have approached fifteen clinical departments, and ten have invited us to present on Reflection Practice as a Lifelong Learning Tool as a grand rounds session. Attendance at each of the sessions has ranged from 35 to 100 participants. We consistently attract an audience that is diverse across disciplines and level of clinician. We can only assume we are reaching students, residents, faculty, and other health professionals during these presentations, which meets our goal of being interprofessional. This educational strategy has connected our working group to the larger health system as a resource that is available and willing to assist in content preparation and delivery. Individuals have expressed interest in introducing reflection as a pedagogical approach in their educational settings. Other examples of impact include the implementation of reflective practice activities in traditional graduate medical education residency programs; new nursing initiatives (both educational and administrative); and Humanism in Healthcare, our narrative rounds presentation series, modeled after Columbia University's Narrative Medicine program, in which prominent scholars and faculty present on a broad range of medical humanities topics. In 2012, we introduced *Narrateur: Reflections on Caring*, our annual art and literary review journal, as part of our Humanities in Medicine Program/Osler Society.[3]

We believe we have successfully created a recipe to stimulate reflective moments that support both "reflection-in-action" and "reflection-on-action," as described by Donald Schön.[4] Most importantly, we have started to bring our school of medicine's core value of reflection "alive" in our health-care system's clinical environments. We are continually planning next steps to further integrate reflection as a lifelong learning tool across clinical departments in our health system and medical school. A new effort is our reflective writing groups, which are offered monthly to all health-system employees. We anticipate that this initiative will become part of the health system's Corporate Wellness Program.

In order to grow our CORP, we are also involved in institutional research efforts to connect reflective practice to patient care and to legitimize the outcomes both as an education effort and as a direct impact on the quality of patient care delivered. Two previous Institutional Review Board–approved clinical research projects led by clinicians in our community of practice include (1) In Their Own Words, which is focused on gathering the patient's story through an expanded social history and possibly improving patient satisfaction with hospital care; and (2) Narrative Medicine in a Nephrology Division: Linking Education, Professional Development, and Quality of Patient Care, which assesses the impact of semistructured writing time in decreasing burnout, improving interpersonal communication among care providers, and fostering more humanistic approach to the care of patients on dialysis.

Our On the Road journey to shift a health-system culture toward reflective practice has had its challenges and barriers, but the efforts described here are stepping-stones toward success. The presence of an open interprofessional community of reflective practice that brings like-minded individuals together to pursue their passions is a reality in diverse initiatives. The evidence of our efforts continues to grow and touch more professionals and, ultimately, we hope, patients and their families.

NOTES

We are pleased to acknowledge Michael Grosso, MD, who suggested the name On the Road, which we adopted for our community of reflective practice.

1. Hofstra North Shore-LIJ School of Medicine, "Values," accessed Mar. 4, 2014, http://medicine. hofstra.edu/about/about_missionvalues.html#reflection.

2. Tabor Flickinger, "In Line at the Hospital Coffee Stand," *Pulse: Voices from the Heart of Medicine,* June 8, 2012, http://pulsemagazine.org/archive/poems/241-in-line-at-the-hospital-coffee-stand.

3. The literary journal is available online at www.narrateur.org, and the Humanities in Medicine Program/Osler Society is at http://medicine.hofstra.edu/about/osler/index.html.

4. Donald A. Schön, *Educating the Reflective Practitioner: Toward a New Design for Teaching and Learning in the Professions* (San Francisco, CA: Jossey-Bass, 1987).

PART 8

New Media

Using the Documentary Sicko to Explore Health Systems

An Online Teaching Innovation to Foster Reflection

LYNN CORCORAN AND JANANEE RASIAH

John Dewey, in his classic text *How We Think,* suggests that reflective thinking is always troublesome "because it involves overcoming the inertia that inclines one to accept suggestions at their face value." He noted that, "Reflective thinking . . . means judgment suspended during further inquiry; and suspense is likely to be somewhat painful."[1] This observation highlights both the complexity and the importance of reflection. Educators in the health professions, and nursing in particular, have adopted a belief in the importance of reflection as a learning strategy that helps learners connect new learning with previous learning. With this as context, the following is a description of an innovative teaching approach designed to foster reflective thinking with the goal of developing reflective nursing practice.

The Challenge—From Classroom to Computer (Lynn's Story): When I teach, I like to teach in the here and now. I connect what is being learned in the classroom with real-life, close-at-hand examples. I use stories, popular culture, and social media to foster reflection and, ultimately, engage students in learning about the role of reflective practice in nursing. In the past few years, my teaching practice has changed and I teach almost exclusively online. Some have wondered if it is possible to teach in an engaging manner using stories, popular culture, social media, and real-life examples in a virtual, online classroom. What follows is an account of one teaching innovation involving use of the documentary film *Sicko* (2007) to address issues in nursing and health care that shifted seamlessly, from in person to online.

In his documentary *Sicko,* Michael Moore highlighted the health systems of various countries (for example, Canada, Britain, and France) and compared them with the health-care system in the United States. The images and dialogue of the people in this film offered rich portrayals of the range of health-care programs and services in the contexts of for-profit, privatized, and not-for-profit, socialized systems. In our brick-and mortar classroom, spirited discussions ensued following the presentation of video clips from the film. Opinions were expressed for and against every imaginable possibility on the spectrum of health-care system models. Class discussions focused on personal and family experiences, receiving health care abroad, and the professional experiences of student nurses.

As different clips were shown over the course of several weeks, student nurses connected concepts and examples from former video clips to those shown later in the term. The energy in the discussions and the diversity of opinions expressed by students indicated affective engagement in this learning and a beginning grasp of the complex issues connected to health economics that influence health-system access and health-care outcomes.

Shifting this teaching innovation to the online environment involved creative use of the same content, while considering the online learners working independently through the course material. Students were presented with a variety of learning activities, aims, and objectives. Our first learning activity focused on economic issues relevant to health-care systems. Advances in knowledge and technology, increases in the cost of delivering health care, and changes in how the system is financed (public versus private, or a combination of these) are a few of the many issues challenging the health-care system. The documentary *Sicko* focuses on the economic structures and organization of different health-care systems across the world. Various approaches to dealing with similar health-care challenges in different countries are highlighted in the stories of individual people.

Students were encouraged to consider and debate the economics influencing the health concerns of the people profiled in the following scenes from *Sicko:* (1) Canadian Waiting Room (2) What Hospital Bills? (Britain), and (3) Life in France.[2] As an optional activity, we suggested that students locate the *Sicko* (2007) "film footnotes" related to the Canadian health system,[3] and present their reflections and perspective in the discussion forum.

The Pedagogy—Reflection, Context, Learners, and Learning: As this activity shifted from a brick-and-mortar university classroom to the online world, it was important to ensure a substantive, rich, and reflective learning experience. The four pedagogical approaches underlying this teaching innovation include (1) understanding that reflection is pivotal for growth as a student nurse and novice practitioner, (2) adapting the way in which reflection can be encouraged in an online environment, (3) focusing on the issues in nursing from a broad context, and (4) knowing the type of learners in the online community. Reflective practice encompasses discovering one's values, biases, strengths, and limitations; fulfilling the expectations of regulatory and professional nursing bodies; and enhancing individual nursing practice on an ongoing basis.[4]

Video clips from the documentary *Sicko* were effective in showcasing relevant and controversial issues in health care, and in fostering reflection. The video clips and web resources offered stimulating triggers for reflective online discussion among the diverse group of students, who provided a variety of perspectives on economic issues in health-care systems. This teaching innovation fostered deep reflection. Student nurses questioned the status quo and, in doing so, their awareness and understanding of the complexity of the health-care system and the sociopolitical contexts of health-care delivery increased.

In the online world, identifying the generation of learners (Millennials, Generation Xers, or Baby Boomers) taking the course is always an important consideration. For example, Millennial learners are accustomed to new technologies and favor the use of social media. Baby Boomers prefer to learn through in-person lectures but may be open to online learning, whereas Generation X learners are keen to embrace online learning.[5]

As educators, our role is to engage all learners—Millennials, Generation Xers, Baby Boomers, and all those learners not yet labeled—to reflect on various issues relevant to health care in an innovative manner in online education environments. Using storytelling, popular culture, current events, and social media are a few ways to entice students in the health professions to reflect, formulate and share opinions, debate issues, derive new insights and understandings, and engage in a meaningful learning experience.

NOTES

1. John Dewey, *How We Think* (Boston: D.C. Heath, 1910), 14.
2. See www.youtube.com/watch?v=rQ1lPPTPSR4; www.youtube.com/watch?v=V2sFT7TO mCs; and www.youtube.com/watch?v=6UwQ2fyEgz0.
3. See www.michaelmoore.com/books-films/facts/sicko.
4. Community Health Nurses Association of Canada, "Canadian Community Health Nursing: Standards of Practice (2008)," accessed June 5, 2015, www.chnc.ca/documents/chn_standards _of_practice_mar08_english.pdf.
5. Cathy Sandeen, "Boomers, Xers, and Millennials: Who Are They and What Do They Really Want from Continuing Higher Education?" *Continuing Higher Education Review* 72 (Fall 2008): 11–31.

"The Elephants in the Medical Encounter"

Reflecting on Systems Thinking with Blogging

MICHELE BATTLE-FISHER

Since participating in the 2012 Institute on Systems Science and Health funded by the Office of Behavioral and Social Sciences Research, National Institutes of Health, I have continued to be fascinated by systems thinking and social networks. Systems thinking involves an approach to understanding that recognizes the nonlinear, complex relationships of elements, or component parts, that exist within systems. It is an approach that requires that we see the world as it is, in all its messiness and complexity. In relation to health, the relative support afforded by a patient's social network can influence their health status outcomes.

I teach a graduate level course titled Social Networks and Health to advanced master of public health students at Wright State University, Boonshoft School of Medicine in Ohio.[1] The popularity of blogging to reach populations that may not come in contact with the peer-reviewed literature is a largely untapped resource for disseminating public health research. As part of this course, I offer an opportunity for students to use social media and blogging to reflect on supportive social networks, complex systems, and systems thinking in relation to health as mentored contributors to the Orgcomplexity Blog.[2] In using blogging as a teaching tool, I ask students to meld available research evidence to a real problem they believe is best framed by using systems thinking to understand it and to articulate this within the public domain. Students are asked to identify and make sense of systems issues underlying complex health questions and concerns with a view to influencing public health policy and initiatives.

My students often come to public health due to their own or a loved one's illness. Students typically select a topic that interests them, that they have background knowledge of, or that they feel comfortable discussing. This topic is submitted to and approved by me as course instructor and mentor. For example, a student was interested in learning about facilitators and impediments to medication adherence among the chronically ill. In particular, he wanted to explore how the composition of a patient's social network might affect the patient's adherence to prescription medication.

When students have little or no exposure to blogging, I have found that it is helpful to provide information and guidelines for navigating the standards, expectations, and realities associated with the blogosphere. I provide an overview of social media as a means of online communication and describe ways in which blogs can be leveraged for maximum exposure. Blog posts are more likely to gain traction if the topic relates to an issue of current interest or is on the cusp of exploding in popularity. Concise, descriptive titles that include key, easily indexed words are more likely to get picked up by search engines. I advise students that they should write something that they would feel comfortable having widely circulated, while maintaining the privacy and confidentiality of those whose experiences may have led to insights.

I emphasize that blogging as a vehicle for credible, academic writing requires good judgment and commitment to conveying accurate information. I advise students to be aware of "gaps in the literature" relating to various social, organizational, and political influences as well as individual factors that are part of the complex systems that affect health and well-being. I ask my bloggers to remain grounded in scholarship but not to be constrained by it. What do I mean by this? I have found that students often forget that much can be learned about life from the arts and humanities, politics, and even personal experience. Given this tendency to restrict themselves, I ask students to step out of their comfort zone, take a leap of faith, and consider different disciplinary perspectives and forms of knowing.

I suggest a maximum word count of 1,000 words for each blog post. Posts over 1,000 words tend to lose readers who are surfing the web or who turn to blogs to escape wordy articles. I also suggest a guideline of three or four references per blog post. "Gray literature," such as blog posts, is allowed as long as these sources are supported by peer-reviewed articles. Students are reminded that copyrighted material must be appropriately cited.

Mastering a blogging voice that is both scientifically sound and generally engaging is a difficult task. Understanding even the simplest social systems can be challenging. To ensure responsible blogging, we spend considerable time understanding systems thinking. Reading previous posts on the Orgcomplexity Blog has helped students to enhance their understanding of systems thinking and social network analysis while also providing examples of engaging posts that include both bioscientific and humanistic perspectives. I advise my students to read and reread their posts, edit their posts, and then edit again, to ensure readability. Brevity and clarity are best. As the course instructor and forum moderator, I upload blogs only after assessing the post in relation to the quality criterion noted above (for example, systems-informed presentation of a personally compelling or relevant public health issue, or readability).

The Patient Protection and Affordable Care Act, which was enacted to enhance the quality and affordability of health in the United States, focuses attention on systems-based thinking as an integral aspect of health-care policy and planning. For example, Nan Lin found a connection between social support and social ties, noting that social resources are "embedded in the ties of one's [social] networks."[3] The support of families, friends, and communities is an integral, if often invisible, aspect of the health-care system. It is important to understand the structure of the social support networks of patients as a web of parts that may change over time.

How does this apply in the context of patient care? Medical care requires a physical (or in the case of telemedicine, a digital) encounter between the patient and the clinician. But what about the other invisible players whose influences are left out of this examination, such as the young girl who makes sure that her grandmother gets to the pharmacy to buy new lancets, the emergency room attendant who seeks to piece together the patient's health narrative under duress, or even the televangelist who promises bodily healing with each dedicated tithe to the ministry? Each person within a patient's social network—family members, friends, and other caring members of the community—will offer different kinds and degrees of support that may be helpful to the patient. A clinician may not be privy to these potential caregivers who may influence a patient's health outcomes and quality of life. Being aware of patients' social network can inform helpful interventions related to their health concerns, perhaps yielding better outcomes than might otherwise have resulted (for example, by easing the relative burden of illness, increasing health-care utilization, and reducing financial and emotional burdens).

Documentation of practical applications of systems-based thinking is necessary further understanding of complex processes, and to support addressing issues related to health and well-being based on this perspective. My student bloggers are learning and experiencing public health from an exciting point of view. Creating blog posts has offered my students a learning experience that has grounded the course in a practical, public health–focused fashion. It is rare for students to explore compelling health-related questions, which are often personally relevant, using systems thinking. I have hoped to address this absence in this course, in part through the use of social media. Engaging students in blogging not only has contributed to a process of reflection and learning but also has offered students opportunities to connect with a wider audience, including the expansion of their own potential academic and health policy networks, through active scholarship.

NOTES

1. The class syllabus can be found at Sante Fe Institute's Complexity Explorer at www.complexity explorer.org/explore/syllabi.
2. *Orgcomplexity Blog,* archive, https://orgcomplexity.wordpress.com.
3. Nan Lin, "Inequality in Social Capital," *Contemporary Sociology* 29 (2000): 785–95.

Digital Storytelling in Primary Care Nurse Practitioner Education

MELODY RASMOR AND SARAH KOOIENGA

Primary care is the first contact for most people's health-care needs; and at its best, it offers coordinated, comprehensive patient care. Primary care is founded on a sustained lifelong partnership with patients and families who are recognized as part of a larger community. Nurse practitioners (NPs) are ideally suited to be primary care practitioners as their educational background embraces holistic human values. In the primary care setting, nurse practitioners are confronted with a variety of health-care issues compelling them to address their own beliefs and values in listening to others' stories. The stories of patients and their families help NPs make sense of their world, providing insights to the past, present, and future. These reflective thinking skills increase the practitioner's capacity to see others and their personal and contextual experience of illness, as well as to address their own attitudes, perceptions, and beliefs.[1]

In advanced practice nursing education, the NP students are constructing a new identity as primary care providers as they evolve from a registered nurse role. Development of a new professional identity is a dynamic process that involves challenging and broadening one's perspectives and outlook. Sharing narratives about student experiences can facilitate self-awareness and identity formation. Narrative stories shared throughout an intensive two-year training program can help student NPs explore the question "Who am I becoming?" In this essay, we explore the use of digital stories as a means to educate students to focus on the patient's story as well as to reflect on their own professional identity formation as a response.[2]

A key element of NP education is the development of history-taking and physical assessment skills. The advanced physical assessment class is an introductory course in all family nurse practitioner curricula, so confidence building and identity formation are developed early in the program. This foundational class focuses on patient-centered communication, listening, and pattern recognition skills.

Using the digital story is an innovation within nursing education. Digital stories are defined as storytelling with the addition of art forms. Using multidimensional ways of sharing—through images, music, narration, text, and video clips—suggests that the intensive work of combining the narrative with technology creates a clearer, fuller vision.[3] It also provides the opportunity for greater understanding of a new world of media in which students must continue to grow, learn, and succeed, enhancing their media literacy.

One way of getting students to pay close attention to the construction and impact of personal essays is to get them to write, share, and analyze their own stories. In the physical assessment course, the students used an autobiographical theme to do a self-introduction digital story. The purpose was to have students start thinking about themselves and the future impact that others have had in our lives. It is a critical thinking exercise to welcome diversity and understand everyone has a story to tell. Most of the decisions that we make as nurse practitioners are based in part on our philosophies of what we believe works best, and our philosophies of what we generally believe is the right thing to do. Rarely, however, do we take the time to reflect upon who we are as a person. Students were instructed to prepare a three-minute, autobiographical digital presentation describing their personal and nursing/professional background. It was also suggested students explore their identity, positionality, and the impact their background, values, and beliefs have on the way that they view the world. Students often included a discussion of family, ancestors, and the impact of family on their attitudes and beliefs toward diversity, multiculturalism, and learning. Finally, students reflected on how these experiences and beliefs translated into their overall experiences and desire to work as a nurse practitioner. These stories utilized programs like PowerPoint, iMovie, or Movie Maker. Pictures either belonged to the students or were "found" pictures. Most students wrote a script and added a voice overlay rather than narrate the story as they presented their three-minute digital story.

The outcomes of this learning exercise impacted this group of students and extended beyond this one physical assessment course. Most students are well versed in technology and embrace the digital revolution. Some nursing faculty need to develop greater media literacy and were assisted in doing so. Due to the students' ability to utilize more than one type of software, the digital story exercise introduces a number of different modalities that strengthen both students and faculty awareness of digital images as a tool to enhance learning. The assignment helped faculty see the possibilities for using technology to enhance reflexivity in other clinical courses.

The digital story is an autobiographical assignment that combines creating, developing, presenting, and listening activities. It has myriad learning outcomes, including new understandings about self, other, religion, culture, and family. The ability to self-evaluate and reflect on one's personal history in a safe, respectful environment was enhanced. The digital story exercise helped promote team building, healthy boundaries, and the development of a cohort. A sense of cohesion and community was created within a class, which prior to the digital storytelling was very task-oriented and individually focused. The assignment begins a process that will continue throughout the primary care nurse practitioner curriculum of developing self-reflective, empathetic, and person-centered practitioners.

The potential for digital storytelling in primary care practitioner education and clinical practice is endless. Providing that patient privacy is rigorously protected, the digital story could be used in a case study learning approach in which patient cases are presented. The digital medium could foster a more holistic view of the patient beyond medical diagnosis or management of chronic health conditions. In a clinical setting, to improve practice and enhance clinical learning, patient testimonials or the telling of patient-centered experiences could be presented as a digital story, fostering the education of both patients and providers and improving the quality of care offered. A potential curricular innovation might be a capstone project at the end of a nurse practitioner program, encompassing the student's clinical challenges, vulnerable groups or populations they encountered, and their personal growth and development as a professional. These stories could be hosted digitally in a protected web-based salon (to protect patient/provider confidentiality).

In conclusion, the digital story is an educational approach that embraces both the thousand-year-old tradition of storytelling and the digital technology of the twenty-first century. This technological and narrative focus can facilitate the development of authentic and empathetic practitioners who view patients as individuals within a community and culture and who value and champion their humanity and unique story.

NOTES

1. Joe Lambert, *Digital Storytelling: Capturing Lives, Creating Communities,* 4th ed. (New York: Routledge, 2013); Bernard R. Robin, "Digital Storytelling: A Powerful Technology Tool for the 21st Century Classroom," *Theory into Practice* 47 (2008): 220–28.
2. Angela Christiansen, "Storytelling and Professional Learning: A Phenomenographic Study of Students' Experience of Patient Digital Stories in Nurse Education," *Nurse Education Today* 31 (2011): 289–93.
3. Lambert, *Digital Storytelling;* Robin, "Digital Storytelling."

How I Learned Reflective Practice from a Simulator Mannequin

LISA RICHARDSON

I want to introduce you to Harvey, the cardiopulmonary simulator. Harvey® is a mannequin torso, aged thirty-five plus, with blue eyes, fair (white) skin, and an ill-fitting auburn wig. He lies on a stainless steel surgical stretcher tucked into a windowless office at Toronto Western Hospital; he shares the space with a disheveled desk, a computer, and a coffeemaker. Harvey does not speak. His eyes are perpetually open. But when he is turned on, Harvey's heart beats vigorously and his chest moves with the respiratory cycle. Using the stethoscope attached to his digital viscera, I listen to his heart sounds, including the closure of heart valves and the turbulent flow of blood across them. As a high-fidelity cardiopulmonary simulator, Harvey reproduces findings in blood pressure and pulses as well as the heart and lung sounds found in various medical conditions. Medical trainees learn and practice their cardiac examination skills with Harvey.

I gather around the steel stretcher with five medical students and resident physicians to teach them how to listen to the heart and to interpret the sounds that they hear. I teach them the practices of cardiac auscultation. Paradoxically, in this pedagogical session with a speechless plastic torso, I create a space for reflective practice. In this short reflection, I will describe how I learned my own principles for reflection from a mannequin simulator.

I am a general internal medicine specialist at Toronto Western Hospital and a teacher in the Faculty of Medicine at the University of Toronto. I am also a critical theorist with a background in Science and Technology Studies. As a theorist, I am conscious of the standardizing and often objectifying practices of medicine and medical education. As we articulate our own identities and bodies as physicians, we learn to observe, parse, measure, decipher, and codify the bodies of our patients. In *The Birth of the Clinic: An Archaeology of Medical*

Perception, Michel Foucault depicts the development of an anatomo-clinical gaze in medicine at the end of the eighteenth century. A physician's anatomo-clinical gaze is a multisensory, external deciphering—one that plunges to the depths of a patient's body to provide a "clinical reading" of it.[1] Cardiac auscultation forms one of the techniques of a physician's gaze. Prior to the development of auscultation in the nineteenth century, physicians diagnosed disease by listening to the narratives of patients and by visually assessing them; there was little attention to physical examination, except palpation of the pulse.

Given my background as a theorist, I was dubious about using Harvey to teach my students. I worried that if students learned skills from a pristine plastic mannequin, they would become similarly cyborgian in their interactions with real patients. They would not learn how to listen to a patient's story or attend to a patient's comfort. Although his idealized and unblemished exterior contains a computer that mimics rare and severe cardiac conditions, Harvey cannot talk to students. Just as he lacks the stubble, wrinkles, cellulite, tattoos, moles, or tobacco stains that remind us of his body's individuality, he also lacks history, experiences, and emotions.

In order to explore my interactions with the simulator from my contra-dictory standpoints as a teacher, learner, and theorist, I engaged in a critical "autoethnography" of Harvey. Through this process, I came to realize how my physician's body has been entrained and articulated during ten years of rigorous training. I revealed my own medical practices that objectify patients (reducing a person's lived experience of illness to a numerical valve or dismissing a person's narrative account of an illness due to temporal pressures or utter exhaustion). Finally, I drew upon my guides from the world of critical theory and feminist theory to position myself alongside Harvey and imagine new perspectives and "fresh sources of analysis."[2] These fresh perspectives actually engendered three tenets of my own reflective practice.

First, my analysis forced me to account for all the bodies and relationships enmeshed with Harvey. Researchers, sound engineers, technicians, artists, and educators created the simulator. The heart sounds and murmurs in Harvey's computer entrails are sounds recorded from real patients. Students and physicians listen to and learn from him. The cardiac findings of real patients in clinics and hospitals around the world are compared to his. Harvey's network of creators, users, and patients reminds me that our patients do not exist in isolation. They too are enmeshed in a network of families, friends, health-care providers, technological devices, diagnoses, institutions, etc. A reflective prac-titioner strives to understand a patient situated within a network of experiences and relationships, both human and nonhuman.

In my reflection on how I learned the highly interpretive listening skill of auscultation, I also learned that medical education actually encompasses an entertainment of the senses and an articulation of my physician's body. I draw upon Bruno Latour's meaning of articulation as the process of "learning to be affected."[3] He develops the notion of articulation through his description of students training for the perfume industry. The perfumers' bodies and body parts (like the nose) take shape as they learn to articulate difference. Just as perfumers are gradually able to distinguish more and more finite differences in smell, a clinician's ear incrementally learns to recognize more subtle findings. By drawing attention to my own senses and hence my physicality as a physician, my medical gaze becomes embodied rather than disembodied. My sensorium and my faculties of reason are integrated. I am no longer a detached, objectivizing, and observation-bound scientist, but a caring, sensing, embodied practitioner. A reflective practitioner recognizes the integration of the physical and psychological experiences of health/illness and medical practice.

Finally, during my analyses of the simulator, I observed that trainees interacting with Harvey often have and display strong affective responses to him. Some users are wondrous of the technological innovation, while others are humored by the mannequin's toupee. Some are dismayed by the glassy eyes, while others admire the ideal physique. Some are nervous about performing for students, while others delight in the opportunity. The recognition of affect in interactions with Harvey highlights my own emotional responses in clinical encounters. It enables me to create either a literal or figurative space to identify my responses and those of my students and patients. This space may be a dedicated discussion to debrief an overwhelming experience such as a Code Blue event or a simple acknowledgement to my team that I am frustrated or saddened by a particular encounter. A reflective practitioner identifies and acknowledges her own emotions as well as the affective moments in her practice.

My initial dismissal of Harvey as a teaching tool led me to deeper analysis through which I was able to reconcile my contradictory standpoints as a physician, teacher, and theorist. Ultimately, the voiceless mannequin helped me to elucidate the cornerstones of a reflective practice. I now routinely use Harvey to teach cardiac auscultation. More importantly, Harvey reminds me to pause during a busy clinical day and acknowledge that clinicians are not detached, deciphering, and disembodied clinical machines—we are interactive, embodied, and affected health-care providers with our own stories and experiences.

NOTES

1. Michel Foucault, *The Birth of the Clinic: An Archaeology of Medical Perception*, trans. A. M. Sheridan (New York: Vintage, 1994).
2. Donna J. Haraway, *Simians, Cyborgs, and Women: The Reinvention of Nature* (New York: Routledge, 1991), 165.
3. Bruno Latour, "How to Talk about the Body? The Normative Dimension of Science Studies," *Body & Society* 10 (2004): 205–29.

Using Electronic Portfolios to Record Reflection

Supporting the Supervisors of Primary Care Physicians in Training

JONATHAN FOULKES AND SAMANTHA SCALLAN

Our account reports a reflective educational session with the "educational supervisors" (ESs) of primary care physicians in the UK. An educational supervisor is responsible for teaching and assessing a doctor in training. In the United Kingdom this is, in part, achieved through the trainee maintaining an online electronic portfolio that includes reflective writing in a diary of learning (the "Learning-Log") within the ePortfolio. These entries can be of several different types, but all have a set format that provides a structure to help the trainee "unpack" and reflect upon the event that the entry describes. The ES is also required to provide written feedback to the trainee within the ePortfolio at the end of each log entry.

The introduction of the ePortfolio in 2007 and the need to maintain a reflective learning diary have been met with mixed opinion among educational supervisors.[1] Concern has been expressed that trainees are writing descriptive entries merely to satisfy a summative assessment process rather than to formatively support and develop their learning. It would seem that trainees now undertake introspection prior to writing their reflective accounts of learning, instead of framing their reflection through dialogue with their ES. As a way of examining these issues, we developed a three-part educational session for educational supervisors.

The aim of the session was to explore the experiences of ESs completing reflective log entries with trainees and to try to expose the difficulties they were encountering in this process. To do this, we purposively planned to use an approach to learning that would be familiar and comfortable, that of "problem case analysis." By drawing on ESs' well-established skills, in particular those of discussion and reflection, we hoped to bring the issues to the fore and to facilitate their addressing them. We wanted to help them to rediscover that their long-standing and well-established educational skills were still relevant and perhaps even more important in an era of the structured ePortfolio. We also wanted to help supervisors establish an educational rather than a managerial dialogue with their trainee, which would be focused on learning and not assessment.

Prior to the session, participants were asked to identify a clinical case that had given them cause for concern—their "problem case." The session was divided into three parts: Telling, Writing, and Narrative-based Reflection. Each part of the session took place over the course of about an hour.

Telling: The first part of the session focused on dialogue and the use of discussion as a way to reflect in depth on their clinical cases. The educational supervisors were encouraged to consider their problem cases in pairs, teasing out the issues as these emerged through discussion with a peer. To close this part, participants fed back their views on what they thought characterized the dialogue and what it had achieved for them. Feedback suggested that the supervisors valued this dialogue as (1) it provided an opportunity to share a difficult experience with a GP colleague, who was viewed as a peer (rather than an expert) sharing common uncertainties or worries; (2) it created time to stop and examine professional behavior and to "be heard" while offering a safe, private space for sharing emotional experiences and exploring alternate viewpoints and possibilities; and (3) it offered a dynamic process involving active listening, questioning, and challenge, all jointly constructed. This was felt to reveal a greater number of learning points than introspection.

Writing: Over the course of about an hour, the ESs were asked to write about their dialogue, foregrounding what they had learned from the discussion, what they might do differently, and what learning needs arose for them and their clinical practice. We hoped the process would help them identify the value of discussion and its role in the process of reflection and, more particularly, to recognize that they already possessed and used these skills. The pairs exchanged written accounts and reflected further on the relationship between the oral and written modes of discourse. Feedback from the supervisors about their views on the value of writing about their cases contrasted with the earlier feedback; their views were divided—showing that some appeared to be comfortable writing and others found it challenging.

Narrative-based Reflection: The final part of the session brought all participants together to consider the links between the dialogue and the written accounts and to discuss how each of these had shaped their thinking. We then drew conclusions about the value of facilitating reflection and how this impacted their trainees' learning. To close the session, the group looked at the learning log templates and considered how these might be used to capture the learning that was occurring within the reflective process. This aimed to bring together the ES/trainee dialogue and the log templates in order to identify the elements of the former that could be represented in the latter.

It was through this third part of the session that it emerged that trainees' learning log entries tended to be written by them in isolation from their ES, even though the two worked closely on a daily basis. The opportunity for valuable discussion and feedback between supervisor and trainee was being lost, and consequently the portfolio entries were seemingly of limited educational value for both supervisor and trainee. Trainees wrote descriptive portfolio entries to satisfy what they saw as a need to pass a summative assessment rather than writing reflectively to help themselves learn. Set in this context, it was clear that the supervisors would struggle to find evidence of reflection and professional development on which to comment in their trainees' logs, resulting in feedback that was brief and general.

A week later, we gathered follow-up written feedback on the session, which was positive and reiterated the views expressed during it. For some supervisors who were less inclined to write, the opportunity to explore written reflection led to a reevaluation of the role of writing in learning; for others, just thinking about the issues had led them to reconceptualize the reflective process and its recording in the ePortfolio. Participants reported that they welcomed the time to consider their practice as educators and to share their experiences and difficulties. Some reported that they would encourage trainees to write their portfolio entries after an ES/trainee discussion to promote reflective writing as a learning experience and not just as an exercise to pass an assessment.

Having brought a number of issues to the surface, our session was intended to highlight the importance of dialogue, reflection, and feedback in the process of learning; to reestablish the role of the supervisor in this; and to show that supervisors already possessed significant educational "skills" (e.g., engaging trainees in reflective dialogue), which were not only relevant to present-day training but important to recognize and reuse. The significance of feedback to development is well evidenced in medical education literature.[2] The role of the person giving feedback—in this case, the ES—is critical, if not instrumental, to the learning process. Without such input, learning can remain introspective and insular. It is little wonder, therefore, that when there is no communication between the supervisor and the trainee writing the log entries, the trainee can feel unsure about what to record—often providing too much description and not enough analysis. Feedback seems to be the missing link that makes "assessment for learning" possible and provides the context for high stakes summative decisions regarding a trainee's progression, something demonstrated by our workshop participants through their dialogues.

In addition to emphasizing the need for discussion and feedback, the educational session also demonstrated the value of writing as an aid to reflection for supervisors. This is acknowledged in the educational literature but has been less frequently used as a way of reflecting on experience. Trainees are now required to formalize "professional conversations" and use them as a basis for reflection and as evidence for learning. However, our session demonstrated that writing can be uncomfortable and a struggle for some educational supervisors and probably their trainees too. Taken as a whole, it is not surprising that both trainees and educational supervisors were frustrated by it in practice. Through our session, we demonstrated that by once more foregrounding the "professional conversation" as a fundamental feature of learning, the link between reflecting on cases and writing entries in the ePortfolio can be reestablished.

NOTES

1. Jonathan Foulkes, Samantha Scallan, and Richard Weaver, "Educational Supervision for GP Trainees: Time to Take Stock?" *Education for Primary Care* 24 (2013): 90–92.
2. Noah Ivers et al., "Audit and Feedback: Effects on Professional Practice and Healthcare Outcomes," *Cochrane Database of Systematic Reviews* (2012), doi:10.1002/14651858.CD000259.pub3.

Using Online Student Journaling as an Approach to Reflection

A Creative, Arts-Based Strategy

KATHERINE J. JANZEN, HEATHER MACLEAN,
AND MARY ANN WIEBE

Reflection has long been a cornerstone for nursing practice and professionalism and is considered a requisite skill by many nursing regulatory bodies. It is essential that reflection be introduced early in the learning trajectory for student nurses in order to provide opportunities to develop this skill. Students are different, bringing personal histories that shape their unique interpretations of their developing practice, and so creating opportunities for reflection provides a means for meaning, learning, and sense making for student nurses.

The idea for the online reflective journal site for first-year nursing students came to us after an online journal site for instructors was successfully tested in 2011. In addition, our faculty had just recently embraced use of creativity across the curriculum for undergraduate nursing students as a means of reflection. Our approach to developing our online reflective journal site was informed by the Peshkin approach to reflection and by the use of creative, arts-based teaching strategies. Peshkin outlined the use of using the subjective "first person" to record reflective experiences,[1] and Perry, Janzen, and Edwards affirmed reflection was enhanced with the use of creative arts-based strategies.[2]

With the help of our Academic Development Centre, we created an online site for the introductory professional practice course (NURS 1214) we offer to nursing students at Mount Royal University. A journal site was created for each instructor and each of the eight respective first-year nursing students in their first clinical experience assigned to that instructor. All clinical instructors were introduced to this mode of reflection first, as it was important to enhance their acceptance and use of the process before introducing the online site to the students. The instructors at first were tentative about the process, but after additional explanation and discussion they were eager to give the online student journal site a try.

As part of their orientation to their first-year clinical course, all students were introduced to the online reflective journal site. The syllabus we created for the course included instructions for using the online site. Students were aware that only their instructor could see their reflections and, although students were required to complete a weekly entry, there was no grade attached to this component of the course. What students posted would not be evaluated. Students were also briefed on the benefits of reflection. We suggested that online journaling would provide an opportunity to share "thoughts, feelings, and experiences that they [had] had each clinical week, finding their voice, . . . discovering the nurse [they were] becoming as [they moved] through [their] clinical year practicum, encouraging dialogue with their instructor, [providing] a safe place to share what puzzled [them] or perhaps scared [them], and a space to celebrate [their] triumphs and challenges."

The reflective writing entries of our students took many forms. The students were encouraged to be creative, resulting in entries that were as creative and individual as each student. Some students recounted an experience they had during clinical. Others shared pictures or poems and then explored how they were feeling or what they discovered about themselves. Still, others posted a musical piece and then discussed online how this applied to their practice. A first-year nursing student recorded this journal entry in narrative form: "Every day is a new adventure here and I quite love that. I am so terrified of meeting my patients each week because I don't know what to expect but I am thankful to care for such amazing people to learn not only about my patient's conditions and emotions but also about myself as a learner and as a human being."

Her clinical instructor responded to her entry, saying:

> Sometimes the greatest lessons we learn in clinical are about ourselves. We learn about our hopes and dreams and face our fears. You are making a difference too. Your presence is making a difference and your kind heart and compassion. Some people get burned out in nursing, but I think that it is because they lose that wonder and awe in meeting people/patients all the time. Yes, the conditions and co-morbidities remain the same, but no patient is ever the same twice. It can remain an adventure all your life if you let it. It is so rewarding when it all comes together and you know you made a difference that day or that shift. So as you head into your last two shifts of clinical keep making that difference that you always do.

Another student demonstrated her creativity in a different way. This journal entry included a photo of her messy bedroom to convey that she wished to "clean up" and related that "this past clinical was the worst for me so far. I did all that I needed to do, vitals and assessments, but it was really . . . Messy."

The impact of the online reflective journal site was elucidated in the impact of the two-way dialogue that grew as each week progressed. Students and instructors enriched each other's lives. Importantly, students risked again and again as they shared their thoughts and feelings with their instructors. The experience of reflecting gave the students the opportunity to build not only confidence but also trust.

Students also exhibited incredible growth as clinical progressed through online reflective journaling. For instructors it was inspiring to see the students embrace their developing roles and sense of becoming a nurse. In the end, they were learning the art of nursing as they reflected. That was a gift that they gave to their instructors each week—a gift that their instructors would treasure forever.

Online reflective journaling can help students gain self-awareness, insight, and understanding about their experiences in clinical. Reflection helps students to link what they are learning in theory to their practice and the experiences they are having. Equally important, online reflection gives students a voice. It is about the students and what they are learning. In the end, nursing is both an art and a science. Reflection is about the art of nursing and what matters to students as they develop that art within themselves.

NOTES

1. Caroline Bradbury⬚Jones et al., "A New Way of Reflecting in Nursing: The Peshkin Approach," *Journal of Advanced Nursing* 65 (2009): 2485–93.
2. Beth Perry, Katherine J. Janzen, and Margaret Edwards, "Creating Invitational Online Learning Environments using Art-based Learning Interventions," *eLearning Papers* 27 (2011): 1–4, www.slideshare.net/elearningpapers/creating-invitational-online-learning-environments-using-art-based-learning-interventions.

Mapping Well-Being

Reflections on the Role of Place in Healthy Human Functioning

SARAH L. HASTINGS AND JACLYN L. MULLINS

One of the topics I explore with my students is the role of place in well-being. We see variations on this theme in recent research examining health outcomes across geographic regions. The Robert Wood Johnson Foundation, for example, publishes an annual online ranking of health data in counties across the United States,[1] which allows users to select a particular state and examine counties assigned various shades of colors depending on the health rankings of residents. I find myself fascinated by these maps, examining shaded clusters of healthy and less healthy counties and wondering about the patterns they suggest. My students and I hypothesize about what the distributions might mean, what factors contribute to health outcomes, and what role interstate highways, population density, climate, or geographical barriers play. We talk about access to educational institutions and medical centers, and those who have lived in these different regions share their experiences of these places. This discussion always serves as a springboard to explore both the many barriers to accessing health care and the ways we can develop cultural competence working with the diverse patient populations characterizing these regions.

This relationship between geography and health outcomes spurred me to think about the role of place in relation not only to traditional measures of health but also to well-being. Well-being is broadly defined to include dimensions of physical health, emotional health, belongingness, and security. How many of us have lived in a variety of places, knowing some were a better "fit" than others? I came across some research examining this very topic while teaching a course in positive psychology.[2] For those unfamiliar with the area, positive psychology examines those aspects of human functioning that reflect the "better side" of human nature. What is it that makes life worth living? How do people overcome challenges? How do we identify and nurture the healthy psychological aspects of a person or, for that matter, of an organization? Further, although researchers, for example, routinely examine how people make a living, how they seek out relationships, and how they pursue pleasurable activities, studies largely overlook the role of place in providing opportunities to do these things.

There is actually a fairly large body of literature, both scholarly and popular, examining national differences on dimensions of well-being and happiness.[3] Fewer studies have examined local differences or obtained the level of specificity found in the Robert Wood Johnson County Health Ranking. The exercise I developed invites student clinicians to examine the role of place in relation to their own sense of well-being. Students reflect on the places they have lived and consider their experience of well-being in relation to these various locations. I begin by giving students handouts of two maps. One map is of the United States and the other is of the world. I ask students to spend a few minutes placing a mark on the areas where they have lived. Some students have many marks on their pages, while others have only three or four.

Next, I ask the students to create a chronological list of these places starting from their early years up until the present. For each location, I ask students to assign a number on a 10-point scale with 1 representing a perceived sense of poor well-being, and 10 representing a perceived sense of high well-being. Then I ask them to list factors—physical and emotional, real and symbolic—they believe contributed to their experience of each place. Finally, we talk about what the students have written. Students take some time to review their maps and to recount their impressions to the class. It can be helpful, if equipment is available, to project students' maps on a screen while they talk about their experiences living in different places.

The place and well-being exercise has been useful by providing an opportunity for students to process aloud the factors that contributed to their well-being, or lack thereof, in the various places they have lived. In some cases, students struggled to disentangle the contributions of very personal events (nuclear family changes, for example) and the contributions of place (access to a strong peer group, schools that provided a sense of belonging, or extended family, for example). From a professional development standpoint, students were able to reflect on the aspects of a place that brought them contentment in their childhood or adolescence versus what they were looking for at the present time, such as living in a location that will allow them to fulfill their professional goals or find a life partner.

One student (coauthor Jaclyn L. Mullins) reflected on the difficulties she experienced when she moved away from her family to pursue an appealing job and a warmer climate. The student described an internal "tug-of-war" between wanting to adhere to family tradition by living close by and embracing new opportunities by moving away. Even though the move proved to be fruitful and she was satisfied in her new location, the student still felt a sense of loneliness related to being far away from her family. She also eventually found herself discontented with the lack of advancement opportunities at her job and wanted to return to graduate school. Her situation grew more complicated when she became engaged to get married. Suddenly, she had to consider not only her own wants and needs but those of her partner as well, and what once seemed like a temporary move began to feel more permanent. She began imagining what it would be like to live there forever. She feared that she would never return to graduate school and would continue to see her family only a few times a year. It was obvious that, for this student, maintaining family ties and achieving her educational goals were things she valued very much, and she ultimately called off her engagement, returned to school, and relocated closer to her family. This student described the place and well-being exercise as reaffirming. While she had previously felt that her reasons for calling off her engagement were inadequate, after participating in the exercise and processing her feelings with her classmates, she felt justified in her decision.

The program where I teach trains students to, among other things, provide behavioral health care for underserved people in rural areas. Geographically, we are located on the edge of the Appalachian region, and we work with our students to develop cultural competence in treating rural populations. This exercise helps student clinicians consider the contributions of place not only to their own well-being but to that of their patients. It helps them think about the degree to which the environment enables patients to meet their basic human needs and the extent to which it provides opportunities for enhancing health and well-being. How readily does a particular environment offer cultural resources and facilities for youth to pursue activities and to meet the demands of their developmental stage? Obviously, the role of place in well-being is subject to many individual and community variables. I have found over several years of using this reflection that it provides a valuable opportunity to have students evaluate the relative contributions of individual, familial, and cultural factors, as well as the "fit" of person and environment to producing optimal health and well-being.

NOTES

1. Robert Wood Johnson Foundation, "County Health Rankings & Roadmaps," accessed Dec. 13, 2013, www.countyhealthrankings.org.
2. Richard Florida and Peter J. Rentfrow, "Place and Well-Being," in *Designing Positive Psychology: Taking Stock and Moving Forward,* ed. Kennon M. Sheldon, Todd B. Kashdan, and Michael F. Steger (New York: Oxford Univ. Press, 2011), 385–95.
3. Eric Weiner, *The Geography of Bliss: One Grump's Search for the Happiest Places on Earth* (New York: Hachette Book Group, 2008).

Google Mapping

Developing Reflective Perspectives on Health and Place

PAMELA BRETT-MACLEAN, CATHERINE RODER,
SHAYNA MCNEILL, MAUREEN ENGEL, AND HEATHER ZWICKER

There is increasing interest in inquiring into spatial dimensions of narratives.[1] We recently piloted an online mapping exercise using Google's My Maps application to help medical students reflect on the influence of place and location on health and health care. We closely modeled this exercise on an assignment developed by Drs. Heather Zwicker and Maureen Engel for their capstone English 486 multimedia course in which students depict urban spaces using Google's digital mapping tool.[2] The first two years of our four-year undergraduate medical education curriculum includes a variety of foundational teaching methods, such as lectures, anatomy instruction, and problem-based learning, which our program calls *discovery learning* (DL). Recognizing that knowing or understanding is always informed by one's perspective, this activity has been designed as a collaborative, reflective learning exercise. As Gillie Bolton has observed, assumptions "that clients, patients, students, members of the public share practitioners' viewpoints, for example, are likely to be dangerously wrong, yet such assumptions are made every day."[3] To help point to such assumptions, students work in pairs and reflect on each other's maps, inquiring into different aspects that may be informing their cartographic representations of paper-based, DL patient cases.

Google's My Maps tool provides a means for creating digital, customized maps that can be edited, updated, and shared. My Maps allows users to dynamically represent geographically referenced information in a visually engaging way. Various multimedia forms, such as "pin" icons, links to websites, and digital media (photography, video, audio), along with written personal reflections and invited online commentary, can all be incorporated. Instructions for using

Google mapping to augment the abstract presentation of patient illness experience, adapted from Zwicker and Engel, are provided below.

DEVELOPING REFLECTIVE PERSPECTIVES ON HEALTH AND PLACE

Part 1—The Map: Using Google's My Maps tool (https://www.google.com/mymaps), create a customized map that relates to the patient's story described in your paper-based DL case. Focus on a specific geographic area or time period that captures a compelling episode or aspect of the patient's story. Do not document the patient's entire life story or history of care. Your story map can be a collection of conceptually linked points or an actual route (A to B to C). Include information that is relevant to the patient's illness and their experience of receiving health care. Include visual and narrative annotations and other multimedia links. Include 10 to 15 points and a minimum of 10 visual images and 10 narrative annotations. Save your map and e-mail the URL to your partner and your DL facilitator by [date, time].

Part 2—Collaborative Reflection: After receiving your partner's map, take about twenty minutes to closely consider the patient's journey. Reflect on aspects of space and place your partner has profiled as influencing the patient's health status, including health-care options that may (or may not) be available where the patient lives. Open to inquiring into your partner's perceptions of lived-in-place, experiences of illness, and health care. Make notes as you reflect on the graphic markings and other visual and narrative content included in the map. Record your initial impressions. Pay attention to how you think about your partner's map after some time has elapsed. Attempt to visit some of the places your partner included on the map (virtually, if not physically). When you return to your partner's map, consider the following: What is missing? What else might be represented in the space depicted? Is there a perspective or practice that is missing? Consider the extent to which your partner's map invites you to understand connections between the lived experience of health and place. Write a short commentary (maximum five hundred words) in which you reflect on what you have come to appreciate, having viewed your partner's map, and also what you wondered about, observed, or reflected on that your colleague may not have captured. E-mail a copy of your reflection to both your partner and DL facilitator by [date].

Part 3—Revisioning: As you read your partner's reflection on your map, appreciate that someone put a great deal of time and care into thinking about your work. Consider new ideas you may not have thought of on your own. Does your partner's reflection help you to recognize preliminary individuals, or culturally conditioned perceptions that informed the map you created? Does it help you to think about your map differently? Consider ways in which you might want to revise your map. You may want to include new insights, things you hadn't thought of before but are aware of now, given your experience of reflecting on your partner's map. There may be additional visual or narrative aspects you feel are important to include at this stage, given a close review of your partner's reflective commentary regarding the map you shared with them. You are free to integrate these as well. Write a short reflective summary (a maximum of two hundred fifty words). E-mail both the URL for your final revised Google map and your final reflection to both your partner and DL facilitator by [date, time].

We piloted this exercise in relation to fictional DL patient cases that our medical students encounter in their first year. Students have shared that this exercise heightened their appreciation of a patient's lived experience. The experience of creating their initial map, considering each other's map, and then reconsidering their map through the lens of their colleague's reflective comments enhanced their understanding of factors that contributed to each patient's presenting health concerns, factors supporting or compromising adherence to treatment regimes, and challenges associated with accessing health care.

Rather than simply seeing patients as "cases," the students imagined their DL patients as embodied beings, living within specific spatial and social contexts. They considered each patient in relation to the fullness of their lives, as people who had families, and when they were employed, had jobs located in places that could potentially influence their health in detrimental ways—as was the case for the fictional Ms. Sweet, a fifty-six-year-old woman who worked as a cook in a lumber camp and lived at a far distance from a major health-care center. See Image 8 for the map Catherine Roder created to depict the illness-related experiences of Ms. Sweet.

After closely reviewing Catherine's map, Shayna McNeill noted a pervasive element of sadness that she felt accurately conveyed how depression can literally "follow" a patient throughout their lives. Shayna suggested including additional points of reference, such as the location of grocery stores with fresh fruits and vegetables, as well as local fitness and health-care centers, to emphasize the challenges that people living in rural areas sometimes face when attempting to maintain "a healthy lifestyle and responsible disease management." Catherine shared that this exercise encouraged her "to think through different locations that were important to Ms. Sweet's life, and critical to telling *her* story, and not the story of just anyone with diabetes and diabetic neuropathy. . . . [It] made the DL case feel like it was more 'life-like,' that it could be about a real

Catherine
Roder's story
map.

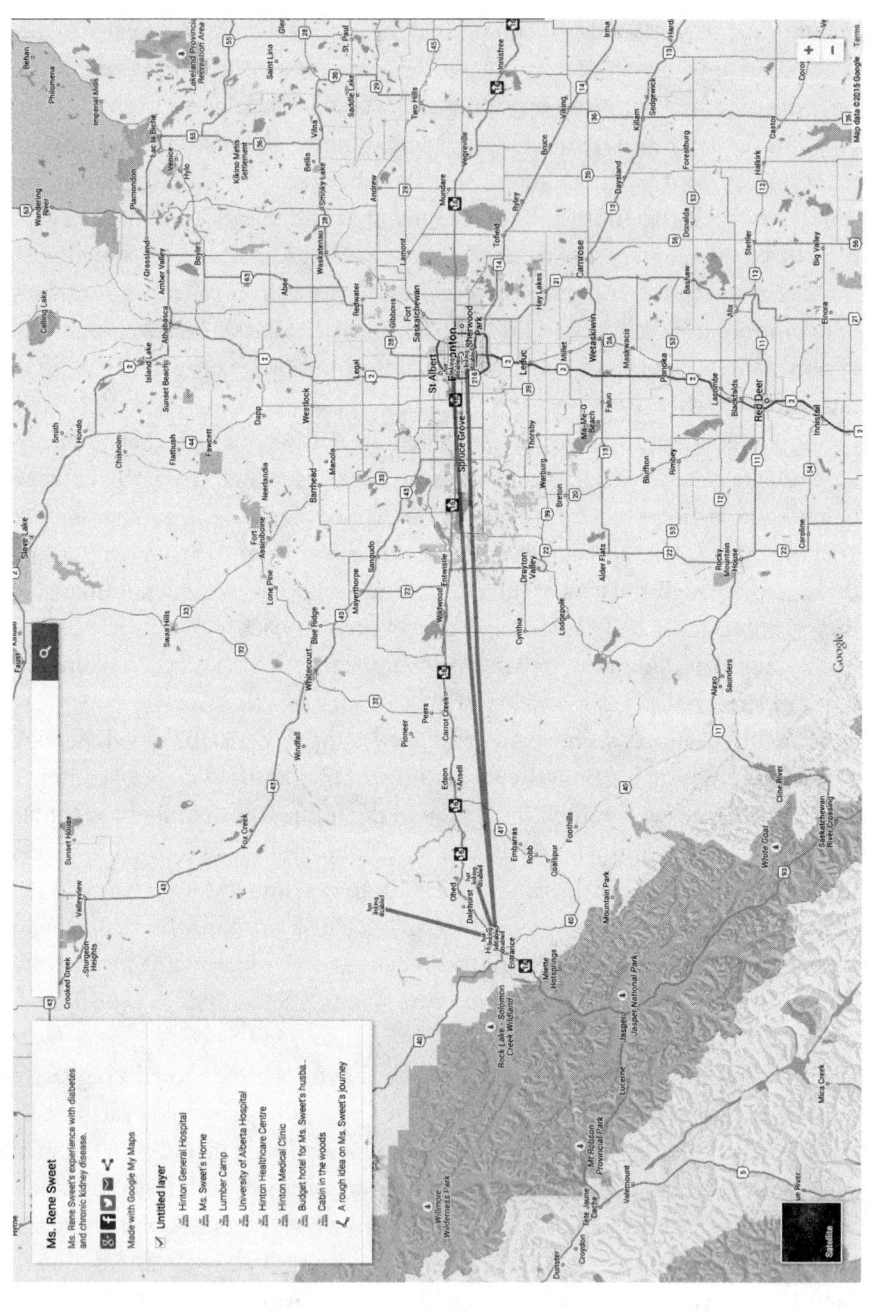

person." For example, creating the map helped Catherine not only imagine the three-hour drive to the city but also recognize that Ms. Sweet would need to find temporary accommodation when receiving dialysis treatment.

Increasingly, online technologies are being adopted to augment teaching focused on the human side of medicine. This reflective exercise is designed to promote awareness of the ways in which a patient's life story and illness experience are situated in different locations and spaces. It is designed to foster enhanced empathic understanding and commitment to providing effective care for real patients who struggle with health challenges in different physical settings. This exercise also helps to remind our preclerkship students that they will soon be caring for real patients, each with unique values, concerns, and resources.

We believe that Google mapping can foster reflection on health and place in a variety of health professions educational programs and contribute to imagining future possibilities in support of better health for all in relation to the spaces and places in which we live. Other variations might include collective mapping of health-care resources or health-seeking experiences within specific locations; mapping of interprofessional, team-based care associated with specific health-care conditions; and mapping of learning experiences focused on exploring social determinants of health (locally and globally). We look forward to learning about innovative variations you may introduce in your setting over time (e-mail pbrett@ualberta.ca).

NOTES

1. Sébastien Caquard, "Cartography 1: Mapping Narrative Cartography," *Progress in Human Geography* 37 (2013): 135–44.
2. Heather Zwicker and Maureen Engel, "Putting Edmonton on the (Google) Map," poster presented at Digital Humanities 2010, London, UK, July 7–10, 2010, http://dh2010.cch.kcl.ac.uk /academic-programme/abstracts/index.html. For the scoring rubric used to assess the original student assignment, e-mail heather.zwicker@ualberta.ca.
3. Gillie Bolton, *Reflective Practice: Writing and Professional Development* (Los Angeles: Sage, 2010), xx.

Video Interactive Guidance

A Reflective Pedagogical Tool for Enhancing Learning Goals and Compassion in the Context of Clinical Communication Skills Education

ELVIRA PEREZ VALLEJOS, DEBORAH JAMES,
AND DICK CHURCHILL

Video Interactive Guidance (VIG) is a type of positive video feedback successfully used in a wide variety of contexts.[1] It is a relationship-based intervention focused on promoting attunement, empathy, and well-being in participants, with a special emphasis on communication. VIG has been effective in supporting the training of health-care professionals and also in clinical supervision. Video feedback provides a unique opportunity for *reflection* on specific aspects of communication but also for *reflexivity* beyond a specific, targeted behavior.[2] Formal VIG training and supervision can be accessed, and it is regulated by the Association of Video Interactive Guidance in the UK.

All undergraduate medical students in the United Kingdom are required to undertake training in clinical communication skills (CCS) as part of their curricula in order to meet the registration requirements of the General Medical Council. Many medical schools adopt the Calgary-Cambridge Consultation Model, which emphasizes aspects such as developing rapport, active listening, promoting empathy, and building trust. In order to facilitate these learning outcomes, medical students in Nottingham take part in a two-hour practical session in which a ten-minute medical history is videotaped while the student gathers relevant information from simulated patients. Students review their video clips in groups of up to twelve students. Feedback is provided by peers, more senior clinicians, and/or CCS facilitators. CCS facilitators receive training to keep sessions safe and supportive (for example, asking students "What went well?") and are instructed to identify the students' own agenda and specific aspects on which they would like feedback. Consequently, the feedback sessions often focus less on strengths and more often on aspects of verbal and nonverbal communication and communicative skills that require improvement.

While these sessions are very powerful in allowing students to review and reflect on their performance, the reliability and effectiveness of this teaching technique can potentially be enhanced with VIG, specifically within the context of revalidation and remediation for students having difficulty. VIG is a plausible pedagogical tool that can easily be adapted to medical school curricula because the technology required (video recording and playback) is already present in the clinical skills facilities usually based in medical schools. VIG is effective as it creates an optimal, safe, and compassionate environment where students feel confident to perform at their best. After group-based VIG sessions, students often report feeling empowered and more in tune with the ideal doctor within themselves. VIG can also facilitate transformative learning by creating disorientating dilemmas.

VIG AS A TOOL FOR REMEDIATION WITHIN CLINICAL COMMUNICATION SKILLS: A CASE STUDY

In the context of remediation, VIG can be delivered in a one-to-one, conventional format in which the VIG guider and health-care professional engage in a process of change by defining specific goals around CCS. The transformative learning journey of a mature medical student who had failed the CCS module over the two previous years is offered as an example. Contrary to the student's expectations, both the student and VIG guider defined new shared co-constructed goals. Previous video footage and newly created scenarios with simulated patients were used. The VIG guider edited the film, selecting very short clips of the most successful moments. During the shared video review sessions, the student and guider engaged in a compassionate and attuned dialogue. Together they reflect on successful moments captured on the video recording that facilitated insightful "learning conversations" and promoted the student's confidence. After three VIG sessions, the student's performance improved significantly and he passed his CCS exam. The student attributed this transformation to his newly gained confidence. He shared, "I think I do feel more confident in myself generally . . . now it is easy for me to step into the role of being a doctor . . . I can see I am more structured now . . . I feel as if I am getting there, to where I want to be."

Recognition of the importance of mindful presence, kindness, and compassion are slowly influencing the current health-care models and helping to restore humanity to medicine.[3] The importance of communication and compassion as integral clinical skills has recently been highlighted in the UK by the Department of Health. While communication skills have been an integral part of most undergraduate medical curricula for many years, there is a need to enhance and develop these skills further to meet the needs of doctors of the future through teaching and research.

NOTES

1. Hilary Kennedy, Miriam Landor, and Liz Todd, *Video Interactive Guidance: A Relationship-based Intervention to Promote Attunement, Empathy and Well-being* (London: Jessica Kingsley Publishers, 2011).
2. Rick Iedema, "Creating Safety by Strengthening Clinicians' Capacity for Reflexivity," *British Medical Journal* 20, Suppl. 1 (2011): 183–86.
3. Paul Gilbert, *The Compassionate Mind: A New Approach to Life's Challenges* (London: Constable & Robinson, 2009).

Beyond Information Giving

Use of a Blended Approach to Reflection to Promote Skill Development in Physiotherapy

LESTER E. JONES

As is the case in other health professions, physiotherapy programs risk being overloaded with content. This is driven by the collective expectations of professional bodies, clinical partners, and teaching traditions. Change is difficult to enforce, and new learning and teaching strategies are treated with suspicion. Yet this is exactly what is needed to ensure that professions maintain relevance, especially those professions with diverse roles and changing standards of professional practice, such as physiotherapy. The relevance of physiotherapy in contemporary and future health care will depend on its ability to adapt to the changing health-care environment. Essentially this means shifting the profession's underlying paradigm from a primarily biomedical model to a more holistic model of health and well-being.[1] Educators thus have an obligation to facilitate this change by creating learning and teaching activities that encourage engagement with broader human experiences and promote deeper thought processes, rather than rote learning of biomedical data or mimicry of manual therapy skills.

Students have never been as resource-rich as they are today. Online anatomy tools allow the human body to be rotated and dissected. Manual therapy skills can be presented in the form of recorded videos that can be reviewed at any time and often from multiple angles. There is also exponential growth of online texts and journals. The amount of information available to students via diverse media is quite simply amazing—so much so that traditional approaches to sharing information, such as by lecture presentation, are essentially becoming obsolete. New learning technologies are changing how we deliver content in health professional education. However, it cannot be assumed that providing students with access to online content is sufficient. Exposure to information does not guarantee good learning outcomes. The key to learning is engagement and depth of understanding.

Clinical skill development is an essential part of physiotherapy training. The following commentary reports on the development of a blended learning approach for teaching core manual therapy skills. Our approach incorporated use of e-learning technologies and online resources. In addition, principles of reflective practice were incorporated as part of our curriculum design (see figure below). Emphasizing active learning, rather than rote learning or mimicry, we needed to inform students about the need to have a more engaged role in their learning compared to traditional didactic approaches. This was equally important for tutors who were most comfortable with their role as experts demonstrating "how" clinical skills should be performed, rather than facilitating a trial-and-error approach to learning.

We incorporated the use of "authentic assessment for learning" along with timely verbal and written feedback.[2] As part of an iterative skill development cycle, learning activities and assessments were structured to enable students to utilize feedback. Students engaged in an ongoing learning process that included tutor feedback, peer assessment, and individual self-assessment and reflection. An online Personal Learning Space (PLS) provided by the university allowed students to collect and organize various learning artifacts (video recordings,

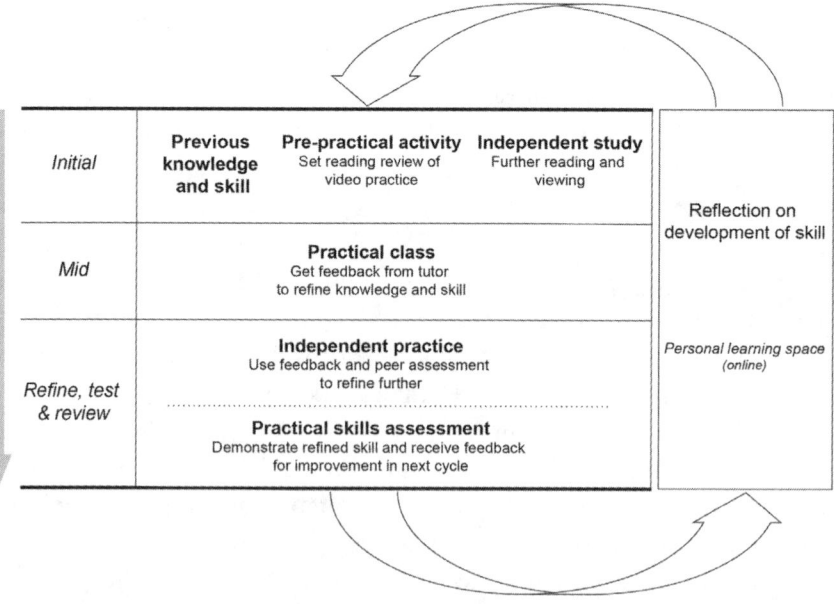

Incorporating reflection in the process of skill development in physiotherapy training.

etc.), as well as upload private recordings of their personal reflections. Use of the online PLS occurred primarily in relation to a specific assessment task—the skills diary. Based on previous work by the author,[3] the skills diary was designed as an introduction to reflective practice. The key purpose of the skills diary was to support self-monitoring of ability and competency in the application of specific manual therapy skills. The skills diary was used by students to reflect on the development of four skills of their choice.

Marking criteria included reward for structuring reflective assignments using a recognized skills development framework and using guides for determining and resolving learning needs, such as SWOT analyses and SMART goal setting. These prompts required students to categorize and, in some cases, rank their experiences so at the very least they promote a superficial level of reflection. For some students, this was as far as they got. The more impressive responses to the task involved students' response to evidence of their skill development. Evidence of skill development was based on tutor feedback, peer assessment, and self-assessment.

Tutor feedback was drawn mainly from the formal skills assessment, which occurred three times across the course, but just twice before submission of the skills diary. In their responses, students often referred to the transformative influence of the initial feedback they received from the tutor on their learning, with skill acquisition confirmed at the subsequent assessment. Peer assessment came from class practical sessions or informal practice and was often standardized by adopting the same marking criteria used by the tutors. Self-assessment was most often presented in the form of narrative reflection, or storytelling. Students often described connections between what they were learning and previous learning or associated life experiences (for example, work at a sporting club). They also used structured formats for reflection, such as the significant learning incident form, which required a description of an incident, including the actions and motivations of those involved, and an evaluation of what this means for the future. While structured templates are not always viewed as appropriate for deep reflection, as they potentially insert too much input and structure into the process, the primary aim here was to capture evidence. Ideally, students engaged in a reflective process in which they considered the accumulated evidence.

An online resource was used to provide students with a definition for reflection and guidance on reflective writing, including examples of different levels of reflection.[4] Students who demonstrated deeper levels of reflection presented submissions that offered more individualized and complex descriptions regarding their experiences of skill acquisition. When done well, student reflections highlighted and interrogated variations between external assessments and their own self-evaluation. They accepted that acknowledging their difficulties and challenges and not just their successes was important in developing a plan to enhance specific clinical skill areas. More superficial examples described a representative physiotherapy student experience without exploring any individual contribution or response to the experience.

By focusing on the process of skill development, the skills diary directed students to be actively engaged in their own learning. By encouraging students to consider external evidence regarding their skills, they were forced to make sense of disparities and reflect on the validity of their own self-assessment. In this way, we used reflective practice to promote realistic self-appraisals. The most dangerous physiotherapist is the one who thinks that he or she is great but who is, in fact, the opposite. We believe that by having our second-year students write about themselves, supported by guidance on reflective writing, they will be better prepared to respond to future reflective opportunities, formal and informal, to further develop this essential skill.

Reflective practice is seen as an effective way of managing change and uncertainty. It is important that students training to work in the health professions are well prepared for its challenges, including possessing skills in reflection. Educators and educational designers can facilitate this by thoughtful and strategic design of curriculum. In recognition of the abundant online resources available, this may mean reducing didactic delivery of content and engaging students in analytical tasks that support lifelong learning, ongoing self-monitoring, and skills in self-assessment. It is our hope that this curriculum innovation will contribute to a culture in support of skill refinement through ongoing reflection and practice.

Our curriculum was designed to introduce students to an ongoing process of reflective skill development that they could use beyond the course. By providing access to the online PLS and skills diary for learning and assessment in their clinical fieldwork placements, we extended the process of reflection into a real-world context. In addition to providing a means for physiotherapy students to reflect on and to document their learning, use of the online skills diary can also help them demonstrate how their learning has enabled improvements in their skills. We believe this engagement with evidence-informed self-appraisal will lead to enhanced development and application of their clinical skills.

NOTES

1. Gillian Webb et al., "Physiotherapy in the 21st Century," in *Contexts of Physiotherapy Practice,* ed. Joy Higgs et al. (Chatswood, NSW: Churchill-Livingstone, 2009), 1–19.

2. D. Boud et al., *Assessment 2020: Seven Propositions for Assessment Reform in Higher Education* (Sydney: Australian Learning and Teaching Council, 2010).

3. Lester E. Jones, John A. Hammond, and Jean-Pascal Beaudoin, "Clinically-Based Learning Portfolios for Guiding Reflection and Professional Development," in *Innovations in Allied Health Fieldwork Education: A Critical Appraisal,* ed. Lindy McAllister et al. (Rotterdam: Sense Publishers, 2010), 131–40.

4. See "Reflective Practice in Health Sciences," Library Guides, La Trobe University, last modified Apr. 13, 2016, http://latrobe.libguides.com/reflectivepractice.

Introducing Narrative Reflective Practice in a Family Medicine Clerkship

A Blended Online Approach

MARIE-THERESE CAVE AND AMY TAN

Anticipation of any transition can never fully prepare one for the reality of what is to be faced. Many times throughout a journey we try to make meaning of what is happening. If we are fortunate, there are those with whom we are able to share stories, yet it is still difficult to explain to those who were not part of the experience. So it is for many students of medicine. The transition from the lecture hall to the clinical setting represents a liminal threshold that serves to heighten students' experience of uncertainty as they are exposed to the practice of medicine.

As educators, we understand that learning begins at times of uncertainty, and reflection is required to make meaning of those experiences, yet there is little space for reflection in clerkship. The learning is practical, an application of abstract knowledge of diseases to patients' illness experiences. Students are encouraged to be *patient centered,* a term that itself conveys that professional knowledge and meaning making are to be focused on the "Other." Clerkship is also the time when the hidden curriculum comes to the fore. Learners are influenced, for good or ill, by preceptor behaviors. The challenge of addressing the impact of these clinical experiences on the person of the learner physician, and how that might play out in terms of their overall professionalism and professional identity, is an educational goal that seems elusive.

Similarly, teaching professionalism is challenging. Students often resent, if not resist, formal curricula on professionalism, believing it to be artificial and of limited value. Many believe that it is not necessary to teach professionalism, as they associate professional attributes with tacit knowledge and character traits, a perception that challenges the requirement for structured curricula directed to promoting the development of professionalism. This was the context in which we set out to implement narrative reflection on practice in the Family Medicine Clerkship at the University of Alberta.

We began by using Rita Charon's "parallel chart" strategy,[1] a narrative genre created to help student interns inquire into their stories of practice. After a short presentation on the origins and purpose of narrative reflective practice (NRP) and parallel charting, students are then given the instructions to write an anonymous narrative of a patient encounter that affected them personally. They write about those things that "don't belong in the medical chart but need to be written somewhere." It is the first of three parallel charts they write during the clerkship; however, this one is different in that it is written hastily, in the moment, all in seven minutes. After reading a couple of random selections for this writing session, a demonstration of the facilitated narrative reflective inquiry process follows.

Inquiry into narratives selected during orientation is somewhat different from the process used in the two subsequent facilitated NRP small groups during the Family Medicine Clerkship rotation. The students bring a written chart to these later small groups, where they each read aloud their own chart. Reading aloud is an opportunity for further reflection, as the author is appreciatively asked if they have further thoughts to add before their peers begin to contribute to the inquiry.

It is in the group inquiry process that we differ slightly and epistemologically from Charon's pedagogy. Dr. Charon is a physician who imagined that close reading of parallel charts with a literary inquiry process would help students appreciate more fully what patients endure and also to consider their journey through medicine. We, as medical educators and researchers, are interested also in how medical learners access tacit knowledge, experience professional education, and develop a professional identity, so we have adopted a research methodology, the three-dimensional narrative inquiry approach.[2] The inquiry "wonderings" are within the three dimensions of temporality, sociality, and place. We imagined that reflection on practice would help our medical learners in the construction of personal, practical, and professional knowledge and professional identity.

Both inquiry approaches enable medical learners to think narratively and to think with the story, which Dr. Charon endorses as a necessary clinical competency for practice. A further commonality between these two NRP pedagogies is that both offer several layers of reflective inquiry. The three-dimensional narrative inquiry approach also stresses that learning is both incremental (one experience building on another) and relational. Early findings indicate that learning around professional identity formation is reciprocal for both student interns and physician facilitators. The facilitation is proving to be a continuous professional development experience for our faculty.

While other narrative reflective processes are employed in medical education, these two pedagogies offer something more—the opportunity for sequential reflection and the benefit of multiple peer perspectives. The inquiry for each chart lasts just twenty minutes, but the reflection continues as subsequent charts in the life of the group incrementally build on the early reflections. As learning is a relational activity, we welcome the diversity of perspectives that a group inquiry affords. We have observed that the experience of coming together to inquire into the parallel charts helps to create a community of practice (CoP).

We learned how important CoPs were to our clerkship students and faculty when in 2011 scheduling changes allowed us to experiment with a combined on-line/in-person NRP small-group approach.[3] After inquiry into parallel charts at orientation, the students joined password-protected "Google Groups," four students and a facilitator. During the rotation, each student posted a digital video of themselves reading their chart. Over the course of a week, their peers in the online small group shared their written responses asynchronously. During an eight-week rotation, there was enough time for each student to share one significant clinical encounter with their small group and for their peers to respond. On the final day of the rotation, student interns returned to the university (with their third parallel chart) and participated in a face-to-face parallel chart inquiry process with members of their virtual NRP group.

Born of necessity, this dual approach to the narrative reflective inquiry, involving in-person and online access, provided some interesting results. Longer reflection time enhanced the reflexivity of responses, but there was less spontaneous dialogue within the group, despite the efforts of facilitators. Both facilitators and students appreciated the flexibility in timing that the asynchronous online groups afforded, as well as the time to mull over the posted video for commentary. Themes identified in the narratives and subsequent discussions were similar for both in-person and online parallel chart groups. While both groups appreciated the benefits and drawbacks of each modality, they reported an overall preference for the in-person method, specifically for the naturally spontaneous interactions that can occur in face-to-face discussions. This preference prevailed in spite of the perceived increased time commitment and coordination challenges involved in organizing in-person small-group sessions. We have now reverted to in-person parallel chart discussion groups but may revisit the online groups in the future.

Throughout the implementation of the NRP pedagogy in the Family Medicine Clerkship, learners have provided narrative evaluations of our parallel chart inquiry process.[4] They value opportunities to hear each other's points of view and appreciate the sense of community and safety that develops over time. Typically, over 90 percent of student interns have found narrative reflective practice relevant to their professional formation during their family medicine rotation.

If clerkship is a period of uncertainty, then a parallel chart inquiry process offers alternate ways of viewing clinical experience and addressing uncertainty and ambiguity in medicine. As student interns with different personal and professional experience inquire into narratives, the tacit becomes explicit and new knowledge is created. Our facilitators (who have written their own parallel charts during faculty development sessions) have discovered that their students' inquiries create new insights for them as facilitators, particularly regarding their own practice as a physician. Students, faculty, and researchers are learning to think *with* the stories rather than *about* the stories. Together, we are all learning to think narratively.

NOTES

1. Rita Charon, *Narrative Medicine: Honoring the Stories of Illness* (New York: Oxford Univ. Press, 2006).
2. D. Jean Clandinin and F. Michael Connelly, *Narrative Inquiry: Experience and Story in Qualitative Research* (San Francisco: Jossey Bass, 2000).
3. Amy Tan, Marie-Therese Cave, and Shelley Ross, "A Novel Asynchronous Format to Implement Narrative Reflective Practice into Family Medicine Clerkship Education," poster presented at the annual meeting of the Canadian Conference for Medical Education, Quebec City, Apr. 20–23, 2013, www.proreg.ca/events/ccme/archive_2013/schedule_abs.php?id=90571.
4. Ibid.

Afterword

Keeping Reflection Accountable

LOUISE ARONSON

A popular truism holds that medicine is the marriage of art and science. For decades, teaching the art of medicine—humanism and professionalism, critical reasoning, patient-clinician communication, and self-regulation—relied heavily on lectures, electives, and role modeling. The well-documented decline in trainee empathy during clinical training, the hidden curriculum, health disparities, and ongoing challenges in patient safety provide ample evidence that this strategy is inadequate. Fortunately, recent regulatory body requirements and initiatives from within the health professions have called for training that better meets patient and societal needs—in other words, for training that is more accountable to both learners and patients. This has led to the recognition within medical education that some attitudes, skills, and competencies—many of which fall squarely in the "art of medicine" camp—cannot be taught or evaluated by traditional methods of instruction, testing, and supervision. This in turn has prompted the addition of a broader range of pedagogical strategies to health professions education.

Reflection is one such recent addition, at least as an explicit topic and cultivated skill. As John Dewey identified nearly a century ago, reflection is the means by which humans convert experience into learning. As such, it must be among the core competencies for twenty-first-century health professionals, who can never fully master the gargantuan, ever-evolving content of medicine or have sufficient skills to optimally address all the complex, unique, and very human situations that present to them daily. In health professions education, however, there remains tremendous variability, and even some debate among scholars, on what is meant by reflection. Indeed, in medicine, *reflection* is a word with many definitions and uses. In anatomy and surgery, it means the folding back of a part upon itself. In ophthalmology and radiology (not to mention physics and photography), it signifies the return of light after striking a surface. Colloquially and in medical education, it most commonly describes "a thought occurring in consideration or meditation" or an exercise that elicits self-awareness, thoughtfulness, or mindfulness.[1] Finally, following the lead of seminal educators, including Jack Mezirow and David Boud, it is one component of *critical reflection,* which moves beyond thoughtful practice to challenge assumptions, metacognitive analysis, and transformative learning. An essential first step, then, in making reflection accountable within health professions education is being explicit about which "reflection" one aims to address.

The articles in *Keeping Reflection Fresh* describe curricular innovations in thoughtful practice and critical reflection. They demonstrate remarkable diversity in methods, learning objectives, learner type, and curricular locus. Moreover, as Alan Bleakley points out in his foreword, they do this in no small part by bringing unique aesthetic and intellectual perspectives to learning. The potential for these reflection-based "art of medicine" strategies to improve both training and patient care stems from three of their common and defining characteristics: (1) a focus on the individual human being, whether trainee, clinician, or patient; (2) a view beyond medicine to the humanities, education, and the social sciences for alternate ways of understanding human experience, improving thinking and communication, and evaluating learners; and (3) the provision of cognitive and emotional tools to help health professionals acknowledge and cope with ambiguity, complexity, and the coexistence of multiple, equally valid interpretations of educational and clinical experiences. In so doing, they are certainly fresh, but are they accountable? Indeed, what does and should accountability mean in reference to reflective learning in the health professions?

Donald Schön defined a reflective practitioner as one who, in attending to and puzzling over essential professional problems, challenges self-evident "truths" and their own prior understandings. According to Schön, the reflective practitioner deliberately "carries out an experiment which serves to generate both a new understanding of the phenomenon and a change in the situation."[2] A reflective practitioner seeks feedback not only to enhance personal professional development, then, but also potentially to inform systems change (through a process of "collective 'reflection–in-action'").[3] By these standards, promoting the development of reflective health-care providers should increase our accountability to ourselves, each other, and our patients. But how do we determine whether our educational efforts meet this important goal?

Although many in the medical humanities have argued that medicine is overly positivist, we cannot deny that funders, learners, and patients are entitled to some proof that their money, time, and faith are meeting their intended aims. Yet demonstrating the benefits of a curricular intervention on patient outcomes has proven nearly impossible. Medical training takes years and involves countless components, many of which change along the way and none of which are delivered in a wholly uniform way to even one cohort of learners. Given these realities, how do we establish our accountability? How do we know a given exercise or activity meant to foster reflection actually does? And how do we increase the odds that such reflection leads to learning that improves patient care and patients' lives?

In my own work at the University of California–San Francisco (UCSF), I have taken what might be described as an algebraic approach to increasing the accountability of our reflective curricula. By algebraic, I mean inferring a larger association by virtue of a series of component associations, as in "If a=b and b=c, then a=c." In essence, we strive to increase the accountability of our reflective curricula by targeting objectives, which in other contexts already have been associated with or are have been proven to contribute to improved learning and patient care. I adopted this approach intentionally in my role as critical reflection curricular leader and scholar, and by fortuitous accident in my work in narrative advocacy.

At UCSF, although both approaches are used, we distinguish between reflection and critical reflection. We define critical reflection as "the process of analysing, reconsidering, and questioning experiences and of making an assessment of what is being reflected upon"[4] for the purpose of learning and improving future professional behavior and outcomes. In contrast to reflection, it requires learners to go beyond creating a representation of experience in the form of an anecdote, artwork, or other product. A critical reflection must include more than personal opinion, even from the most thoughtful of trainees, since feedback is essential to learning and a multiplicity of perspectives is necessary for the frame shift of transformative learning. Critical reflection further requires identifying one or more learning issues and creating a learning plan and/or alternate approach to try the next time the issue is encountered. While the vast majority of meaningful experiences yields a multiplicity of learning issues, we and others have shown that choosing one of immediate relevance—critically reflecting on it in this way and producing a plan for which the learner is accountable—dramatically increases learning and the likelihood of behavioral change. The fact of documentable learning increases our accountability to the trainee, while the behavioral change increases the exercise's accountability to patients, society, and the profession.

Narrative advocacy may seem at first only vaguely related to reflection. We quickly learned, however, that in order to provide "expert advice to society on matters of health,"[5] our students and residents first had to witness, represent, interpret, and analyze some of their most moving, challenging, and traumatic experiences—that is, they had to reflect. In retrospect, this should not have come as a surprise. Narrative advocacy draws its credibility from stories based in clinical experience. These stories, when linked to key issues in health and health care, have the power to change minds, hearts, behaviors, and policies. Perhaps not surprisingly, then, our trainees unanimously report that sharing and harnessing such experiences for the greater good improved their empathy for themselves, their patients, and each other, and it improved their self-efficacy as public professionals. Equally important, narrative advocacy promotes accountability by using reflection for concrete social and professional ends. Learners must link their clinical experiences to key issues and challenges in patient care. As an added benefit, the work produced not only teaches its author and his or her peers, but, in a sizeable minority of cases, influences patients, colleagues, and legislators. Our trainees' narrative advocacy articles have been published in medical journals, health-care blogs, and newspapers, locally and nationally. This is truly transformative learning—experience converted into action, development of new skills with ongoing utility, and generation of products with the potential to educate, inspire change, influence policy, and give a voice to society's most vulnerable.

My work in these areas has convinced me that we can increase the accountability of our reflection curricula by doing three things. First, we should focus our educational efforts more on critical reflection and less on reflection in the broader, more pedagogically amorphous sense. While both require training and practice, critical reflection is a complex skill with greater potential to educate and produce behavioral change. Second, reflective curricula should incorporate methods known to increase attainment of desired educational results. These include structured (as opposed to unstructured) reflection, personal learning plans, and faculty trained to provide feedback that supports both learning from experience and development of learners' reflective skills. Third, reflection will more easily secure its rightful place in the curriculum if it is explicitly linked to skills and competencies with established value and to outcomes that increase our professional accountability to patients and society.

Keeping Reflection Fresh contains a wealth of articles by educators who have developed creative, innovative curricula that keep reflection fresh and develop learners' skills in the art of medicine. This freshness inspires not only trainees but also educators, and it enriches medicine. The next step for those of us committed to this work is to challenge ourselves to find ways of retaining this freshness while also increasing the accountability of the work. Moving in that direction will help reflection secure a firmer foothold in the curriculum and, more importantly, ensure our work truly and significantly benefits those who matter most: our learners and patients.

NOTES

1. Dictionary.com, s.v. "reflection," accessed Nov. 30, 2015, http://dictionary.reference.com/browse/reflection.
2. Donald Schön, *The Reflective Practitioner: How Professionals Think in Action* (New York: Basic Books, 1983), 68.
3. Ibid., 250.
4. Louise Aronson et al., "A Comparison of Two Methods of Teaching Reflective Ability in Year 3 Medical Students," *Medical Education* 46, no. 8 (2012): 809.
5. Medical Professionalism Project, "Medical Professionalism in the New Millennium: A Physician's Charter," *The Lancet* 359, no. 9305 (2002): 520–22.

Contributors

DEBBI ANDREWS, MD, is a developmental pediatrician, medical educator, and writer. She is an associate professor and divisional director of developmental pediatrics in the Faculty of Medicine & Dentistry at the University of Alberta, Canada. Her stories and poems have been widely published.

JENNIFER ADAEZE ANYAEGBUNAM, MS, is an MD degree candidate at the University of Virginia School of Medicine. She is a graduate of the Narrative Medicine program at Columbia University.

SUSAN ARJMAND, MD, is a family practice physician in Chicago. She has a master's degree in health professions education from the University of Illinois College of Medicine, where she teaches narrative medicine and reflective writing. She is also a professional classical musician and performs with Chicago-based opera companies.

LOUISE ARONSON, MD, MFA, is professor of medicine at the University of California–San Francisco, where she holds an Arnold P. Gold Professorship, directs the UCSF Medical Humanities, and is chief of geriatrics education. Her research is focused on reflective learning and geriatrics education. She is the author of *A History of the Present Illness* (2013), as well as numerous articles, essays, and stories in medical, lay, and literary journals.

CLAYTON J. BAKER, MD, CM, is clinical associate professor of medical humanities and bioethics at the University of Rochester School of Medicine and Dentistry. He is also a practicing internist and writer. His work has been published in journals such *JAMA, Annals of Internal Medicine, NEJM,* and *Academic Medicine,* and in anthologies.

SYLVIA BARTON, RN, PhD, is associate professor and associate dean at Global Health, Faculty of Nursing, University of Alberta, Canada. Her academic expertise in community, indigenous, and global health is focused on critical social and cultural influences that shape experiences of illness and well-being in rural and urban settings.

JAY BARUCH, MD, associate professor of emergency medicine at Alpert Medical School at Brown University, is an emergency physician, educator, and writer. His fiction includes *Fourteen Stories: Doctors, Patients, and Other Strangers* (2007) and *What's Left Out* (2015), both published by the Kent State University Press.

MAREN BATALDEN, MD, MPH, is a practicing general internist and senior director of Inpatient Quality at Cambridge Health Alliance. She is an assistant professor in medicine at Harvard Medical School.

MICHELE BATTLE-FISHER, MPH, MA, is a clinical assistant professor at the Wright State University Boonshoft School of Medicine. Her research areas are health policy and systems theory. She is the author of *Application of Systems Thinking to Health Policy and Public Health Ethics: Public Health and Private Illness* (2014).

RACHAEL BEDARD, MD, is a fellow in geriatrics and palliative care at the Icahn School of Medicine at Mt. Sinai. She completed her residency and chief residency at Harvard Medical School/Cambridge Health Alliance.

DEIRDRE BENNETT, MB, MA, MPH, is a senior lecturer in the Medical Education Unit in the School of Medicine at the University College Cork, Ireland.

JEANNE BEREITER, MD, is a child and adolescent psychiatrist and clinical associate professor at the University of New Mexico School of Medicine, where she also teaches reflective writing to premedical students, medical students, residents, and faculty.

SUSAN BIDINOSTI, AOCA, is a research associate at Western University. She is also an artist, print designer, and graduate of the Ontario College of Art and Design.

AMY R. BLAIR, MD, is associate professor of family medicine at the Loyola University Chicago Stritch School of Medicine and director of the Center for Community and Global Health. She has been involved in medical service to domestic and international underserved communities throughout her career.

JULIE BLASZCZAK is a medical student at the University of Michigan Medical School.

ALAN BLEAKLEY, DPhil, is professor of medical humanities at Falmouth University and emeritus professor of medical education at Plymouth University Peninsula School of Medicine in the UK. His recent books include *Patient-Centered Medicine in Transition: The Heart of the Matter* (2014) and *Medical Education and Medical Humanities: How the Medical Humanities Can Shape Better Doctors* (2015).

RONNA BLOOM, MEd, is a poet and psychotherapist. She has published five books of poetry and is the poet in residence at Mount Sinai Hospital and poet in community at the University of Toronto.

JONATHAN BOLTON, MD, MA, is an associate professor of psychiatry at the University of New Mexico School of Medicine. He has taught psychiatry and anthropology at Harvard Medical School, Brown University, and University of New Mexico.

LYNDSEY BOREHAM, MB, is a GP registrar at Cornerways Medical Centre in Hampshire, UK.

J. MICHAEL BOSTWICK, MD, is professor of psychiatry, Mayo Clinic College of Medicine, and senior associate dean for admissions, Mayo Medical School. He created the Disruptions in Development curriculum in 2005 for first-year medical students and continues to adapt it to address new patient challenges and health-care issues.

J. DONALD BOUDREAU, MD, is an associate professor in the Faculty of Medicine at McGill University. He chairs the Physicianship Curriculum Committee and is a core member of the McGill Centre for Medical Education. He is also an Arnold P. Gold Foundation Associate Professor of Medicine.

PAMELA BRETT-MACLEAN, PhD, is associate professor in the Department of Psychiatry and director of the Arts & Humanities in Health & Medicine Program in the Faculty of Medicine & Dentistry at the University of Alberta, Canada.

LUCY BRUELL, MS, is an instructor in the Division of Medical Humanities and editor-in-chief of the Literature, Arts and Medicine Database at the New York University School of Medicine, where she also is a facilitator in the Humanistic Aspects of Medical Education seminars.

PIER BRYDEN, MD, MPhil, is a staff psychiatrist at the Hospital for Sick Children and associate professor in the Department of Psychiatry in the Faculty of Medicine at the University of Toronto.

ROBERT J. BULIK, PhD, devoted his life as a professor to academic medicine for almost twenty years, during which time he developed the structure and scoring rubric for the Patient's Story. He is currently a consultant to major health-care organizations preparing proposals to Centers for Medicare/Medicaid Services.

MARIE-THERESE CAVE recently retired as a faculty member in the Faculty of Medicine & Dentistry at the University of Alberta. Previously, she created and coordinated curricula in reflective practice. She continues to be actively involved in inquiring into the value of narrative reflective practice in the professional development of medical practitioners.

L. C. CHAN, MB, PhD, was a hematologist and clinical professor in pathology. He was codirector of the Centre for the Humanities and Medicine and also codirector of the Medical Ethics and Humanities Unit at Hong Kong University. He passed away in 2015.

MELISSA CHAN, MD, is a classically trained artist and former Georgetown University Medical Centre Arts-in-Medicine Fellow. She is currently a practicing family physician in California who enjoys the integration of the visual arts with medicine.

RITA CHARON, MD, PhD, is a general internist and literary scholar at Columbia University. She originated the field of narrative medicine at Columbia University in 2000 and serves as executive director of the Program in Narrative Medicine.

JULIE CHEN, MD, FCFP, is a family doctor and assistant professor in the Department of Family Medicine and Primary Care at Hong Kong University, where she is co-coordinator of the medical humanities curriculum for medical students.

NEVILLE CHIAVAROLI, MPhil, MEd, is senior lecturer in medical education in the Department of Medical Education, University of Melbourne.

DICK CHURCHILL, DM, is clinical associate professor and director of clinical skills at the University of Nottingham Medical School (UK). His research interests are focused on adolescent health.

MARGARET B. CLARK, DMin, is an instructor in practical theology at St. Stephen's College (Edmonton, Canada). Her areas of expertise include collaborative inquiry, clinical pastoral education supervision, spiritual assessment, and spiritual care.

AMY CLEMENTS-CORTES, PhD, RP, MT-BC, MTA, is a senior music therapist and practice adviser at Baycrest Centre (Toronto), assistant professor at University of Toronto, and instructor and supervisor at Wilfrid Laurier University. She is president of the World Federation of Music Therapy and director of Notes by Amy (www.notesbyamy.com).

ORIT COHEN CASTEL, MD, MPH, is a family physician and a preceptor for students and family medicine residents at the Rappaport Faculty of Medicine, Technion, Israel. She is lecturer at the Department of Nursing, University of Haifa, where she teaches teamwork and communication skills and conducts workshops for teachers in the health professions.

INGRID COLOGNA is a registered art therapist and social worker at Women's College Hospital (Toronto). She continually seeks new ways of incorporating the visual arts within her practice with clients and in furthering student education.

LYNN CORCORAN is a faculty member at Athabasca University in the bachelor of nursing program (Canada). She is a registered nurse with over twenty years of experience in the areas of nursing education, women's health, and community health.

JACK COULEHAN, poet, physician, and medical educator, received the 2012 Nicholas Davies Award of the American College of Physicians for "outstanding lifetime contributions to the humanities in medicine." His most recent poetry collections are *Bursting with Danger and Music* (2012) and *The Wound Dresser* (2015).

MARCEL D'EON, PhD, is faculty lead for teaching and curriculum development in the College of Medicine at the University of Saskatchewan, Canada. He is also the current editor of the *Canadian Medical Education Journal.*

PAUL DAKIN is a GP trainer in North London, UK, and honorary secretary of the Association for Medical Humanities (UK). His research interest is the representation of deafness in literature.

SAYANTANI DASGUPTA, MD, MPH, is a faculty member in the Program in Narrative Medicine, and cochair of the Seminar in Narrative, Health and Social Justice at Columbia University, New York. Learn more about her work at www. sayantanidasgupta.com.

KAREN DEVON, MD, MSc, is an endocrine surgeon and assistant professor of surgery at the University of Toronto. Her academic focus is surgical ethics and medical education. She can be followed on twitter at @specialkdmd.

ANJALI DHURANDHAR, MD, is an associate professor in the Department of Medicine at the University of Colorado, Denver, and also the associate director of the Arts and Humanities in Healthcare Program for the Center for Bioethics and Humanities.

JACALYN DUFFIN, MD, PhD, is a hematologist and historian; she has occupied the Hannah Chair of the History of Medicine at Queen's University since 1988. Author of eight books, she researches the history of disease, technology, and religion.

KATE ECCLES is a creativity educator and psychoanalyst in training in Zurich, Switzerland.

MARGARET EDWARDS, RN, PhD, is professor and dean in the Faculty of Health Disciplines at Athabasca University, Canada.

ANGELA ELSTER is senior vice president, Research and Education at the Royal Conservatory of Music in Toronto.

MAUREEN ENGEL, PhD, is assistant professor and director of Humanities Computing and director of the Canadian Institute for Research Computing in Arts at the University of Alberta.

JANET FINLAY is professor of English and communications at St. Clair College (Windsor, Canada). She is also facilitator of the Reflective Practice/Narrative Competency Seminar in the Palliative Medicine Residency Program at Western University (London, Canada).

MICHELE FLEIGER, MFA, is an award-winning actor and theater instructor. She is committed to exploring the potential of theatrical principles in enhancing creative awareness across a wide range of learners and professional groups.

ALICE FORNARI, EdD, RD, is professor of science education, population health, and family medicine, and associate dean of Educational Skills Development at the Hofstra North Shore-LIJ School of Medicine, New York. She is also assistant vice president of faculty development at the North Shore-LIJ Health System.

JONATHAN FOULKES, BM, FRCGP, has worked in general practice for over thirty years. He is medical director of Quality Management and Training Standards in the Royal College of General Practitioners, London, UK. He is also an associate GP dean of Health Education Wessex and an honorary fellow at the University of Winchester.

PATRICIA FRAIN, MEd, MPS, was the director of Spiritual Health Services (2003–13) at Winnipeg Health Sciences Centre (HSC), during which time she created the Spiritual Diversity Program. She currently contributes to the Winnipeg HSC, the largest health and trauma care center in Manitoba, Canada, as a staff consultant.

JONATHAN FULLER is an MD/PhD student in the Faculty of Medicine at the University of Toronto.

KENNETH FUNG, MD, MSc, is a staff psychiatrist and associate professor, Department of Psychiatry, University of Toronto. He is also clinical director of the Asian Initiative in Mental Health Program, University Health Network. His interests include cultural psychiatry, spirituality, and psychotherapy.

PIPPA GARDINER, MB, is a GP trainee in Southampton, UK.

ELIZABETH GAUFBERG, MD, MPH, is an associate professor in medicine and psychiatry at Harvard Medical School and the Jean and Harvey Director of the Arnold P. Gold Foundation Research Institute. She also directs the Cambridge Health Alliance Center for Professional Development and leads the patient-doctor course for the Harvard Medical School, Cambridge Integrated Clerkship.

PAUL GEORGE, MD, MHPE, is assistant professor of family medicine and director of second-year curriculum at Alpert Medical School at Brown University, Rhode Island.

GORDON GIDDINGS is a physician who practices palliative medicine in Ottawa, Canada, and Hamilton, New Zealand. He is also an associate editor with the *Canadian Medical Association Journal*.

ERIKA GOBLE, PhD, recently completed her doctorate with the Department of Secondary Education, University of Alberta, and is manager of research at NorQuest College (Edmonton, Canada). Her research focuses on the ethics and aesthetics of health care, images in teaching, research, and practice, and aesthetic experience.

KAREN GOLD is a social worker and educator at Women's College Hospital (Toronto), with a special interest in arts-based and narrative methods. Her doctoral research focused on practitioner writing, and she has published on narrative in professional practice, training, and inquiry.

WILL GOODISON, MD, recently graduated from medical school, is currently working as a junior doctor. Will was involved in the direction and production of "Cancer Tales" for four years at the University of Bristol.

WENDY A. HALL, RN, PhD, is a professor in the School of Nursing at the University of British Columbia (Canada). She has worked with community members in action research and workshops for many years.

DEBRA HAMER, MD, is a fifth-year psychiatry resident at the University of Toronto.

RACHEL HAMMER is an intern in medicine and psychiatry at Tulane University in New Orleans, Louisiana. She earned her MD at the Mayo Clinic College of Medicine, where she taught medical students humanities and creative writing after earning an MFA in creative nonfiction at Seattle Pacific University.

PAM HARVEY is a physiotherapist who joined School of Rural Health at Monash University in Melbourne, Australia, in 2007. She is involved in medical and health professional education, working mainly with clinical educators.

SARAH L. HASTINGS is professor of psychology at Radford University, Virginia. Her areas of research include psychological well-being and health, professional practice, and gender.

WARREN HERSHMAN, MD, MPH, is director of Student Education, Department of Medicine, and professor of medicine at Boston University School of Medicine.

BARBARA HIRSCH, MD, MS, is a clinical assistant professor in the Department of Medicine/Hofstra North Shore-LIJ School of Medicine, New York. She is a practicing endocrinologist at North Shore Diabetes and Endocrine Associates (www.nsdea.com).

CAROL S. HODGSON, PhD, is the J. Alan Gilbert Chair in Medical Education Research in the Faculty of Medicine & Dentistry at the University of Alberta, Canada. She has more than twenty years of experience in curriculum development, evaluation, and research in medical education.

ROBERTA JACKSON is an instructor in the Department of English at the University of Calgary, Canada, and a member of the University of Calgary Narrative Research Group.

JOY JACOBSON is a poet and a senior fellow at the Center for Health, Media, and Policy at Hunter College, New York, where she teaches narrative writing to students of the health professions and practicing clinicians.

DEBORAH JAMES, PhD, is reader in Child and Family Communication at Northumbria University. She works across health, education, and social care using video feedback to support change in families and workforces.

KATHERINE J. JANZEN, RN, MN, is an assistant professor in the Faculty of Health and Community Studies at Mount Royal University, Canada. She is interested in student engagement and the use of creative arts-based teaching strategies.

LESTER E. JONES has been involved in the pre- and post-registration of physiotherapists and other health professionals in London, England, and, since 2007, in Melbourne, Australia. In 2011 he was awarded a La Trobe University Citation for Outstanding Contribution to Student Learning.

THERESE JONES, PhD, is director of the Arts and Humanities in Healthcare Program for the Center for Bioethics and Humanities and is associate professor in the Department of Medicine at the University of Colorado, Denver. She is the editor of the *Journal of Medical Humanities.*

JESSE KANCIR, MD, MSc, is currently an MPhil candidate studying public policy at the University of Cambridge, UK.

KHALED KARKABI, MD, MMH, is a clinical assistant professor and chair of the division of family medicine at the Rappaport Faculty of Medicine, Technion, Israel. He has an MA in medical humanities and teaches literature and medicine, compassion, and reflective competence using arts and narratives to medical professionals.

MARTINA KELLY, MB, is an associate professor and clerkship director in the Department of Family Medicine at the Cumming School of Medicine at the University of Calgary, Canada.

MONICA KIDD is a family physician and clinical associate professor at the University of Calgary, Canada. Kidd is also the author of several books of poetry, fiction, and nonfiction and is a former journalist with CBC Radio.

ELIZABETH ANNE KINSELLA, PhD, is an associate professor in the Faculty of Health Sciences and a researcher in the Centre for Education Research & Innovation in the Schulich School of Medicine & Dentistry at Western University, Canada. Her research investigates ethics, phronesis, reflection, reflexivity, and the arts in health professional education and practice.

KERRY KNICKLE, LLM (ADR), is an academic educator at the Standardized Patient Program, University of Toronto, with twenty years of experience in experiential learning and simulation methodology. Her dispute resolution focus highlights how assumptions, judgments, and poor communication inform personal and professional interactions.

MARTIN KOHN, PhD, is director of the Program in Medical Humanities in the Center for Ethics, Humanities and Spiritual Care, Cleveland Clinic, and associate professor of medicine, Cleveland Clinic, Lerner College of Medicine of Case Western Reserve University, Ohio.

SARAH KOOIENGA, PhD, FNP-BC, is an assistant professor at the University of Wyoming (Laramie). Sarah embraces narrative pedagogies as a means to promote excellence in primary care. As an educator, she focuses on developing and mentoring reflective future nurse practitioners.

ARNO K. KUMAGAI, MD, is professor of internal medicine and medical education and director of the Family Centered Experience and Longitudinal Case Studies Programs at the University of Michigan Medical School.

AYELET KUPER, MD, PhD, is a Wilson Centre Scientist and internist at Sunnybrook Health Sciences Centre, based at the University of Toronto.

ANASTASIA KUTT, BSc, coordinates education programs for the CARE Program for Integrative Health & Healing at the University of Alberta, Canada.

MARK LACHMANN, MD, MHSc, is a geriatric psychiatrist at the University of Toronto.

JENNIFER L. LAPUM, PhD, RN, is an associate professor at Ryerson University, Canada. As a poet and arts-based researcher, she is focused on advancing the use of art in health science research. Her goal is to ensure that the 7,024th patient does not feel like the 7,024th patient when entering and exiting the health care system.

NANCY LOO is a professional concert pianist, teacher, and prison ministry volunteer. From 2012 to 2014, she was the artist in education at the Absolutely Fabulous Theatre Connection in Hong Kong.

JEROME LOWENSTEIN, MD, is a professor of medicine at New York University School of Medicine. He is the founder of the Humanistic Aspects of Medicine Education program, the founder of the Bellevue Literary Press, and the nonfiction editor of the *Bellevue Literary Review*.

SUE MACDONALD is coordinator of Consumer Involvement and Initiatives at Vancouver Coastal Health in British Columbia. She has extensive experience advocating for the inclusion of patient voices in mental health service delivery.

HEATHER MACLEAN, RN, MN, is a registered nurse and associate professor in the Faculty of Health and Community Studies at Mount Royal University in Calgary, Canada. Her interests include student engagement and use of creative arts-based strategies in education.

D. STEWART MACLENNAN, NP, holds a joint appointment as faculty lecturer with the Faculty of Nursing, University of Alberta, and Alberta Health Services (Edmonton, Canada). He teaches health assessment and pharmacology and also provides health-care services to individuals in forensic environments.

M. MICHIKO MARUYAMA, MD, graduated from the UBC Northern Medical Program in 2015. She is currently a cardiac surgery resident at the University of Alberta (Canada). Prior to medicine, she completed a degree in industrial design and remains actively engaged in exploring connections between medicine, art, and design (see www.artoflearning.ca).

VIRGINIA MCCARTHY, MDiv, is assistant director of the Center for Community and Global Health at Loyola University Chicago Stritch School of Medicine. She guides experiential reflection for students at all levels of training, locally and internationally.

IRENE MCGHEE, MD, is assistant professor in the Department of Anesthesia at the University of Toronto, with a focus on interprofessional communication and collaboration at Sunnybrook Health Sciences Centre in Toronto.

NANCY MCNAUGHTON, MEd, PhD, is an associate director with the Standardized Patient Program at University of Toronto, where she has worked for thirty-one years. Her research focuses on the role of emotion in health professional education.

SHAYNA McNEILL is currently a fourth-year medical student at the University of Alberta, Canada. She previously completed a BHSc from the University of Calgary in Health and Society and has a keen interest in how social factors affect health and health-care delivery.

ALEXA MILLER, MA, is founder of Arts Practica, a medical education consultancy helping health-care providers be more mindful observers of art. A cocreator of Harvard Medical School's "Training the Eye: Improving the Art of Physical Diagnosis" course, Miller writes and consults on the alignment of medical training with visual art.

JACLYN L. MULLINS is a doctoral student in the counseling psychology program at Radford University, Virginia. Her research interests include posttraumatic growth, forensic issues, and rural mental health.

CATHERINE MYSER, PhD, is a bioethicist and medical anthropologist. She has more than twenty years of experience in ethics, social science, global health research, education, and service at medical schools and hospitals in Africa, Asia, Australia, the Caribbean, Europe, the Middle East, and North America.

ALIM NAGJI, MD, BHSc, is a family and emergency medicine physician practicing in Ontario. He has had a longstanding interest in, and has been actively involved in, introducing theater approaches in medical education.

AMY NAKAJIMA, MD, is an obstetrician-gynecologist in Ottawa, Canada. She has a special interest in working with vulnerable patients and provides care at Bruyère Continuing Care and the Wabano Centre for Aboriginal Care. As a clinical educator, she is focused on teaching patient safety and quality improvement in undergraduate and postgraduate medical education.

STELLA NG, PhD, FAAA, is an assistant professor of speech-language pathology at the University of Toronto. She is also director of research in the Centre for Faculty Development, an education scientist in the Centre for Ambulatory Care Education, and a cross-appointed scientist with the Wilson Centre.

JEFF NISKER, MD, PhD, is a professor of obstetrics and gynecology at the Schulich School of Medicine & Dentistry at Western University, where he was coordinator of the Medical Ethics and Humanities Program from 1995 to 2011.

LARA NIXON is a family physician and assistant professor in the Department of Family Medicine at the University of Calgary (Canada), where she works clinically in team-based inner-city care. Her interests include vulnerability, relationship-centered care, and medical education. Lara is also a member of the University of Calgary Narrative Research Group.

JULIE G. NYQUIST, PhD, is a professor in the Department of Medical Education at the Keck School of Medicine of the University of Southern California.

SIUN O'FLYNN, MB, is head of the Medical Education Unit, School of Medicine, at University College Cork, Ireland, and a consultant physician at Cork University Hospital.

JOANNE K. OLSON, RN, PhD, is a professor in the Faculty of Nursing, University of Alberta (Canada). Her areas of expertise include teaching and learning, interpersonal communication, interprofessional education, nurse-client communication, nursing and health promotion, spirituality, and faith community nursing.

CHRISTOPHER OWEN, BM, MChem, MRCP (UK), is a physician trainee in Sydney, Australia.

LAURIE PERELES, MD, is a family physician, and a clinical associate professor in the Department of Family Medicine at the University of Calgary. She is also a member of the University of Calgary Narrative Research Group.

ELVIRA PEREZ VALLEJOS, PhD, is a senior research fellow at the CaSMa project (Horizon Institute for Digital Economy Research) at the University of Nottingham, UK. She is an accredited video interaction guider practitioner interested in improving mental health communication among young people and the clinical communications skills of junior doctors.

BETH PERRY, RN, PhD, is a professor in the Faculty of Health Disciplines at Athabasca University, Canada. Beth teaches health discipline students online and is interested in creating arts-based teaching strategies.

ALLAN PETERKIN, MD, is professor of psychiatry and family medicine at the University of Toronto, where he is the humanities lead for undergraduate medical education and head of the Program in Health, Arts and Humanities. He cofounded the literary journal *Ars Medica* and is the author/editor of fourteen books for adults and children.

CHRISTINA PHAM, MD, is a dancer and practicing general internist at the University of California–San Francisco, focusing on women's health primary care. She completed her residency in internal medicine at Harvard Medical School/ Cambridge Health Alliance.

SHANON PHELAN, PhD, is an assistant professor in the Faculty of Rehabilitation Medicine at the University of Alberta (Canada). Her research interests include reflexivity, childhood disability, and ethics.

NATALIE RADOMSKI, PhD, is a senior lecturer in the Monash University, School of Rural Health, in Australia. She is involved in educational development and educational research. Natalie's research interests include workplace-based learning, curriculum design, and community-based medical education

LINDA S. RAPHAEL, PhD, is director of the Medical Humanities Program at George Washington University School of Medicine and Health Sciences. She has authored numerous works, including *Narrative Skepticism: Moral Agency and Representations of Consciousness in Fiction* (2001), and, most recently, a chapter in *Pain and Emotion in Modern History* (2014).

JANANEE RASIAH, MN, RN, is a faculty member at Athabasca University, Canada, in the bachelor of nursing program, where she teaches and is involved in research related to family nursing.

MELODY RASMOR, EdD, FNP-BC, COHN-S, is an assistant clinical professor at Washington State University. Her research focuses on educational uses of the digital story in nurse practitioner education to demonstrate the importance of history taking and listening to patients' stories.

CHRISTY A. RENTMEESTER, PhD, is associate professor, Center for Health Policy and Ethics in the Creighton University School of Medicine in Nebraska. Her recent scholarship focuses on justice issues related to vulnerable patient groups. She teaches ethics in both undergraduate medical education and graduate courses.

LISA RICHARDSON, MD, MA, is a clinician-educator in the Division of General Internal Medicine and assistant professor of medicine at the University of Toronto.

JEFFREY M. RING, PhD, is a health psychologist and principal at Health Management Associates, as well as a clinical professor of family medicine in the Keck School of Medicine at the University of Southern California.

CATHERINE RODER is currently a fourth-year medical student at the University of Alberta, Canada.

TOM ROSENAL is an associate professor emeritus in the Department of Critical Care Medicine at the University of Calgary (Canada). He is a member of the University of Calgary Narrative Research Group and works in the fields of health-care humanities, professionalism, and clinical informatics.

TAMAR RUBIN, MD, completed training in general pediatrics at the University of Alberta and is currently a clinical immunology and allergy fellow at the University of Manitoba (Canada). Her academic interests include medical education, narrative reflective practice, and enhancing patient-centered care through the humanities.

RON RUSKIN, MD, is an associate professor in the Department of Psychiatry at the University of Toronto and director of the Three-Day Program at Mount Sinai Hospital. He is a member of the Toronto Psychoanalytic Society and the Toronto Institute for Contemporary Psychoanalysis. He is also a founding editor of *Ars Medica*.

SUSAN J. SAMPLE, PhD, MFA, is course director for the elective "Writing the Doctor-Patient Relationship" in the Division of Medical Ethics and Humanities at the University of Utah School of Medicine. She also teaches medical discourse to undergraduate students and leads poetry workshops for patients, their families, and caregivers.

MICHELE SARRACCO, LCSW, is in private practice in New York City. She is a facilitator in the Humanistic Aspects of Medical Education seminar.

LYNN-BETH SATTERLY, MD, is a family physician and medical educator. She is founding medical director of Amaus Medical Services of the Cathedral of the Immaculate Conception and associate director of the Physician Assistant Program at Lemoyne College in Syracuse, New York. She also has a master's degree in instructional design, development, and evaluation.

BETH SAWATSKY, BTH, BRS, MA, is director of Spiritual Health Services and the Spiritual Diversity Education Program at Winnipeg Health Sciences Centre, a large trauma and health-care center in Manitoba, Canada.

SAMANTHA SCALLAN, PhD, is a senior lecturer in medical education at the University of Winchester (UK) and the Wessex School of General Practice Educational Research Lead.

MARK SCARBECZ, PhD, received his doctorate in sociology from the University of Arizona. He is a professor and the assistant dean for Institutional Affairs at the University of Tennessee College of Dentistry, where he teaches courses in behavioral science.

CAROL SCHILLING completed her PhD in literature and currently teaches in interdisciplinary courses in the Health Studies Program at Haverford College in Pennsylvania. Her teaching focuses on health and humanities, health and social justice, bioethics, and disability.

SARA K. SCHNEIDER, PhD, supports health-care providers, law enforcement, teachers, and clergy in the spiritual, cultural, and learning dimensions of their professional practice. A faculty member at National Louis University, she is the author of three books on performative aspects of the body (see www.sarak schneider.com).

JASNA K. SCHWIND, PhD, RN, is an associate professor at Ryerson University (Canada). Using arts-informed narrative inquiry, she explores humanness of care in person-centered contexts in education and practice.

MARCIA S. SEEBERG, MS, LMHC, is a mental health counselor and instructor at the University of Tennessee College of Dentistry. She counsels students using a patient-centered approach.

AUDREY SHAFER, MD, is professor of anesthesiology, perioperative, and pain medicine at the Stanford University School of Medicine and the Palo Alto Veterans Affairs Health Care System. She directs the Stanford Medicine and the Muse Program. She is author of *The Mailbox* and is a published poet.

SEEMA SHAH, MD, MSPH, has incorporated her interest in the arts and health into various activities, including her community educator role in workshops for health science students.

JOHANNA SHAPIRO, PhD, is professor of family medicine and director of the Program in Medical Humanities & Arts at the University of California Irvine

School of Medicine. Her research and scholarship focuses on medical student–patient relationships, including interactions with "difficult," stigmatized, and culturally diverse patient populations.

JONATHAN LOUIS SMITH, BM, BS, is a trainee in the Portsmouth General Practice Specialist Training Scheme, Wessex, UK. His clinical interests are focused in the areas of pediatrics and ophthalmology.

PENELOPE SMYTH, MD, is a neurologist and multiple sclerosis clinician, as well as an associate professor in the Department of Medicine at the University of Alberta, Canada. Her interest in medical education and professionalism developed in relation to her various contributions to residency programs in neurology over the course of her career.

JENNIFER SOTSKY is an MD degree candidate at the Columbia University College of Physicians and Surgeons. She is also a graduate of the Narrative Medicine program at Columbia University in New York City.

MAURA SPIEGEL, PhD, is associate director of the Program in Narrative Medicine at Columbia University. She teaches literature and film at Columbia University and Barnard College.

LISA MARIE STERR has a BA in psychology and is a peer support worker for people experiencing mental illness. She lives in Vancouver, British Columbia, Canada.

MARGARET L. STUBER, MD, a child and adolescent psychiatrist, is the Daniel X. Freedman Professor and vice chair, Education in the Department of Psychiatry and Biobehavioral Sciences at the University of California, Los Angeles. She is also assistant dean for Well-being and Career Advising in the UCLA David Geffen School of Medicine.

BRANDON SULTAN is an MD degree candidate at the Howard University College of Medicine. He has master's degrees in bioethics and narrative medicine, both from Columbia University in New York City.

AMY TAN, MD, MSc, is associate professor and undergraduate education director in the Department of Family Medicine and is also the Year 1 and 2 physician-ship course director in the Undergraduate Medical Education program at the University of Alberta (Canada).

BEV TAYLOR, PhD, is emeritus professor of nursing at Southern Cross University. Her career has centered mainly on reflective practice. She was part of the original team of academics who introduced reflective practice to Australian clinicians and students in the 1980s.

JULIE SCOTT TAYLOR, MD, MSc, is senior associate dean, Clinical Sciences, and professor of behavioral and clinical medicine at the American University of the Caribbean School of Medicine, Sint Maarten. She is also an adjunct professor of family medicine at the Alpert Medical School of Brown University in Providence, Rhode Island.

ULRICH TEUCHER, PhD, began his career as a pediatric nurse on a cancer ward. He completed his dissertation, "Writing the Unspeakable: Metaphor in Cancer Narratives," in comparative literature and psychology and is currently associate professor in culture and human development at the University of Saskatchewan (Canada).

TREVOR THOMPSON, MD, PhD, is a family physician and reader in healthcare education at the University of Bristol. He has helped champion the place of the arts in the medical curriculum as a route to more person-centered care in the UK.

KELLY THRESHER is a GP program director with the Southampton GP Education Team, Health Education Wessex. She teaches foundation trainees and general practice specialty trainees at Southampton University Hospitals NHS Trust, UK.

STEVE TRUMBLE, MD, MBBS, is a general medical practitioner and head of the Department of Medical Education at the Melbourne Medical School, University of Melbourne, Australia.

ANDERSON TSANG, MBBS, is a clinical assistant professor in neurosurgery in the Department of Surgery at the University of Hong Kong. He also facilitates the performance arts workshops in the medical humanities curriculum.

SUNITA VOHRA, MD, MSc, is a professor in the Faculty of Medicine & Dentistry and the School of Public Health at the University of Alberta. She is also the founding director of the Complementary and Alternative Research and Education (CARE) program, the PedCAM Network, and the Integrative Health Institute at the University of Alberta, Canada.

HEDY S. WALD, PhD, is clinical associate professor of family medicine at the Alpert Medical School of Brown University (Rhode Island), where she directs the Family Medicine Clerkship reflective writing (RW) curriculum. She conducts faculty development workshops internationally on RW-enhanced reflection in support of professional identity formation and resilience.

SHELLEY WALL, PhD, MScBMC, AOCAD, is an assistant professor in the Biomedical Communications program, Institute of Medical Science, and in the Department of Biology, at the University of Toronto. She is also the inaugural illustrator in residence in the Faculty of Medicine at the University of Toronto.

DELESE WEAR, PhD, is professor of family and community medicine at the Northeast Ohio Medical University in Rootstown, Ohio.

CAROLINE WELLBERY, MD, PhD, is professor of family medicine at Georgetown University Medical School, where she runs an arts-in-medicine program. Her medical humanities website can be accessed at imh.georgetown.edu.

FRED WERTZER, EdD, MSW, MS, is a facilitator in the Humanistic Aspects of Medical Education (HAME) seminar. He has been affiliated with HAME for nearly thirty years.

MARY ANN WIEBE, MN, RN, is an associate professor in the Faculty of Health and Community Studies at Mount Royal University in Calgary, Alberta, Canada. Her academic interests include the use of creative arts-based teaching strategies to engage students from diverse cultural backgrounds.

RUTH WONG works as a medical librarian in the Hong Kong University library system.

VENUS WONG is the honorary lecturer in the Centre on Behavioral Health and co-coordinator of the mindful practice component of the medical humanities curriculum at the University of Hong Kong.

DOROTHY WOODMAN, PhD, is a contract instructor at the University of Alberta (Canada). Her teaching and research interests include race, gender, and illness; neoliberalism and biomedicine; and superheroes and survivors in comics.

GOPAL YADAVALLI, MD, is an assistant professor of medicine at the Boston University School of Medicine, where he is program director for the Internal Medicine residency program.

LYNN YAU is an arts educator and CEO (Planning & Arts Learning) at the Absolutely Fabulous Theatre Connection in Hong Kong. She has been instrumental in developing a range of learning projects across sectors through the arts that are recognized locally and abroad.

OLIVE YONGE, RN, PhD, is a professor in the Faculty of Nursing and Vargo Teaching Chair at the University of Alberta (Canada). Her academic work is focused on teaching, learning, and interpersonal communication.

JOSEPH ZARCONI, MD, is system vice president for medical education and chief academic officer at Summa Health System (Akron, Ohio) and professor and associate dean for clinical education at the Northeast Ohio Medical University.

MATEUSZ ZUROWSKI, MD, MSc, is an assistant professor and staff psychiatrist in the Department of Psychiatry at the University of Toronto. He directs the Neuropsychiatry Clinic in the University Health Network. His interests include movement disorders and chronic pain.

HEATHER ZWICKER, PhD, is a professor of English and film studies in the Faculty of Arts, as well as dean in the Faculty of Graduate Studies and Vargo Teaching Chair at the University of Alberta (Canada).

Index

LITERATURE AND MEDICINE

Michael Blackie, Editor • Carol Donley and Martin Kohn, Founding Editors